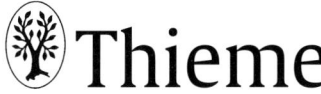

The Post-traumatic Vegetative State

Giuliano Dolce, M.D.
Professor and Chief Neurologist
Institute S. Anna for
Intensive Care and Rehabilitation
Crotone, Italy

Leon Sazbon, M.D.
Senior Lecturer
Sackler School of Medicine
Tel Aviv University
Former Director
Intensive Care Unit for
Vegetative Patients
Loewenstein Rehabilitation Center
Raanana, Israel

With contributions by
M. Gil, H. Hacker, O. Keren, C. Koren, A. Pincherle, M. Quintieri, L. Rahmani, J. E. Resnik,
W. G. Sannita, E. Schmutzhard, P. Scola, S. Serra, A. Shilansky, R. Weitz, M. R. Zylberman

33 Illustrations
17 Tables

Thieme
Stuttgart · New York

To Inge and Nelly
– for a life of love and patience.

Library of Congress Cataloging-in-Publication Data
The post-traumatic vegetative state / [edited by] Giuliano Dolce, Leon Sazbon ; with contributions by M. Gil ... [et al.].
   p. ; cm.
 Includes bibliographical references and index.
 ISBN 1-58890-116-5 – ISBN 313130071X
 1. Persistent vegetative state. I. Dolce, Giuliano. II. Sazbon, Leon.
 [DNLM: 1. Persistent Vegetative State.
 WB 182 P857 2002]
 RB 150.C6 P67 2002
 616.8'49--dc21

2002020323

© 2002 Georg Thieme Verlag,
Rüdigerstraße 14, D-70469 Stuttgart, Germany
http://www.thieme.de
Thieme New York, 333 Seventh Avenue,
New York, N. Y. 10001 U.S.A.
http://www.thieme.com

Cover design: Renate Stockinger, Stuttgart
Typesetting by Satzpunkt Bayreuth, Bayreuth
Printed in Germany by Gulde Druck, Tübingen
ISBN 3-13-130071-X (GTV)
ISBN 1-58890-116-5 (TNY)   1 2 3 4 5

Important Note: Medicine is an ever-changing science undergoing continual development. Research and clinical experience are continually expanding our knowledge, in particular our knowledge of proper treatment and drug therapy. Insofar as this book mentions any dosage or application, readers may rest assured that the authors, editors, and publishers have made every effort to ensure that such references are in accordance with **the state of knowledge at the time of production of the book.**
 Nevertheless, this does not involve, imply, or express any guarantee or responsibility on the part of the publishers in respect to any dosage instructions and forms of applications stated in the book. **Every user is requested to examine carefully** the manufacturers' leaflets accompanying each drug and to check, if necessary in consultation with a physician or specialist, whether the dosage schedules mentioned therein or the contraindications stated by the manufacturers differ from the statements made in the present book. Such examination is particularly important with drugs that are either rarely used or have been newly released on the market. Every dosage schedule or every form of application used is entirely at the user's own risk and responsibility. The authors and publishers request every user to report to the publishers any discrepancies or inaccuracies noticed.
 Some of the product names, patents, and registered designs referred to in this book are in fact registered trademarks or proprietary names even though specific reference to this fact is not always made in the text. Therefore, the appearance of a name without designation as proprietary is not to be construed as a representation by the publisher that it is in the public domain.
 This book, including all parts thereof, is legally protected by copyright. Any use, exploitation, or commercialization outside the narrow limits set by copyright legislation, without the publisher's consent, is illegal and liable to prosecution. This applies in particular to photostat reproduction, copying, mimeographing or duplication of any kind, translating, preparation of microfilms, and electronic data processing and storage.

Contributors

Mali Gil, M.A.
Head, Department of Speech, Language and
Swallowing Disorders
Loewenstein Rehabilitation Center
Raanana, Israel

Hans Hacker, M.D.
Professor Emeritus
Johann Wolfgang Goethe Universität
Frankfurt am Main, Germany

Ofer Keren, M.D.
Lecturer, Tel Aviv University
Sackler School of Medicine
Clinical Director
Clinical Neurophysiological Unit
Deputy Director
Traumatic Brain Injury
Loewenstein Rehabilitation Center
Raanana, Israel

Cecilia Koren, M.A.
Deputy Head, Department of Speech, Language
and Swallowing Disorders
Loewenstein Rehabilitation Center
Raanana, Israel

Alessandro Pincherle, M.D.
Clinical Neurophysiologist
Università degli Studi di Genova
Genova, Italy

Maria Quintieri, M.D.
Clinical Neurophysiologist
Institute S. Anna for Intensive Care
and Rehabilitation of Brain Injury Patients
Crotone, Italy

Levy Rahmani, Ph.D.
Associate Professor of Psychology
Tel Aviv University, Medical School
Division of Health Professions
Specialist in Clinical and Rehabilitation Psychology
Former Head of Psychology
Loewenstein Rehabilitation Hospital
Raanana, Israel

Jacqueline Elise Resnik, B. App. Sci. P.T.
Director, Department of Physiotherapy
Rehut Medical Center
Tel Aviv, Israel

Walter G. Sannita, M.D.
Professor and Director
Unit of Neurophysiopathology
Department of Motor Science and Rehabilitation
Università degli Studi di Genova
Genova, Italy
Associate Professor of Psychiatry
State University of New York
Stony Brook, New York, USA

Erich Schmutzhard, M.D.
Professor, Univ.-Klinik für Neurologie
Neurologic Intensive Care Unit
Innsbruck, Austria

Paolo Scola, M.D.
Otorhinolaryngologist
Institute S. Anna for Intensive Care
and Rehabilitation of Brain Injury Patients
Crotone, Italy

Sebastiano Serra, M.D.
Clinical Neurophysiologist
Institute S. Anna for Intensive Care
and Rehabilitation of Brain Injury Patients
Crotone, Italy

Anat Shilansky, M.S.W.
Head, Department of Social Work
Loewenstein Rehabilitation Center
Raanana, Israel

Rosemarie Weitz, B.S.W.
Department of Social Work
Loewenstein Rehabilitation Center
Raanana, Israel

M. Rachele Zylberman, M.D.
Neurology and Psychiatry Specialist
Head, Department of Neuro-Rehabilitation
Osp. San Gionvanni Battista
Rome, Italy

Foreword

In the 30 years since Plum and I described and named the vegetative state, there has been widespread interest in the medical, ethical and legal aspects of this strange condition.

It is therefore not surprising that at least three books on this topic, from different countries, are soon to be published. This one reviews the available medical data and emphasizes how much remains to be found out about the pathophysiology of the condition, and how limited is our understanding of the mechanisms underlying consciousness. Consistent with its claim to be "the first systematic presentation of a new phase in the history of neurorehabilitation," this book is optimistic about the chances of good recovery from the vegetative state. It details in practical terms the many complexities of the medical management of these patients and will be a useful source for those dealing with patients who are temporarily vegetative. It deals with how to ensure that such patients can make the most of their capacity for recovery, and will not be further handicapped by avoidable complications. It acknowledges that various countries hold differing views about the appropriate management of patients who are permanently vegetative. In North America and several countries in Northern Europe, an ethical and legal consensus has emerged that continuing treatment that is considered to be of no benefit to such patients may not be justified.

Its withdrawal is therefore regarded as an ethically and legally acceptable option, and is claimed not to infringe the European Convention on Human Rights (B. Jennett, *The vegetative state: medical facts, ethical and legal dilemmas,* Cambridge: Cambridge University Press, 2002). Mediterranean countries are not part of this consensus, but little has been published about their viewpoint. It is therefore valuable to have the opposing view set out here, even if many of us from elsewhere would reject the supposed contrast between "a policy of abandonment" and "compassionate care." We also believe that we are being compassionate, although we interpret this differently. It is therefore likely that this book, as well as providing practical guidance for rehabilitationists, will be a useful contribution to the debate that is bound to continue about the ethical and legal issues surrounding this perplexing condition.

Fortunately, survival in a permanent vegetative state is the outcome for only a few of the many patients who, thanks to the technologies of resuscitation and intensive care in the acute stage, now survive episodes of severe brain damage that would previously have proved rapidly fatal.

Bryan Jennett CBE, MD, FRCS
Emeritus Professor of Neurosurgery
University of Glasgow, Scotland

Preface

Traumatic brain injury is the primary cause of death in the first 45 years of life. Mortality during the early post-traumatic phase has been significantly reduced in developed countries, thanks to scientific and technological advances in emergency care and reanimation. However, severe post-traumatic disabilities are increasingly frequent. Notably, cases of "vegetative state" lasting anything from a few days to many months have been progressively increasing in frequency. Vegetative state can persist over long periods of time, or may become permanent. These terms are generally applied when the condition lasts for more than 1 year, although they are discouraged in the International Working Party's report on the vegetative state (London, 1996). The estimated incidence is five new cases per million population per year.

The diagnosis of vegetative state and, more specifically, the management of patients in such a condition, require the appropriate expertise and a multidisciplinary approach. The vegetative state requires maintenance of life in the absence of contact between the patient and the outside world, as well as procedures aimed at minimizing the impact of common yet potentially severe complications and aiming to provide the necessary conditions to promote the recovery of motor and higher brain functions. Patients in the vegetative state suffer from serious and diffuse primary and secondary brain lesions and present with deficits reflecting pathophysiological states that may be highly peculiar to the individual injury or injuries. Practical experience is therefore required in order to devise patient-specific therapeutic strategies, while defining precise rules to help the patient progress from an emergency state to a condition of controlled stability.

Unlike long-term coma in steady conditions and with no chances of recovery, patients in the vegetative state show a great many signs and signals which the therapist must identify, help elicit, and then interpret. Besides partial or complete recovery of mental and neurological functions, on the one hand, or outcome as a chronic condition, on the other, another development of the vegetative state has attracted interest in recent years: the state of the minimal responder. This form of life represents a new condition in human existence about which little is yet known, but which needs to be discussed in order to assist those involved in the care of patients in post-traumatic vegetative state.

In the present handbook, combining theoretical and practical approaches, the authors summarize three decades of experience in recuperative care for patients in the vegetative state. The goals are to help bridge a gap in the specialist literature; to provide anesthesiologists, neurologists, physiatricians, internists, and therapists with the expertise they need; and to assist them in improving the treatment of these patients. A second but equally relevant aspect – the relationship between the attending physician and the patient's family during many months of personal contact – is also considered, with the focus on how the physician should relate to the families of patients who lack mental activity and for whom a definite prognosis is not easy to establish. The organization and the structural/technological facilities required when planning and operating a unit dedicated to the treatment of patients in the vegetative state are also discussed, with particular attention being given to the meeting of regulatory requirements.

Giuliano Dolce and Leon Sazbon

Acknowledgements

The Authors wish to thank Dr. and Mrs. G. Pugliese for their warm and friendly support and encouragement to review a full 40-years of work and experience in a book. This project would have never been accomplished without Mrs. Rossella Casciaro's patience and dedication.

Contents

1 **Introduction** 1
History of the Concept of Vegetative State 1

2 **Preliminary Concepts** 3
Leon Sazbon, Giuliano Dolce
Etiology 3
Epidemiology 4
    Age and Gender 4
    Season and Time of Day 5
    Circumstances of VS 5
    Recovery 5
Neuropathological Basis of the
Vegetative State 6

3 **Neurophysiopathology** 11
Giuliano Dolce, Leon Sazbon
Relationship with the Outer World........... 11
Relationship with the Inner World 15
Working Hypothesis on the Brain's Functional
Organization in the Vegetative State 16

4 **Clinical Picture** 18
Leon Sazbon, Giuliano Dolce
General Considerations 18
Medical Aspects and Complications 18
    Cardiovascular Effects 18
    Respiratory Complications 19
    Urinary Complications 19
    Gastrointestinal Complications 19
    Motor Problems 20
    Periarticular New Bone Formation 21
    Seizures 21
    Ventricular Enlargement 22
    Undernutrition 22
    Water and Electrolyte Balance 22
    Hematological Alterations 23
    Hormonal Disorders 23
    Immunologic Disorders 24
    Infections 24
    Deep Vein Thrombosis 24
    Autonomic Disturbances 25
    Dermatological Changes and Bedsores ... 26

    Complications of Medications 26
    Other 26
Neurological Aspects 26
    Neurological Examination 26
    Posture 27
    Spontaneous and Pathological Movements 27
    Passive Movements and Muscular Tone .. 27
    Behavioral Responses 28
    Ocular Motility 28
    Oral Reflexes and Automatism 29
    Oculocephalic Reflex 29
    Trunk and Limbs 29
    Reflexes 30
Recovery of Conscious Activity 30
Prognostic Value of Neurological Signs 32
Giuliano Dolce, Leon Sazbon
    Basic Glossary and Definitions of
    Relevant Signs 33
Differential Diagnosis 35
Erich Schmutzhard
    Introduction 35
    Locked-in Syndrome 36
    Akinetic Mutism 38
    Paramedian Diencephalic Syndrome
    (Hypersomnia) 39
Prognosis and Outcome 41
Leon Sazbon, Giuliano Dolce
    Survival 41
    Recovery of Consciousness 42
    Recovery of Function 44
Assessment of the Vegetative State 46
Ceclia Koren, Mali Gil, Leon Sazbon
    The Glasgow Coma Scale 47
    The Rancho Los Amigos Levels of
    Cognitive Functioning Scale 47
    The Disability Rating Scale 47
    The Western Neuro-Sensory
    Stimulation Profile 48
    The Coma/Near Coma Scale 48
    The Coma Recovery Scale 48
    The Sensory Stimulation Assessment
    Measure 49
    Prognostic Model of Emergence from
    Vegetative States 49

The Coma Exit Chart 50	Procedure for Body Weight Monitoring ... 94
The Sensory Modality Assessment and	Feeding: Routes of Administration 94
Rehabilitation Technique 51	Treatment in the Gym 94
The Preliminary Neuropsychological	Respiratory Treatment 96
Battery 51	Verticalization 97
Loewenstein Communication Scale for the	Hydrotherapy 98
Minimally Responsive Patient 51	Positioning the Patient on the
	Wheelchair 100
	Treatment of Swallowing Disturbances .. 102
5 Ancillary Examination 60	Evaluation and Treatment of Spasticity .. 104
Leon Sazbon	Management of Tracheostomy Patients
Laboratory Findings........................ 60	in the Vegetative State..................... 107
Neuroimaging in the Vegetative State......... 61	*Paolo Scola*
Hans Hacker	Countercannula Disinfection 107
Neurophysiological Assessment of Brain	Inhalation 107
Function in the Persistent Vegetative State 65	Swallowing 108
Alessandro Pincherle, Walter G. Sannita	Fibrotracheal Bronchoscopy 108
Electroencephalography.................. 66	Complications 108
Sleep EEG 67	Cannula Removal 108
Stimulus-Related Evoked Potentials 67	
	8 Minimal Response Syndrome 110
6 Therapy 76	*Ofer Keren, Jacqueline Resnik*
Leon Sazbon, Giuliano Dolce	What is Minimal Response Syndrome? 110
Medical Therapy 76	Significance of the Syndrome 110
Types of Drug Used in the Vegetative State 76	Implications for Health Policy 110
Deep Brain Electrical Stimulation 78	Diagnosis and Assessment Tools 111
Surgical Therapy 79	Incidence and Prevalence 112
Incidence of Hydrocephalus 80	Practical Management Recommendations ... 113
Diagnosis and Treatment 80	Clinical Management 113
Outcome of Surgery 81	Objectives of Treatment 113
Stimulation Techniques 81	Treatment Aimed at "Care" 113
Types and Techniques of Sensory	Treatment Aimed at "Therapy" 114
Stimulation 82	Clinical Treatment Providers 115
Assessment and Outcome 83	Policy and Ethics Related to the Minimally
Other Potential Advantages 84	Responsive Patient 116
Conclusions 84	Conclusions 117
7 Practical Guide to the Management	**9 Ethical Aspects** 120
of Patients in the Vegetative State 89	*Giuliano Dolce, Leon Sazbon*
Maria Quintieri, Sebastiano Serra	
General Considerations 89	
Observation of the General State 90	**10 Treating Families of Patients in**
Survey of Vital Parameters 90	**Vegetative State: Adjustment and**
Pharmacological Therapy and Drug	**Interaction with Hospital Staff** 124
Administration Modes 90	*Anat Shilansky, Rosemarie Weitz*
Procedure: before Drug Administration ... 90	Focusing on the Families 124
Treatment Program 91	Family Assessment 125
Hygiene 91	Typical Psychological Reactions of the
Evaluation of Nutritional Aspects and	Family Members 125
Methods 93	

Focusing on the Staff: Emotional Stress
and Sources of Tension 127
Recommendations and Suggested Strategies . 128

**11 Covert Cognitive Abilities of a Person
with Altered Consciousness** 131
Levy Rahmani

**12 Intensive-Care Unit for Vegetative State:
Management Guidelines** 141
M. Rachele Zylberman
General Organizing Criteria 141
Admission Criteria 142

Discharge Criteria.......................... 143
The Department 143
    Structural Organization 144
Building Materials 145
Equipment and Biotechnology 145
Lying-in Period 145
Gymnasium 146
Sanitary Rooms 146
Human Resources 146

Epilogue and Future Prospects 147
Giuliano Dolce, Leon Sazbon

Index 149

1 Introduction

The progression from unconsciousness and coma to recovered wakefulness – either direct or with a transition through a condition such as the vegetative state – is often characterized by a very complex clinical picture, which is determined by pathophysiological mechanisms that are only known in part. The treatment of patients in this phase – in relation to total or partial recovery of higher brain functions/mental functions – implies detailed procedures, while nursing practices and the many measures required to avoid secondary complications follow precise rules. The recovery of higher brain functions and mental activity requires individualized treatment and relies on an empirical approach, which is usually also based on the creativity, collaboration, and drive of the therapists and family members concerned. Such care cannot replace rehabilitative procedures conceived as part of a scientific plan of treatment. When there are deficits for which detailed identification of the physiopathological basis is lacking, a thoroughly scientifically based therapeutic model must be followed. Experimentation should never be justified in patients who are not in a position to choose treatment or discuss the risks with the attending physician. Although often underestimated, this aspect may generate moral dilemmas for those who are in charge of patients in vegetative state, as these patients present with the most serious of all deficits: the loss of identity. It is also for this reason that, after many years of work with such patients, we have felt the need to carry out close scrutiny and critical evaluation of our experience in order to revise the available clinical outline of the vegetative state and to try characterize the world in which patients in this condition live. This rationale has allowed us to elaborate a new approach to the diagnosis, prognosis, and treatment of patients in the vegetative state.

The driving force behind the preparation of this manual has been not only our immense curiosity and interest in this pathology and its mysterious features, which involve the most highly evolved function of the human being – awareness – but also the love we have felt for those individuals who, through their illness, have contributed to the growth in the quality of our own awareness.

History of the Concept of Vegetative State

The *Oxford American Dictionary* defines "vegetative state" as a condition of living "a merely physical life, devoid of intellectual activity or social intercourse" that is characteristic of "an organic body capable of growth and development but devoid of sensation and thought" [1]. The term "vegetative" is used in the scientific terminology of several languages to signify an "autonomous being."

More than a century ago, in 1899, Rosemblath described the first case of a long-term "chronic" coma in which the patient survived for 8 months on artificial nutrition [2]. The very specific clinical picture of a patient lying passively, akinetic, unresponsive, and with eyes open was described by Kretchmer in 1940 as an "apallic" syndrome, with the term "apallic" being meant to describe the loss of complex functions of the cerebral cortex (pallium) [3]. To the author, this functional decortication signified a "mesencephalic" existence. According to Kretchmer, the loss of cortical function, due either to cortical (and white matter) or brainstem lesions, presents a typical picture of a condition in which there is no contact with the outside world, lack of reaction and recognition, and an attentive look. Kretchmer described this syndrome as an expression of panagnosis and panapraxis. In 1972, Jennett and Plum described this clinical picture in terms of a global disturbance in cognitive function [4].

Following the efforts of several authors, this clinical condition was described in progressively greater detail, and various definitions of it were suggested, including the term "vegetative state" originally proposed by Jennett in 1972 and accepted by the London workshop [5]. Publications by the American Task Force on the vegetative state in 1994 and by the London conference marked a milestone in the study of this serious cerebral pathology, by defining the vegetative state in terms that still apply today. In spite of its negative connotations, the term "vegetative state" does in fact fulfill two requirements in defining the condition: it is universally broad and etymologically correct. The heading "vegetative state" now also includes several syndromes that are often confused with other conditions in the relevant literature, due to the lack of a precise definition based on clinical or anatomical-pathological criteria.

Irrespective of whether its origin is post-traumatic or vascular, a vegetative state may develop after 3–4 weeks of coma, or can occur as a result of progressive, degenerative, or congenital neurological disease. According to the American Task Force, a vegetative state is characterized by concomitant findings of:

- Absence of awareness of self or environment and inability to interact with others
- Absence of sustained or reproducible behavioral or voluntary responses; absence of responses to auditory, visual, tactile, or noxious stimuli
- No comprehension or verbal expression
- Intermittent wakefulness, occasionally observed in the presence of a sleep-wake cycle
- Sufficiently preserved autonomic functions of the hypothalamus and brain stem, allowing survival with medical and nursing care
- Sphincteral incontinence
- Preserved spinal and cranial nerve reflexes (pupillary, oculocephalic, corneal, oculovestibular, and gag)

According to Sazbon, the condition referred to as "vegetative state" is characterized by two cardinal signs – wakefulness and unawareness. Any condition included within this framework is to be considered as a vegetative state, regardless of origin, etiology, duration, course, or outcome. All authors agree with the American Task Force in accepting that two cardinal features characterize the clinical picture: that the vegetative state is one of three possible progressions of coma (although it represents a special condition), and that it manifests a loss of the contents of consciousness even after the recovery of vigilance – as distinct from coma. "Contents of consciousness" is meant to describe both the ability to relate to the outer world (awareness) and the awareness of self. It is apparent that the contents of consciousness are lacking in the vegetative state, as also are sensory functions, attentiveness, and spatiotemporal orientation – that is, all of the functions that make up a conscious experience of the outer world.

We do not regard this point of view as correct, and wish to discuss it from a different angle, based on observations that are expounded in greater detail in Chapter 3, page 16 below. Specifically:

- The vegetative state is an expression of a direct primary brain pathology, and is not an extension of coma. Although existing from the outset of the brain pathology, the vegetative state may be masked by a state of coma, thus hindering a proper diagnosis.
- We believe inappropriate attention has been given to those functions that allow the patient to relate with the inner world, including in addition to imagination, ideas, and will, feelings and memory as well – all functions that allow the continuation of mental life.

References

1. Oxford American Dictionary, ed. Ehrlich E. New York: Oxford University Press, 1980.
2. Rosenblath W. Über einen bemerkenswerten Fall von Hirnerschütterung. Dtch Arch Klein Med 1899; 64: 406–420.
3. Kretchmer E. Das apallische Syndrom. Z ges Neurol Psychiat 1940; 169: 576–579.
4. Jennett B, Plum F. Persistent vegetative state after brain damage: a syndrome in search of a name. Lancet 1972; i: 734–6.
5. Andrews K, Beaumont JG, Danze F, et al. International Working Party report on the vegetative state. London: Royal Hospital for Neurodisability, 1996 (http://www.comarecovery.org/pvs.htm).

2 Preliminary Concepts

Leon Sazbon and Giuliano Dolce

Etiology

Vegetative state (VS) is defined behaviorally as the absence of an adequate response to the outside world and absence of any evidence of reception or projection of information in the presence of sleep – wake cycles. Patients may have periods of wakefulness with open eyes and movement, but responsiveness is limited to primitive postural and reflex movements of the limbs. They never speak, and some never regain recognizable mental function [1]. According to the *Oxford English Dictionary* [2], individuals in VS "live a merely physical life, devoid of intellectual activity or social intercourse; [they are] capable of growth and development but devoid of sensation and thought." The term was coined in 1972 by Jennett and Plum [1] to eliminate the confusion caused by the multitude of disorders in the literature, such as akinetic mutism, apallic syndrome, and prolonged coma, which share the common denominators of wakefulness with unawareness. These clinical criteria for VS were more recently confirmed by the Multi-Society Task Force [3].

Over the years, certain qualifiers have been added to the term VS, often incorrectly. The term "persistent vegetative state" (PVS) has been used by some researchers to refer to any type of VS, and by others to refer specifically to VS of long duration [3–6]. The word "persistent" is defined by *Webster's Tenth Collegiate Dictionary* [7] as "continuing to exist in spite of interference or treatment", and "persistence" is defined by the *COBUILD Collins English Language Dictionary* [8] as continuing "to exist, even after you have tried to make it disappear." The indiscriminate use of "persistent" in relation to VS has led to the misconception that the syndrome is always irreversible, when the term actually refers merely to a disorder that began in the past and is continuing in the present. This problem is exacerbated when (as is not uncommon), "persistent" is replaced with "permanent". The latter term describes to a state that began in the present and will continue through the future – implying a negative and irreversible prognosis. There is a fine line between reversible and the irreversible VS, and a clear clinical definition is still lacking. On the basis of our experience, we consider VS, using practical criteria, irreversible when it has persisted for 1 year in patients after coma of traumatic origin, or for 6 months in patients after coma of nontraumatic etiology. These distinctions have importance for medical decisions regarding the introduction or continuation of therapy and its intensity. The International Working Party [9] has recommended that both terms – persistent and permanent – should be dropped altogether.

VS should be differentiated from coma, which is characterized by an inability to obey commands, utter recognizable words, or open the eyes, and the absence of sleep – wake cycles. Coma is always a transient state. According to Plum [10], comatose patients who survive for more than a few days or weeks will regain cyclic electroencephalographic patterns of arousal/nonarousal with or without their behavioral appearance. These patients may live indefinitely, provided they retain hypothalamic functions and a majority of tegmental brainstem functions [10].

VS is always an expression of a direct primary brain pathology and is not an extension of coma. Although it exists from the start, the VS is masked by the state of coma, thus hindering diagnosis.

The causes of VS may be acute (traumatic or nontraumatic) or chronic (degenerative and metabolic disorders or developmental malformations). Examples of traumatic injury are motor vehicle accidents, gunshot wounds, domestic accidents, and birth injury; nontraumatic causes include hypoxic – ischemic encephalopathy, central nervous system (CNS) infection, CNS tumor, cerebrovascular injury, and CNS toxins or poisoning. Examples of degenerative disorders are Alzheimer's disease, multi-infarct dementia, and Creutzfeldt-Jakob disease, and examples of developmental malformations include congenital hydrocephalus and severe microcephaly. The most common acute causes in adults and children are injury-induced head trauma and hypoxic-ischemic encephalopathy, generally following coma of several days to weeks. In rare cases, VS may occur immediately after traumatic injury (documented, for example, in boxers after a knockout). The duration of VS can vary widely, from only a few seconds to many years.

Epidemiology

The early editions of the International Classification of Diseases (ICD) grouped vegetative state (VS) with acute coma (code 780.01), and it was only 9 years ago that VS was first listed as a distinct entity (code 780.03). No epidemiological studies of VS have been conducted since the new classification, so figures are hard to establish. The estimated annual incidence of brain trauma in the United States varies widely, from 180 to 400 patients per 100 000 population [11–13]. The prevalence of VS is unknown, although in some American publications the suspicion is stated that the numbers range between 10 000 and 25 000 adults and 6000 to 10 000 children [14–18]. Researchers in Japan, France, Italy and other countries have calculated a national annual incidence of 0.9–2 per 100 000 [19–22]. The percentage of patients remaining in VS has been estimated in different studies to range from 0.2% to 14 % of all cases of acute coma in various studies [19,23–28], depending on patient age, etiology, and the temporal criteria used. The actual rate may be even higher, as patients with open eyes are often misdiagnosed as being comatose.

In Israel, until recently, all patients in the country who were in traumatic VS for at least 1 month were referred to the Loewenstein Rehabilitation Hospital. This center therefore provides an excellent setting for an epidemiological analysis of VS in Israel. From 1975 to 1998, a total of 580 patients with VS of traumatic origin were admitted, an average of 23.2 new cases per year. The true incidence may of course be higher, as these figures exclude patients with short-term VS. For the first 8 years (1975–1983), an average of 16.3 patients were admitted per year, whereas in the last 15 years, this number jumped to 30. This increase may be explained by the increased use of intensive life support already at the accident site, the more rapid means of transport to neurosurgical centers, and the accelerated growth of the population. According to Israeli population studies, the incidence of traumatic VS is in the order of 0.4–0.5 per 100 000 inhabitants [29,30]

Age and Gender

The age distribution of patients in VS was calculated in an Israeli series of 580 patients at the Loewenstein Hospital and correlated with recovery [31]. The findings are shown in Table 2.**1**.

There were 446 males and 134 females, a ratio of 3.3 : 1.0. In an earlier series of 134 patients reported by the same authors [30], the mean age was 26.8 ± 14.6 years, with a range of 3–79 and a male/female ratio of 4 : 1. Most of the cases of VS (72.24 %) occurred in patients between the ages of 16 and 45.

Age was apparently related to recovery of consciousness, with the highest recovery rate (about 70 %) being recorded in patients less than 30 years old, followed closely by the 31–45-year-old group. Only 50.5 % of patients aged over 46 years recovered consciousness. The mean age in the recovered group was 28.1 ± 14.2 years, and in the nonrecov-

Table 2.1 Age distribution of 580 patients in the vegetative state (mean 29.95 ± 15.4 years; range 3–78 years; median 25 years) [31]

	Age groups					Total
	3–15	16–30	31–45	46–60	61+	
Recovery	41 (69.49%)	220 (70.96%)	70 (64.22%)	35 (50.72%)	15 (45.45%)	381 (65.68%)
No recovery	18 (30.51%)	90 (29.04%)	39 (35.78%)	34 (49.28%)	18 (54.55%)	199 (34.32%)
Total	59 (10.2%)	310 (53.4%)	109 (18.8%)	69 (11.99%)	33 (5.7%)	580 (100.0%)

ered group, 33.4 ± 16.9 years; this difference was statistically significant ($P > 0.001$) [31]. However, in our experience, children have a poorer functional outcome than adults. Some authors hypothesize that the lesser myelination in the young brain and its lower ability to regulate vascular perfusion make it subject to greater shearing forces during acute injury [32–34]. However, other authors disagree, claiming that the chances for both vital and functional recovery decrease with age [35,36].

Season and Time of Day

The rate of occurrence of new cases of VS shows seasonal variability. The highest frequency has been noted in fall (autumn), followed in order by summer, winter, and spring [30,37]. In the Israeli study by Sazbon et al. [20], the frequency peaked in October and August ($P < 0.003$), coinciding with the school holiday and the Jewish High Holy Days. Time of day is also a factor, with 70 % of patients being injured between 5 p. m. and midnight [30].

Circumstances of VS

Most cases of VS can be traced to traumatic head injury. In Israel, the most common cause of traumatic head injury leading to VS is road accidents (Table 2.2), with a considerably higher rate of blunt injuries (95 %) than penetrating injuries (5 %).

Sazbon et al. [30] studied 70 patients in VS admitted to Loewenstein Rehabilitation Hospital who were victims of car accidents. They found that 39 % had been pedestrians, 36 % passengers in the vehicle, 16 % drivers of the vehicle, and 9 % cyclists. Interestingly, the pedestrians received only 17–21 % of the acute brain injuries and the passengers 19–21 %, whereas the drivers received 37 % of the acute head injuries, but accounted for only 16 % of the VS cases. The pedestrians and cyclists had the worst prognosis, with 56 % and 50 %, respectively, remaining in permanent VS until death. Rates for drivers and passengers were 40 % and 37 %, respectively. These data are in line with the findings of the 1988 *Fédération Française des Associations de Médecins Conseils* (FFAMC) conference [38], organized by consultant physicians of insurance companies in France, which concluded that VS lasted markedly longer in pedestrians hit by cars than in car drivers.

Recovery

Recovery from VS is defined as the ability to establish visual or verbal contact with the outside world [32]. Sazbon and Grosswasser [29] reported a 54 % recovery rate in their earlier series of 134 patients and 65.68 % in the later series of 580 patients [31]. Most patients who regained consciousness did so in the first 3 months. After 1 year, only a handful of the patients still in VS achieved a state of minimal responsiveness. The others remained in permanent VS or died.

Regrettably, no large series of VS patients have recently been published in the medical literature for comparison. Only two studies of VS of traumatic etiology were conducted in the 1970s – those by Vigouroux et al. [39] with 150 cases and Higashi et al. [19] with 100 cases of all etiologies, of which 38 % were of traumatic origin. In the 1980s, studies were conducted by Bricolo et al. [23] (135 cases), Brule et al. [20] (100 cases), Lyle et al. [40] (159 cases), and Braakman and Jennett [27] (140 cases). In the 1990s, Sazbon and Grosswasser [29] published one series of 134 cases of traumatic etiology, followed by Levin et al. [41] (93 cases) and the Multi-Society Task Force on PVS publication, which summarized previous publications [17]. To date, there have been only three studies of patients in VS of nontraumatic origin: Levy et al. [42] (55 cases), Heind and Laub [43] (127 cases of mixed etiology) and Sazbon et al. [44] (102 cases).

Table 2.2 Causes of brain injury in Israel [30,31]

	1975–1983 (n = 134)	1975–1998 (n = 580)
Road accidents	92 (69 %)	480 (79.32 %)
War wounds and army accidents	16 (12 %)	46 (7.93 %)
Miscellaneous[*]	26 (19 %)	74 (12.75 %)

[*] Assaults, falls, domestic mishaps, other accidents. This rate may be lower than in other countries because of the low incidence of alcoholism in Israel [30]. Reproduced with permission from Taylor & Francis Limited, http//www.tandf.co.uK. Brain Injury 6: 359–362, 1992

Neuropathological Basis of the Vegetative State

Research into the neuropathology of vegetative state (VS) has been delayed because of a low level of interest among physicians and the few centers working with this type of patient worldwide.

Patients with VS appear to have a macroscopically normal brain. In 1956, Strich was the first to suggest that diffuse axonal injury (DAI) in the subcortical white matter and descending tracts into the brain stem was the basis of what he termed "severe post-traumatic dementia" [45]. This was later supported by Peerless and Rewcastle [46] and Zimmerman et al. [47]. However, Jellinger [48] and Peters and Rothemund [49] claimed that the axonal damage is secondary ischemia, brain swelling, or high intracranial pressure. In animal studies conducted in the 1980s, Gennarelli et al. [50] and Adams et al. [51] proved that the primary damage was axonal.

Most of our current knowledge on the neuropathology of VS comes from the studies by Adams et al. [52–54], Graham et al. [55], and Kinney and colleagues [56,57]. Recently, Adams et al. [58] conducted a precise and detailed neuropathological brain study of 49 patients in VS who never recovered, including 35 after blunt head injury. They found, in agreement with Kinney and Samuels [56], that VS results from widespread and bilateral damage to the cerebral cortex itself, the thalamus, and many of the intracortical and subcortical connections. This leads to one of three presentations: diffuse destruction of the cerebral cortex, either alone or associated with diffuse damage to the white matter; or diffuse damage to the thalamus only. By contrast, Maxwell et al. [59] claimed that the diffuse axonal damage was in effect a manifestation of a process of secondary axotomy, in which acute brain injury caused focal swelling of the axons and mitochondria, nodal blebs, and a focal decrease in the internodal axonal diameter, followed by loss of axonal microtubules, alterations in neurofilaments, involution of the internodal axolemma, and development of axonal swelling, culminating in axonal separation with axonal retraction bulbs. There may be microcystic spaces, with residual hemosiderin and macrophages [60]. The primary axotomy is identified within 1 h of injury, and the secondary axotomy after at least 4 h.

On the basis of their comprehensive study, Adams et al. [58] distinguished the severity of DAI. In grade 1, the damage is exclusively in the white matter and there are no focal lesions, and in grade 2, the lesion is localized to the corpus callosum. Grade 3, the most severe, is characterized by widespread damage to the white matter axons and local lesions in the corpus callosum and rostral brain stem. Grade 1 DAI is infrequent in VS, but occurs often in minor head injuries, serving as the pathological mechanism for clinical sequelae. The focal damage may be seen macroscopically, but is seldom observed only in microscopic examinations. In their series [58], 71% of the brains had grade 2 or 3 DAI, with structural abnormalities, intracranial hematomas, and sustained moderate or severe ischemia. Some also had diffuse neuronal loss in the cortex, with or without "excessive pallor" of the thalamus and white matter.

In the study by Kinney et al. [57], DAI was also the more common lesion, appearing as damage to the white matter, with hemorrhagic foci in the corpus callosum and the dorsolateral quadrant of the rostral brain stem, adjacent to the superior cerebellar peduncle. Cervos-Navarro and Lafuente [61] reported that the severity of the clinical syndrome and the outcome depend on the total number of damaged axons and their location, as well as the proportion of damaged to undamaged axons. Disruptive damage leads to axotomy, whereas nondisruptive damage is internal. Axonal repair may be attempted with both types, but is usually more successful with the second [61].

In VS, the thalamus is apparently injured via one of two mechanisms: retrograde degeneration as a result of the axonal damage, which takes several months to appear, or neuronal loss as result of ischemia, which becomes apparent a very short time after the event [58]. There is a lower frequency of damage to the cerebral cortex and/or brain stem. In the few patients affected, the lesions tend to occur in the midline, or less often laterally, in the cerebral peduncle [58]. The preservation of the hypothalamus and brain stem is characteristic of VS, as they are necessary to maintain vegetative functions. Of the 49 patients investigated by Adams et al. [58], 28 sustained damage to the thalamus. In most of them, the lesion was diffuse, and it was almost always associated with widespread damage to the white matter, with or without cerebral cortex or brain-stem damage. The importance of the thalamus was underscored by Kinney al. [57] in 1994, in their study of the brain of Karen Anne Quinlan, a 21-year-old woman who remained in VS for 10 years after a cardiopulmonary arrest. The disproportionately greater damage to the thalamus than to the cerebral cortex raised questions about the role of the thalamus in cognition and awareness. Other authors have reported similar findings [48,62].

Ischemia, brain swelling, anoxia, and acidosis play a role in the production of secondary damage after VS of traumatic origin. This includes vascular proliferation in the impact zone, which peaks in the first 3 weeks after injury and diminishes gradually thereafter over months and years, leaving functional small sclerotic vessels [61]. In the series published by Adams et al. [58], ischemic brain damage was present on arterial boundary zones in 43% of cases, and was often accompanied by diffuse signs, indicating a global reduction in cerebral blood flow (CBS). Following the report by Graham et al. [60], they classified the ischemic damage as follows:
- Severe: diffuse or multifocal lesions or infarcts within specific arterial areas
- Moderate: ischemic damage limited to arterial boundary zones, appearing alone or in combination with subtotal infarction in the distribution of arterial territories

Ischemic lesions tend to be more severe in the presence of concomitant intracranial hematomas or extracranial injuries, particularly if the intracranial pressure is high [63].

Some researchers have postulated that over time, the volume and weight of the brain are reduced due to the striking loss of axons and neurons, so that the brain becomes more consistent, with an apparently compensatory enlargement of the ventricles [58,64]. There may also be a secondary astrocytic reaction, which increases over weeks and months, resulting in a glial scar [61]. The role of the glial proliferation is not clear. Ramón y Cajal (quoted in [61]) suggested that glia inhibit axonal regeneration, whereas Reier et al. [65] affirmed that axons can penetrate the axonal web. Other authors have supported the notion that laminin, a growth substrate for brain neurons, is produced by astrocytes following injury, inducing neuron sprouting [66–68].

Another secondary event in trauma is collagen production and fibrosis, especially when the injury occurs in the vicinity of the cortex. Fibroblasts are present around vessels, but usually disappear within a few months [61].

When the sequence of histological reactions stabilizes, a contusional zone remains, resembling an old infarction.

The same lesions seen in humans have been reproduced experimentally in primates by Gennarelli et al. [69], Jane et al. [70], and others [71,72]. The animals were subjected to high-magnitude angular acceleration of the head and long-pulsion (5–10 ms) and controlled head movements without focal loading. The severity of axonal injury depended on all three conditions and on the direction of the head motion. Sagittal acceleration produced DAI grade 1, acceleration in the coronal plane produced DAI grade 3, and horizontal acceleration produced grade 2 [53,73].

References

1. Jennett B, Plum F. Persistent vegetative state after brain damage: a syndrome in search of a name. Lancet 1972; i: 734–736.
2. Oxford English Dictionary, 2nd ed. Simpson JA, Weiner ESC, editors. Oxford: Clarendon Press, 1989. Online: http://www.oed.com/, November 2001.
3. Multi-Society Task Force on PVS. Medical aspects of the persistent vegetative state, 1. N Engl J Med 1994; 330: 1499–508.
4. Sazbon L, Grosswasser Z. Prolonged coma, vegetative state, postcomatose unawareness: semantics or better understanding? Brain Inj 1991; 5: 1–2.
5. Giaccino JT, Zasler ND. Outcome after severe traumatic brain injury: coma, vegetative state and the minimally responsive state. J Head Trauma Rehabil 1995; 10: 40–56.
6. Higashi K, Sakata Y, Hatano M, et al. Epidemiological studies of patients with persistent vegetative state. J Neurol Neurosurg Psychiatry 1977; 40: 876–85.
7. Webster's Tenth New Collegiate Dictionary. Springfield, MA: Merriam-Webster, 1995.
8. Collins COBUILD English-language dictionary. London: Collins, 1985.
9. Andrews K, Beaumont JG, Danze F, et al. International Working Party report on the vegetative state. London: Royal Hospital for Neurodisability, 1996 (http://www.comarecovery.org/pvs.htm).
10. Plum F. Coma and related global disturbances of the human conscious state. Cereb Cortex 1991; 9: 359–424.

11. Klauber MR, Barrett-Connor E, Marshall LF, Bowers SA. The epidemiology of head injury: a prospective study of entire community-San Diego County, California, 1978. Am J Epidemiol 1981; 113: 500–9.
12. Kraus JF, Black MA, Hessol N, et al. The incidence of acute brain injury and serious impairment in a defined population. Am J Epidemiol 1984; 119: 186–201.
13. Whitman S, Coonley-Hoganson R, Desai BT. Comparative head trauma experiences in two socioeconomically different Chicago-area communities: a population study. Am J Epidemiol 1984; 119: 570–80.
14. Ashwal S, Eyman RK, Call TL. Life expectancy of children in a persistent vegetative state. Pediatr Neurol 1994; 10: 27–33.
15. Gillies JD, Seshia SS. Vegetative state following coma in childhood: evolution and outcome. Dev Med Child Neurol 1980; 22: 642–8.
16. Jennett B. Vegetative state; causes, management, ethical dilemmas. Curr Anaesth Crit Care 1991; 2: 57–61.
17. Multi-Society Task Force on PVS. Medical aspects of the persistent vegetative state, 1. N Engl J Med 1994; 330: 1499–508.
18. Tresch DD, Farrol HS, Duthie EH, et al. Clinical characteristics of patients in the persistent vegetative state. Arch Intern Med 1991; 151: 930–2.
19. Higashi K, Sakata Y, Hatano M, et al. Epidemiological studies on patients with a persistent vegetative state. J Neurol Neurosurg Psychiatry 1977; 40: 876–85.
20. Brule JF, Danze F, Vallee D. Etat végétative chronique. Rev Fr Dommage Corpor 1988; 14: 191–5.
21. Blin F. Epidemiologia e costo delle cure. In: Tasseau F, Boucand MH, Le Gall JR, Verspieren P, editors. Evoluzione del coma: stati vegetativi cronici, ripercussioni umane, aspetti medici, giuridici ed etici. Milan: Kailash, 1994: 39–52.
22. Sato S, Inamura H, Ueki K, et al. Epidemiological survey of vegetative state patients in the Tokohu District, Japan: special reference to the follow-up study after one year. Neurol Med Chir (Tokyo) 1979; 8: 327–33.
23. Bricolo A, Turazzi S, Feriotti G. Prolonged post-traumatic unconsciousness. J Neurosurg 1980; 2: 625–34.
24. Granholm L, Svendgaard N. Hydrocephalus following traumatic head injuries. Scand J Rehabil Med 1972; 4: 31–4.
25. Grossman P, Hagel K. Post-traumatic apallic syndrome following head injury, 1: clinical characteristics. Disabil Rehabil 1996; 18: 1–20.
26. Campbell AGM. Children in a persistent vegetative state. Br Med J 1984; 289: 1022–3.
27. Braakman R, Jennett B, Minderhoud M. Prognosis of the post-traumatic vegetative state. Acta Neurochir 1988; 95: 49–52.
28. Kampfl A, Schmutzhar E, Franz G, et al. Prediction of recovery from post-traumatic vegetative state with cerebral magnetic resonance imaging. Lancet 1998; 351: 1763–7.
29. Sazbon L, Groswasser Z. Outcome in 134 patients with prolonged post-traumatic unawareness, 1: parameters determining late recovery of consciousness. J Neurosurg 1990; 72: 75–80.
30. Sazbon L, Costeff H, Groswasser Z. Epidemiological findings in traumatic post-comatose unawareness. Brain Inj 1992; 6: 59–62.
31. Sazbon L. Vegetative state [personal communication].
32. Sazbon L. Prolonged coma. Progr Clin Neurosci 1985; 2: 65–81.
33. Dambska M, Dydyk L, Szretter T, et al. Topography of lesions in newborn and infants' brains following cardiac arrest and resuscitation. Biol Neonate 1976; 29: 194–206.
34. Mahoney WJ, Souza BJ, Haller JA, et al. Long term outcome of children with severe trauma and prolonged coma. Pediatrics 1983; 71: 756–62.
35. Johnston RB, Davis Mellts E. Pediatric coma: prognosis and outcome. Dev Med Child Neurol 1980; 22: 3–12.
36. Bruce DA, Schut L, Bruno L, et al. Outcome following severe head injuries in children. J Neurosurg 1978; 48: 679–88.
37. Thompson GB, Klonoff H. Epidemiology of head injuries. In: Vinken PJ, Bruyn GW, editors. Handbook of clinical neurology, vol 3. Amsterdam: North-Holland, 1975: 23–4.
38. Agustin P, Dujardin M, Fourbier C, et al. Les traumatismes craniens avec coma: analyse descriptive et approche pronostique. Colloque de Rouen FFAMCSA, Janvier 1988. Paris: ADEP/LITEC, 1990: 1–36.
39. Vigouroux PR, Baurand C, Choux M, et al. Etat actuel des aspects séquelaires graves dans les traumatismes craniens de l'adulte. Neurochirurgie 1972; 18 (Suppl 2): 1–260.
40. Lyle DM, Pierce JP, Freeman EA, et al. Clinical course and outcome of severe head injury in Australia. J Neurosurg 1986; 65: 15–8.
41. Levin HS, Saydjian C, Eisenberg HM, et al. Vegetative state after closed head injuries: a traumatic coma bank report. Arch Neurol 1991; 48: 550–85.
42. Levy DE, Knill-Jones RP, Plum F. The vegetative state and its prognosis following nontraumatic coma. Ann NY Acad Sci 1978; 315: 295–306.

43. Heind JT, Laub MC. Outcome of persistent vegetative state following hypoxia or traumatic brain injury in children and adolescents. Neuropediatrica 1996; 27: 94–100.
44. Sazbon L, Zagreba F, Ronen I, et al. Course and outcome of patients in vegetative state of non traumatic etiology. J Neurol Neurosurg Psychiatry 1993; 56: 407–9.
45. Strich SJ. Diffuse degeneration of white matter in severe dementia following head injury. J Neurol Neurosurg Psychiatry 1956;19: 163–85.
46. Peerless SJ, Rewcastle NB. Shear injuries of the brain. Can Med Assoc J 1967; 96: 577–582.
47. Zimmerman RA, Bilaniuk LT, Gennarelli T. Computed tomography of shearing injuries of the cerebral white matter. Radiology 1978; 127: 393–6.
48. Jellinger K. Pathology and pathogenesis of apallic syndromes following closed head injuries. In: Dalle Ore G, Gerstenbrand F, Lucking CH, Peters F, Peters UH, editors. The apallic syndrome. Berlin: Springer, 1977: 88–103.
49. Peters F, Rothemund E. Neuropathology of the traumatic apallic syndrome. In: Dalle Ore G, Gerstenbrand F, Lucking CH, Peters F, Peters UH, editors. The apallic syndrome. Berlin: Springer, 1977: 78–87.
50. Gennarelli TA, Thibault LE, Adams JH, et al. Diffuse axonal injury and traumatic coma in the primate. Ann Neurol 1982;12: 564–74.
51. Adams JH, Graham DI, Murray LS, et al. Diffuse axonal injury due to nonmissile head injury in humans: an analysis of 45 cases. Ann Neurol 1982; 12: 557–63.
52. Adams JH, Doyle D, Graham DI, et al. Microscopic diffuse axonal injury in cases of head injury. Med Sci Law 1985; 25: 265–9.
53. Adams JH, Doyle D, Ford I, et al. Diffuse axonal injury in head injury: definition, diagnosis and grading. Histopathology 1989; 15: 49–59.
54. Adams JH, Mitchell DE, Graham DI, et al. Diffuse brain damage of immediate impact type. Brain 1977; 89: 253–68.
55. Graham DI, Lawrence AE, Adams JH, et al. Brain damage in non-missile head injury secondary to high intracranial pressure. Neuropathol Appl Neurobiol 1987; 13: 209–17.
56. Kinney HC, Samuels MA. Neuropathology of the persistent vegetative state: a review. J Neuropathol Exp Neurol 1994; 53: 548–58.
57. Kinney HC, Korein J, Panigrahy A, et al. Neuropathological findings in the brain of Karen Ann Quinlan: the role of the thalamus in the persistent vegetative state. N Engl J Med 1994; 330: 1469–75.
58. Adams JH, Jennett B, McLellan DR, et al. The neuropathology of the vegetative state after head injury. J Clin Pathol 1999; 52: 804–6.
59. Maxwell WL, Povlishock JT, Graham DI. A mechanistic analysis of nondisruptive axonal injury: a review. J Neurotrauma 1997; 14: 419–40.
60. Graham DI, Ford I, Adams JH, et al. Ischemic brain damage is still common in fatal non-missile head injury. J Neurol Neurosurg Psychiatry 1989; 52: 346–50.
61. Cervos-Navarro J, Lafuente JV. Traumatic brain injuries: structural changes. J Neurol Sci 1991; 103: S3–14.
62. Relkin NR, Petito CK, Plum F. Coma and the vegetative state associated with thalamic injury after cardiac arrest [abstract]. Ann Neurol 1990; 128: 221–2.
63. Sazbon L, Groswasser Z. Outcome of 134 patients with prolonged post-traumatic unawareness, 1: parameters determining late recovery of consciousness. J Neurosurg 1990; 72: 75–80.
64. McLellan DR, Adams JH, Graham DI, et al. The structural basis of the vegetative state and prolonged coma after non-missile head injury. In: Papo I, Cohadon F, Massarotti M, editors. Le coma traumatique. Padua: Liviana, 1986: 165–87.
65. Reier PJ, Stensaas LJ, Guth L. The astrocytic scar as impediment to regeneration in the central nervous system. In: Kao CC, Bunge RP, Reier PJ, editors. Spinal cord reconstruction. New York: Raven Press, 1983; 163–95.
66. Manthorpe M, Nieto-Sampedro M, Skaper SD, et al. Neurotrophic activity in brain wounds of the developing rat: correlation with implant survival in the wound cavity. Brain Res 1983; 267: 47–56.
67. Rogers SL, Letourneau PC, Palm SL, et al. Neurite extension by peripheral and central nervous system neurons in response to substratum-bound fibronectin and laminin. Dev Biol 1983; 98: 212–20.
68. Liesi P, Kaaklola S, Dahl D, et al. Laminin is induced in astrocytes of adult brain by injury. Embo J 1984; 3: 683–6.
69. Gennarelli TA, Thibault LE, Adams JH, et al. Diffuse axonal injury and traumatic coma in the primate. Ann Neurol 1982; 12: 564–74.
70. Jane JA, Osward S, Genarelli T. Axonal degeneration induced by experimental noninvasive minor head injury. J Neurosurg 1985; 62: 96–100.
71. Ommaya AK, Genarelli TA. Experimental head injury. In: Vinken PJ, Bruyn GW, editors. Handbook of clinical neurology. Amsterdam: North-Holland, 1975: 67–91.
72. Erb DE, Povlishock JT. Axonal damage in severe traumatic brain injury: an experimental study in CAT. Acta Neuropathol 1988; 76: 347–58.

73. Gennarelli TA, Thibault LE. Biological models of head injury. In: Becker DP, Povlishock JT, editors. Central nervous system trauma: status report. Bethesda, MD: National Institutes of Health, 1985: 391–404.

3 Neurophysiopathology

Giuliano Dolce and Leon Sazbon

Relationship with the Outer World

From a neurophysiological point of view, the brain structures and functional organization regulating conscious activity and allowing awake humans to express the contents of consciousness (that is to say, awareness of oneself and of the environment) only subsist when four specific conditions are met simultaneously:
- Presence of specific sensory inputs
- Presence of nonspecific, diffuse input from the ascending reticulothalamic activating systems diffusely projecting to the cortex
- Cortical activity with neuronal discharge in the medium-frequency range
- Activation of the primitive ipsilateral and contralateral motor systems, which stabilize spatial relationships and orient the system toward the source, thereby allowing for perception

These functional conditions must have a certain degree of interaction (the "theory of coherence"), and it is therefore insufficient for a certain cerebral area to be activated unless activation occurs to a degree that is appropriate to the activity of the interacting structures or functions. Information processing in the nervous system (which lacks a central pacemaker) becomes comprehensible only when the functional interaction between the activated cortical areas or brain systems is taken into account. This interaction is largely mediated through the thalamocortical system; another example elucidating the theory of coherence is given by the functional relationship between cortex, hippocampus and limbic system. Cortical information processing appears optimal when a theta rhythm of around 5 Hz is established in the hippocampus. This mechanism is considered to be the neurophysiological correlate for the phenomenon occurring (for instance during tests at school) when a strong emotional charge interferes with cortical information recall and causes a black-out of memory functions. It is therefore to no avail to activate a single cerebral structure in order to obtain improvement in performance. It would be necessary to determine the optimal coherence between the various structures to attain the best performance.

For many years, neurologists adhered to the concept that any given clinical picture would reflect the dysfunction (almost invariably a deficit, seldom hyperfunction or malfunction) of a particular structure or system. This induced Plum and Posner [1] to outline a number of different syndromes, characterized by their complex clinical picture and referred to as direct or indirect lesions of the encephalic brain stem, i.e. the syndrome of rostrocaudal deterioration responsible for coma.

The vegetative state, by contrast, results from a great variety of etiologies and pathophysiological mechanisms, in comparison with the relatively uniform clinical picture which, for instance, synthetically represents the "locked-out" syndrome [2]. Laminar encephalitis, selective damage to cortical neurons induced by insulin, several metabolic disturbances, anoxia, multiple or isolated lesions of the hemispheric structures, diencephalon, or brain stem, and lesions of the connections both between or within brain hemispheres, are all pathophysiological mechanisms capable of inducing a vegetative state.

The location, extent, and nature of the pathological anatomic lesions that determine the vegetative state do not correlate with the clinical progression. The fact that the deficit causing the vegetative state does not involve a single functional area alone, but depends on a reduction of the reciprocal connections among several brain structures, explains the lack of a definite anatomical correlate as a reference for recuperation. In our personal experience, we have often observed that patients with relatively inconspicuous morphological damage on brain computed tomography (CT) or magnetic resonance imaging (MRI) scans did not recover awareness, in contrast to unexpected recuperations in post-traumatic patients with multiple extensive lesions characterizing a severe postacute encephalopathy.

This discrepancy is most likely due to a single factor, represented by the degree of functional residual plasticity (very powerful at an age when maturation is incomplete, e.g. before 25 years), which allows a new postlesional organization to form (in general by the sixth month, but most often between the third and fourth months after brain injury), thereby establishing a certain degree of reciprocal activation among the major functional systems regulating the mechanisms needed for awareness to exist.

Following a certain functional hierarchy, the first of these major mechanisms is related to medium-frequency cortical neuronal discharge. Consciousness is not manifested at maximal discharge frequencies, during metabolic coma (e.g. in case of very high insulinemia), or when there are interfering physical factors such as low temperatures. Second, consciousness is almost completely lacking in the absence of specific input, as is seen for instance when sensory deprivation is induced experimentally. Also, conscious activity is not seen with reduced function of the ascending nonspecific activating systems (e. g. in barbiturate coma) or of the reticulothalamic system projecting diffusely to the cortex.

Although the functional anatomy and pathophysiology of these systems have been described and extensively covered in the literature, the motor component, which intervenes in mechanisms permitting contact with the outer world, has not. This contact is completely interrupted in the vegetative state.

The primitive motor systems are responsible for ipsilateral and contralateral movements, described in detail in the German literature [3,4]. We wish to describe these motor systems at this point, because the functional role they play in the pathophysiology of vegetative state is poorly known, although it is as relevant as that of the other systems described above.

Movements toward the right or left determine the spatial displacement of the body. Two distinct systems exist in each hemisphere to execute movements toward the same side (the ipsilateral system) or toward the opposite side (the contralateral system) (Fig. 3.1). The neurons of the ipsilateral system originate in several nuclei of the vestibular area, along the border of the floor of the fourth ventricle. The axons of these neurons rise, without crossing, to the mesencephalic periaqueductal reticular substance, where they terminate. The fibers of a second neuron rise, together with the uninterrupted fibers from the reticular substance, to the ventral intermediate nucleus (VIM) of the thalamus and reach cortical area 6aδ. A second system is represented by fibers from the central medial thalamic nucleus reaching the putamen. If this system is stimulated in the cat or monkey, the head and the body turn toward the stimulated side. A comparable stimulation effect has also been observed in humans. In wakefulness, this system is continuously active and pulls the body to that side when the opposite system is not operative. The erect body posture and straight backward movement known as backward locomotion are achieved in the wakeful state through a physiological level of excitation that is symmetrical in intensity on both sides of the brain stem.

The execution of the movements involved in contralateral turning of the body and eyes involves a far more complex functional arrangement than in the case of ipsilateral movements, the key anatomical structure of which is the "entopeduncular" nucleus of Montanalli – Hassler, or internal pallidum. The contralateral thalamocortical system arises from several thalamic nuclei to reach different cortical areas. The known circuits are:

- From the anterior ventral nucleus of thalamus (receiving afferents from the internal part of the pallidum) to area 6aα
- From the posterior lateral nucleus of thalamus to area 8 and 6spl
- From the anterior nucleus to area 32, within the cingulum

All of these cortical areas project onto the other segments of the pallidum, along with fibers stemming from area 22.8 and probably also area 5. A part of these fibers crosses the internal pallidum, again reaching the anterior ventral nucleus and closing the pallidothalamocortical circuit.

The most important descending portion from the pallidum is the Q-bundle, which crosses the median line and terminates in a periaqueductal zone surrounded by the reticular formation, from which the dorsolateral tegmental tract descends. The effect on the movement of arms, legs and eyes takes place through the descending reticulobulbospinal and vestibulospinal fibers, a portion of which passes through the vestibular nuclei. The contralateral system in the frontal lobe (area 8) and parietal lobe (areas 5 b and 7) also provides fibers that descend directly through the internal capsule and cerebral peduncle to cross the median line at the mesencephalic level and terminate in the reticular formation. In humans, the selective stimulation of the internal pallidum and its efferent systems by stereotactic methods causes sideways movements of the body toward the opposite side and dilatation of the pupils. If the head is immobilized, vicarious movements toward the opposite side of the ocular bulbs can be observed. A weaker response is obtained with stimulation of the external pallidum.

Through GABAergic neurotransmission, the putamen inhibits both the internal and external pallida, with its stimulation provoking an ipsilateral sideways movement. Stimulation of the right putamen, for instance, provokes the same response as stimulation of the left pallidum – i. e., a sideways movement toward the right. These systems for sideways movements toward the opposite side are continuously active in the state of wakefulness. When activity is symmetrical and equivalent in both hemispheres, a tonic, erect position of the body directed frontward, not sideways, is achieved. A forward marching movement (forward locomotion) results when the symmetrical activation of ipsilateral systems is reduced simultaneously.

These subcortical and cortical mechanisms for sideways movement are also particularly important in the processes of apperception. In 1937,

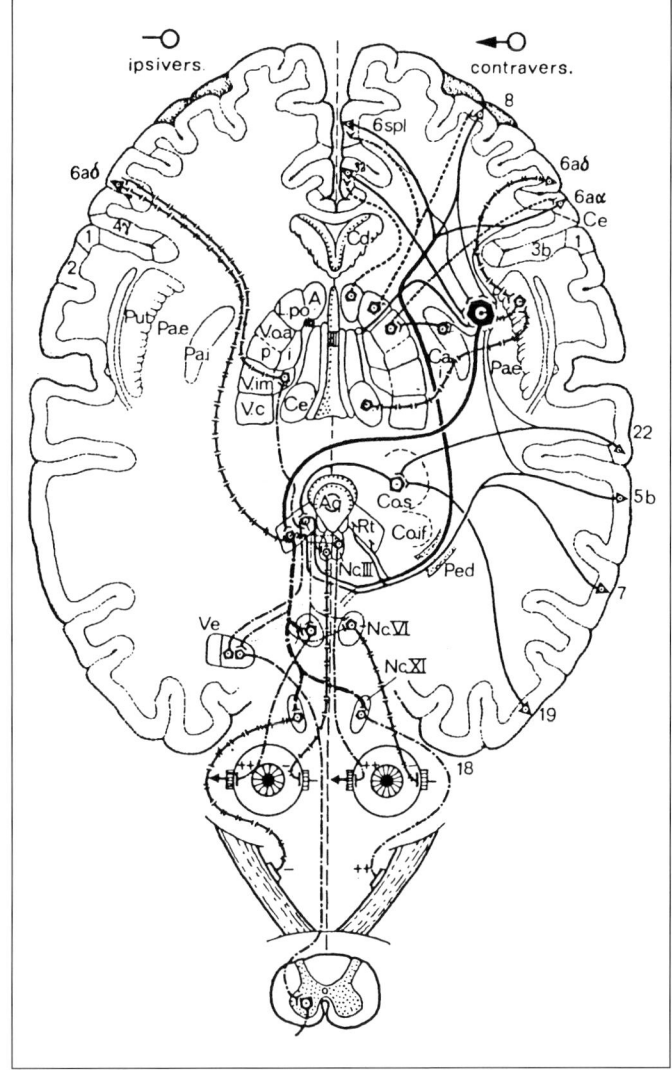

Fig. 3.1 Schematic outline of relevant pathways of the ipsilateral and contraversive primitive motor systems (adapted from HASSLER [4])

Kleist referred to an "optomotorisches System," and also described auditory – motor and olfactory – gustatory – motor systems [5]. Even earlier, Sir Charles Sherrington (1857–1952) and Cécile Vogt (1875–1962) and Oskar Vogt had observed that when the cortical zone adjacent to the primary auditory area is stimulated, a gaze and head movement toward the opposite side appears. The same happens when cortical areas adjacent to the primary visual area are stimulated. Undoubtedly there are motor systems proximal to the primary sensory areas, the function of which is to turn the body toward the source of sensory inputs. Every sensory system, therefore, possesses its own regulatory motor apparatus within the cortex. The most obvious clinical example of the connection between perception and the opposite motor system is the pseudosyndrome of Balint (or congenital bilateral aplasia of frontal area 8), in which perception is not possible and objects are not seen, in the absence of any lesion of the visual system, when the head is immobilized and lateral eye movements are blocked. Clinical studies have also reported patients who are transiently unable to perceive their body and the contralateral hemispace after extended coagulation of the pallidum or thalamic nuclei receiving afferents. In addition, bilateral surgical ablation of the temporal poles (which probably interrupts the pallidal circuits) induces an akinetic mutism syndrome with prolonged loss of consciousness in epileptic patients [6] also in the absence of any lesions of the brainstem structures.

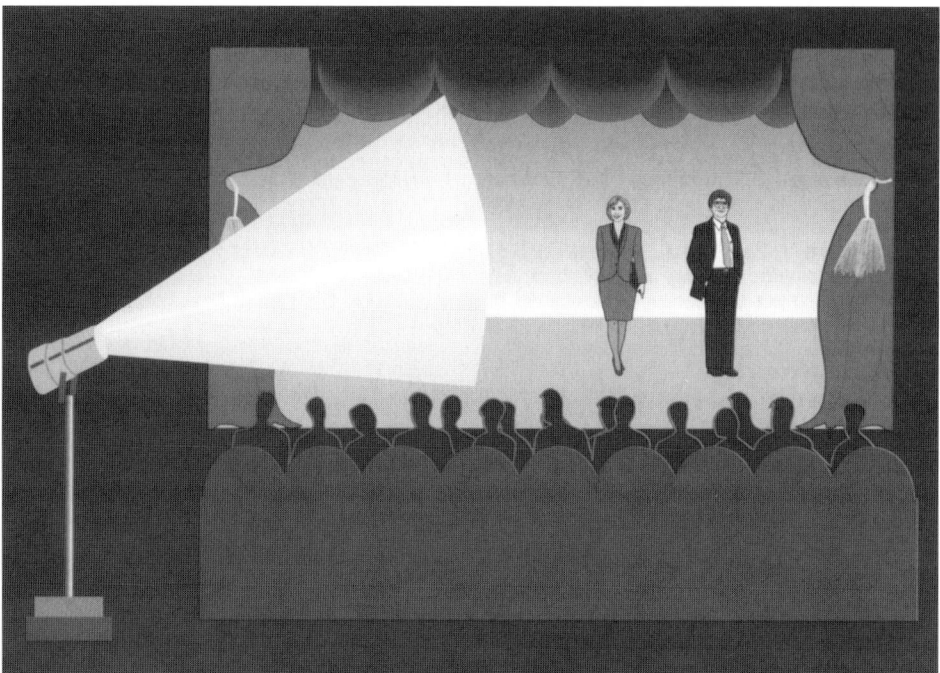

Fig. 3.2 Metaphorical model of consciousness in three of its basic aspects: vigilance, conscious activity, and contents. The audience represents the outside world; the theater, the inside world; the actors, conscious activity; the stage lighting, light; and the text, contents. If the text does not exist, the performance cannot take place. If the actors also (representing the average frequency discharge of cortical neurons) talk too softly, the audience will not be able to understand them. If the light from the stage (vigilance) is too dim or blinding, the performance will not be visible. If the stage lighting is not directed toward the stage (ipsilateral and contralateral motor mechanisms), the actors will be unable to act. Only simultaneous functioning of all of these elements thus allows the performance (conscious state) to take place. A fourth aspect – consciousness of ourselves – is not suitable for inclusion in a neurological function model, as it concerns a specific condition, exclusive of human beings, and goes beyond physiological categories

In conclusion, it is evident that to maintain a state of consciousness that allows operative behavior, reciprocal interaction between several functional structures is required. A certain degree of functional coherence must exist among specific sensory afferents, nonspecific activating afferents from the major subcortical systems (mostly in the mesencephalon and diencephalon) projecting diffusely to the cortex, primitive (ipsilateral and contralateral) motor systems, and cortical neurons discharging at medium frequency. The absence of only one of these factors can induce loss of consciousness (Fig. 3.**2**).

This model allows for a better understanding of the different mechanisms and functional structures responsible for the onset of coma. The post-traumatic vegetative state, similar to a "locked-out" syndrome, is not a primary result of the absence of a single response, but depends on the impossibility of obtaining harmony with the outer world. This occurs mostly due to a lack of synchronous function among the motor components regulating the complex phenomena of perception, with the patient becoming unable to see because he cannot look, and unable to hear because he cannot listen.

From a clinical point of view, two conditions stand out: absolute akinesia (preceding every initiated activity of consciousness, which remains absent for the duration of the ongoing akinesia) and "orientation gaze" (*Zuwendung*, tracking). The latter involves a conjugate, source-oriented gaze caused by auditory or visual inputs recalling some memory (e. g., the face or voice of a particular person) and evoking displacement in the immediate surrounding space. This is almost always the first sign of recuperation, no matter how minimal. The relationship with the outer world, although interrupted during the vegetative state, remains or becomes possible as long as the major functional systems described above are sufficiently active to achieve a certain degree of reciprocal functional coherence. Humans can also use other systems, phylogenetically much older, that help establish contact with the "inner world" and can also maintain a residual function during the vegetative state, in the absence of wakefulness.

Relationship with the Inner World

Under physiological conditions, these two separate systems are very well integrated functionally, but can assume a certain degree of independence, particularly in the post-traumatic vegetative state.

Pierre Broca (1824–80) defined the limbic lobe as including the formations that constitute the cortical gyri, situated in a ring shape around the brain stem and representing the phylogenetically oldest part of the cortex. The limbic lobe includes diverse formations, such as the parahippocampal gyrus, the cingulate gyrus, the subcallosal gyrus, and the lower (and morphologically simple) cortex of the hippocampal formation. The hippocampal formation includes the hippocampus, dentate gyrus, and subiculum. In 1937, James Papez (1883–1958) outlined the way in which these structures are organized into a neuronal functional circuit and first suggested the "Papez circuit" as the anatomic substrate of emotional behavior: as emotions reach the conscious level and influence thought, cognitive functions in turn influence emotions. The concept of a limbic system was subsequently broadened, and direct and indirect relationships with other, especially neocortical structures, were better defined. This system integrates and coordinates the behavioral expression of emotional states or changes and represents the functional structure intended for the normal relationship of the individual with his or her own internal world. The vegetative and endocrine integrated hypothalamic responses to unpleasant or pleasant stimuli prepare the organism for flight, attack, sexual activity, and different behavioral patterns involving adaptation. These internal reactions are relatively simple and do not require conscious control, unlike those that are needed for the individual to adapt to modifications in the outer world. These are much more complex and less predictable and provide a far greater variety in quality and quantity of responses to stimuli. To relate to the outer world, responses are also devised to carry on peculiar projects and strategies. Perhaps this is the condition that led to the notable evolution of consciousness itself in humans, enabling them to meet the enormous complexity of the external environment [7]. The functions that regulate the relationship with the outer world are regulated, as we have seen above, by the major thalamocortical functional systems and through the sensory and motor systems.

Working Hypothesis on the Brain's Functional Organization in the Vegetative State

Higher primates and humans rely on two major (anatomical and functional) arrangements of the brain to maintain contact with the inner world and the surrounding environment.

The main structures that are at the basis of these arrangements (which are interconnected, though to some extent independent) are outlined in Chapter 3, figs. 11–15. The neocortex, thalamus, basal ganglia, and ascending reticular activating system (ARAS) mediate higher brain functions such as perception, awareness, speech, motor skills, and motor planning. The limbic system (also including the hypothalamus) regulates instead the brain functions relating to the inner world of emotions, emotional reactions, mood, rage, fear, etc. that also can occur in the absence of vigilance, as is the case during sleep. Brain functions do not appear to develop from a large number of independent and partly interacting modules (the theory of localized functions), nor do they apparently depend on dynamic connections (the theory of equipotentiality). According to the coherence model, brain function appears instead to depend on the interplay between distinct areas/structures of the brain.

For this interplay to occur, efficient functional connection among active structures is necessary, and is normally provided by the brain's white matter. We can now imagine that the axonal damage following brain injury varies (depending on the dynamics related to rotation, translation, linear or angular acceleration it sets into motion) and may exert different effects depending on the gray matter involved and the length of the axons. In addition to the lower mass compared to the other system, the limbic system is structurally arranged in space to form a "ring" that is located deep inside the brain and protected by the hemispheres and cerebrospinal fluid. Axonal connections are shorter compared to the long axons connecting the neocortex to the thalamus and brain stem, for example. Conversely, any secondary damage due for instance to hypoxia, ischemia, acidosis, intracranial increased pressure, or reduced perfusion should develop without significant topographic differences in the two major systems we have taken into consideration. A different distribution and entity of primary neuronal damage (especially in relation to diffuse axonal injury) is at the basis of and supports the practicability of our hypothesis.

The brain functions that allow contact with the outer world are still partly operative after several months in the vegetative state, and communication can also occur in the absence of vigilance – with vegetative responses (such as tears) being observed to external inputs with relevant emotional content (such as being called by a familiar voice). By contrast, vigilance remains a functional prerequisite for any contact, no matter how feeble, with the surrounding environment.

The limbic system is connected through the Gudden fasciculum (mamillary tegment) to other ascending sensitive (especially taste), reticular, spinal, and autonomic systems. This arrangement helps us understand the way in which the perception and recognition of the voice of a specific person, for example, may be possible via some functional bypassing of a damaged thalamocortical specific sensory system.

All this suggests that the axonal damage immediately following head injury may be less salient than the damage selectively affecting the interconnections among the brain stem, thalamus, and neocortex. Notably, widespread axonal damage of this type should affect long pathways dedicated to the primitive lateral motor systems as well as those mediating in voluntary motility. The akinesia, often generalized, complete, and persistent that is observed in the vegetative state is the clinical result of this pathophysiological arrangement. In agreement with this hypothesis, the reduced extension of the anatomical damage affecting the limbic system and its connections would justify the residual function of brain structures regulating contact with the inner world.

It therefore seems a practicable hypothesis that the pathophysiological conditions causing development into a vegetative state may already come into operation on brain injury, although they are eventually concealed by the concurrent coma. The system regulating vigilance, namely the ARAS, also suffers sudden functional blocking. This blocking, however, is not irreversible, and a discrepancy may underlie another condition peculiar to the vegetative state – i. e., the permanence of vigilance in the absence of any apparent contents. When this condition lasts for a long time (a month or more), a peculiar condition characterized by the lack of any relationship with the surrounding environment in association with a relatively spared emotional life and contact with the inner world (through responses mediated by flushing, mimicry, changes in heart rate, tears, etc.) can develop.

References

1. Plum F, Posner JB. Diagnosis of stupor and coma. Philadelphia: Davis, 1973.
2. Kinner HC, Samuels MA. Neuropathology of the persistent vegetative state: a review. J Neuropathol Exp Neurol 1994; 53: 548–58.
3. Jung R. Aufmerksamkeit und Bewusstsein mit ihren physiologischen Bedingungen in Psychiatrie der Gegenwart, vol I/1A. Heidelberg: Springer, 1967: 612–45.
4. Hassler R. Brain mechanisms of intention and attention, with introductory remarks on other volitional processes. Prog Brain Res 1980; 54: 585–614.
5. Kleist K. Bericht über die Gehirnpathologie in ihrer Bedeutung für Neurologie und Psychiatrie. Z Ges Neurol Psychiatr 1937; 158: 159–93.
6. Terzian H, Ore GD. Syndrome of Klüver and Bucy; reproduced in man by bilateral removal of the temporal lobe. Neurology 1955; 5: 373–80.
7. Kupferman I. L'ipotalamo ed il sistema limbico: la motivazione. In: Kandel ER, Schwartz JH, Jessell TM, editors. Principi di neuroscienze. Milan: Ambrosiana, 1994: 764–75.

4 Clinical Picture

Leon Sazbon and Giuliano Dolce

General Considerations

Patients in the vegetative state (VS) are placed in specialized recovery units after an initial period of days or weeks in reanimation or intensive care. Before the individual medical diagnostic and therapeutic procedures are discussed, the general approach to management needs to be elucidated.

Prevailing medical practices in general apply to specific circumstances that warrant specific and predictable procedures. However, in patients in VS, some aspects of care necessarily diverge from these principles, and the protocol is in several ways independent of the patient's clinical condition. For example, laboratory tests are usually not done unless specifically indicated, while roentgen films are made of all eight major joints during the first 6 months, to allow early detection of periarticular osseous formations. Because it is impossible to formulate a prognosis or predict either the clinical progression or the duration of the VS, the goals of management are twofold: to keep the patient alive and anticipate all possible complications; and to facilitate conscious activity – an indispensable condition for functional recovery. The fundamental rules guiding each step in patient treatment are precise, punctilious adherence to schedule (hours and days of selected interventions), order, and silence. These provide the patient with the requisite therapeutic milieu, minimizing the risk of potentially life-compromising, emergency conditions that can be induced by the grave clinical condition itself.

The clinical picture of the patient in VS consists of two interrelated parts: the internal symptomatology, which is unique in each individual case; and the universal neurological signs and symptoms and their changes over time. Progression of the first can affect the progression of the second. We will describe both of these aspects separately.

Medical Aspects and Complications

The complications and sequelae of VS form a wide spectrum of clinical pictures, affecting practically all biological systems. Medical, neurological, and surgical problems can complicate the rehabilitation process and even pose a threat to life. Some are a direct consequence of the alteration in brain function and its autonomic and hormonal influences [1], and others are nursing-related or iatrogenic. This section describes the most common complications of VS in relation to the organ or system affected.

Cardiovascular Effects

Cardiovascular complications are more frequently observed in the acute phase following head trauma, when the patient is still comatose, although they may carry over into the rehabilitation phase of VS. The rate of patients affected by cardiovascular complications varies from 7% [2] to 32% [3].

Hyperdynamic cardiovascular reactivity to head trauma is manifested by three main clinical symptoms: neurogenic hypertension, changes in cardiac rate, and arrhythmia.
- Moderate degrees of systemic hypertension (160 mmHg systolic or more) in the absence of high intracranial pressure is a frequent finding [4]. Kaliski et al. [3] reported hypertension in 11% of 180 patients with severe head injuries and a mean coma duration of 55 days.
- Changes in cardiac rate are frequently observed. Tachycardia occurs more often than bradycardia, which is a poor prognostic sign [5].
- Among the arrhythmias, ventricular extrasystoles are seldom recorded. Sazbon and Grosswasser [2] and Kaliski et al. [3] also described electrocardiographic findings of nonspecific S – T and T wave changes.

According to Kirland and Wilson [6], the hypothalamus and nucleus of the solitary tract are the brain areas implicated in this type of hyperdynamic cardiovascular response. In addition, patients in VS with associated chest trauma may suffer myocardial damage, with cardiac contusion and subendocardial hemorrhage.

Respiratory Complications

Patients in VS may show normal or periodic respiratory rhythms. Among the latter, it should be emphasized that the presence of central hyperventilation, a well-recognized pattern of periodic breathing, indicates a bad outcome [7]. Another type of periodic respiratory rhythm is ataxic breathing, an absolutely irregular respiratory pattern, which is also associated with very poor prognosis; and adult respiratory distress syndrome, which was observed by Sazbon and Groswasser in 7% of patients [2].

A certain degree of hypoxia, with Po_2 between 60 and 80 mmHg in arterial blood, combined with a certain degree of hypercarbia, is the rule. The coexistence of these two conditions is characteristic of inadequate ventilation due to lung obstruction, lung collapse, bronchospasm, pulmonary edema, mechanical failure, or drug overdose [8,9]. Eisenberg and Levin [10] claimed that in acute comatose patients, the presence of the triad of high intracranial pressure, hypoxia, and hypotension following brain trauma may predict either VS or death. In patients who recover from VS, tidal volume is normal, but both the inspiratory and expiratory phases of vital capacity are markedly reduced, as is forced vital capacity [11].

Tracheobronchial infection or colonization is an almost unavoidable complication in patients who have undergone intubation or tracheostomy. Tracheal granulation also occurs very frequently, which can lead to stenosis. Tracheomalacia, tracheoesophageal fistula, and innominate artery erosion are severe but very rare complications. Parenchymal infections were reported in 37% of 134 patients in one series of patients in VS for at least 1 month, but pulmonary abscess is rare. Atelectasis, fat embolism related to concurrent limb fracture in the earliest weeks, and pulmonary embolism following deep phlebothrombosis, are not uncommon. Macrobronchial aspiration is often fatal, and recurrent microaspiration leads to pneumonia.

Rib fractures and unilateral concomitant traumatic paralysis of the phrenic nerve are cofactors of hypoventilation and recurrent pulmonary problems.

One iatrogenic respiratory complication is pneumothorax, caused by a failed attempt at subclavian vein cannulation.

Associated finger clubbing, unilateral or bilateral, has been frequently observed [12].

Urinary Complications

Lack of sphincter control is an important clinical feature of trauma-induced VS. Clinicians must perform tonus bladder studies to avoid overlooking a neurogenic bladder, which can lead to upper urinary tract impairment. Krimchansky et al. [13] studied bladder function in 17 patients in VS for 1 month and found that all of the patients had neurogenic bladder of the hypertonic type. There were no cases of detrusor – sphincter dyssynergia or unstable bladder. Some authors have tentatively claimed that it is the pons that controls detrusor and external sphincter function [13,14], whereas others localize this function to the precentral lobe of the cortex [15].

The urinary tract is often the site of hospital-acquired infection in patients with VS, with reported incidences of 39% [2] and 37% [3]. Most cases are associated with the use of an indwelling catheter or intermittent catheterization; the longer the duration of catheterization, the higher the risk [1]. In patients with an indwelling catheter, asymptomatic bacteriuria is common; fever, when it occurs, may be due to the urinary infection or another source, and the reason is often hard to determine. Treatment of asymptomatic bacteriuria is strongly discouraged.

The use of absorbent pants or diapers may be associated with maceration of the skin. Penile inflammation, erosions, or ulcerations are also usually related to external sources.

Surprisingly, urolithiasis is very rare (2%), despite the often long-term bedridden status of these patients [16].

Gastrointestinal Complications

Gastrointestinal complications develop in 50% of patients in VS [3]. There is often bleeding from the digestive tract, both in the acute phase and even years after onset. In most cases, the hemorrhage is microscopic, and esophagitis, gastritis, or ulcers may be found on gastroesophageal endoscopy [17]. The mechanism remains unclear [16], since after several weeks and months stress can be excluded as an underlying factor. Gastric pH is usually normal. In patients with gastric acidity, neutralization with antacids or H_2-blockers can cause bacterial overgrowth, which may be a risk factor for pneumonia. Reflux is another major complication, given that all patients in VS are fed by nasogastric tube or percutaneous endoscopic gastrostomy. Fluoroscopic studies show that in the supine position, rapid introduction of the food bolus causes regurgitation and sometimes, in turn, bronchial aspiration. Reflux may be avoided by slowing the food delivery and placing the patient in a reclining (semisitting) position. Gastric reflux is not related to the dietary components, food quantity, or presence of a feeding tube [18].

Patients in VS often have impaired liver function [3]. Biopsy series have reported contradictory results. Aiges et al. [19] noted no liver cell damage or inflammatory reactions, but this finding was not supported by Kaliski et al. [3]. The elevation in liver enzymes may be a consequence of either viral hepatitis following blood transfusion (often done in the acute phase after trauma) or, in the absence of a positive hepatitis serologic screen, administration of anticonvulsant or other drugs. Although vegetative patients are incontinent, constipation due to inactivity is common. At the same time, diarrhea may be caused by hyperosmolar foods or overgrowth of bacteria, particularly *Clostridium difficile*; its severity varies widely.

Motor Problems

The pathology of head injury is heterogeneous, involving diffuse axonal injury, multifocal cortical contusions, and secondary hypoxic damage. This may lead to disorders of movement and to disturbances of motor control and tonus [20].

Spasticity

Upper motor neuron (pyramidal) lesions may manifest clinically as spasticity – that is, hyperreflexia of the stretch reflex, resulting in a velocity-dependent increase in tendon reflexes [21]. The reported rate of spasticity in a Japanese series of VS patients was 32% [22]. Its biological basis is complex and not well understood. Current opinion holds that spasticity derives from an interruption of the corticospinal, vestibulospinal, and reticulospinal tracts and their modulatory influences on the spinal alpha motor neurons [23]. Symptoms may be positive, such as exaggerated nociceptive reflexes and withdrawal, autonomic hyperreflexia, dystonia, and contractures, or negative, such as paresis and fatigability [24]. In bedridden patients, the long-term inactivity can lead to shortening and retraction of the tendons and joint deformities and contractures. Other possible sequelae are bedsores, respiratory infections, osteoporosis, sepsis, deep vein thrombosis, pulmonary embolism, and periarticular new bone formation. Patients in VS may adopt diverse postures, but generally, progressive limb flexion is seen, either in abduction or adduction; the fingers are flexed, with the thumb hidden under the other fingers or emerging between the second and third finger. In rare cases, there may be extension of one or more fingers, usually the second or the fifth; clawing is noted even less often. The head shows a tendency to lean backward owing to hypertonus of the paravertebral muscles, occasionally achieving a position of opisthotonos.

Rigidity

Rigidity is a cardinal sign of extrapyramidal syndrome. Lesions of the basal ganglia in VS have been described by several authors (see Chapter 3). In the Japanese series presented by Higashi et al. [22], rigidity was noted in 62% of patients. Jennett and Teasdale [25], in an autopsy study, noted ischemic lesions in 91% of head-injury patients, 89% of whom had lesions of the basal ganglia. Bricolo [26] and Graham et al. [27] reported that half of the patients in VS had hemorrhage or necrosis of the basal ganglia as a consequence of direct trauma, in addition to ischemic lesions of the putamen and pallidum. In rare cases, there are involuntary movements (hemiballism, chorea or athetosis) and/or disorganized movements. Generally, muscle hypotony is very frequent until the end of the first month of VS, when it begins to decrease gradually while tonus increases, ultimately to the characteristic flexor hypertonus, sometimes accompanied by isolated isometric muscular contractions.

Plegia or Paresis

Plegia or paresis is almost the rule in VS. Feldman [28], in an unpublished series of 117 patients in VS of traumatic origin for at least one month, found a 70% rate of tetraplegia and a 30% rate of hemiplegia. Higashi et al. [22] found that 55% of their patients in VS were tetraplegic, 18% were hemiplegic, and the remainder were triplegic or monoplegic.

Motor Reactivity

Abnormal involuntary movements or normal uncontrolled movements are the result of extensive cerebral lesions causing disturbances of sensory input or of processing or programming by the motor areas. Examples are sucking, chewing, or swallowing, pelvic crural flexion movements, scratching, and slow, search-like movements.

Sazbon and Groswasser [4], in a study of 99 patients in VS, reported a 13% rate of flaccid motor unresponsiveness – 67% decerebrate reactivity and 15% decorticate reactivity. Normal motor reactivity was seen in only 4% of the patients [4]. A mixture of decerebrate and decorticate reactivity is not uncommon in individual patients (e. g., a decerebrate response on one side of the body or in one limb and a decorticate one on the other side, or in the rest of the limbs).

Periarticular New Bone Formation

Periarticular new bone formation (PNBF) is due to abnormal metaplasia of the connective tissue near the joints, in which undifferentiated mesenchymal cells undergo transformation under the influence of unknown factors and form histologically true bone. The reported frequency in VS varies from 11% to 76% in various studies [29–34], probably owing to differences in selection procedures. It is usually noted at the time of a transversal cut, or reported retrospectively. In a prospective radiological of patients in VS for 2–32 months, Sazbon et al. [30] found that PNBF is an expression of a progressive disease, starting about 1–2 months after trauma and peaking at up to 5 months. The process is self-limited, terminating at 14 months or before. PNBF is mainly localized to the large joints, mostly in the shoulder, followed by the hip, and then the elbow and knee. Hand and spinal involvement is rare [35,36]. The clinical picture is divided into three types: pseudoinflammatory, pseudotumoral, and ankylosing. The direct cause remains obscure. Suggested possible etiologic factors, all based on scanty evidence, include long-term immobility, spasticity, paralysis, trophic changes in the affected limb, local trauma to the affected joint, or traumatic effect of physiotherapy [29–31,37]. Sazbon et al. [30] found no correlation between the presence of PNBF and mechanical ventilation in the early stage of coma or recurrent genitourinary infections, and no correlation between its progression and the patient's age or sex, or with the etiology, duration, or outcome of VS. The appearance of PNBF may be identified by a specific L-dopa test and a nonspecific thyrotropin-releasing hormone test, with an increase in growth hormone concentrations in both [38]. PNBF undoubtedly poses a major problem during comprehensive rehabilitation programs.

PNBF is not specific to VS. It accompanies a variety of neural and extraneural insults, of which traumatic lesion of the brain or spinal cord is the most common. It may also be related to poliomyelitis, tetanus, carbon monoxide poisoning, burns, and stroke [38].

Seizures

Epilepsy

Epilepsy is a temporary brain dysfunction consisting of recurrent, unprovoked hyperchronous discharges of cortical neurons [39,40]. Post-traumatic epilepsy is characterized by recurrent seizure episodes in patients with brain injuries that cannot be attributed to any other cause [41]. The reported incidence of post-traumatic epilepsy varies from 1.9% to 53% [3,37,42–55]. Specifically, in VS, Higashi et al. [22] and Feldman [28] both reported an incidence of almost 50%, whereas Sazbon and Grosswasser [4] reported only 32%. The occurrence of epilepsy varies with age (with a greater likelihood in younger adults) [46,55], genetic predisposition, type of injury (penetrating or closed), duration of unconsciousness [39,52,53], formation of intracranial hematomas of any type, presence of intracranial infection or depressed skull fractures, and tearing of the dura mater [27,54]. The epileptic attacks may occur early after the traumatic event (from a few seconds to up to 1 month after), or later (delayed epilepsy). In patients with closed depressed skull fractures, Jennett et al. [55] found no differences in the incidence of late epilepsy between patients who underwent elevation of the fragment bone and those receiving conservative treatment. The attacks may be focal or secondary and generalized; the latter type is more persistent over time. Caveness et al. [56] reported that 25% of their severely brain-injured patients had focal attacks and 50% had both – either separately, or secondary and generalized following focal.

Myoclonus

Myoclonus refers to involuntary rough and very brief muscular contractions, with or without displacement of body parts. The presence of myoclonus usually indicates a metabolic cause or a severe anoxic episode complicating the primary traumatic injury to the brain [57]. Johnston and Sheshia [58] and Snyder et al. [45] reported that myoclonic seizures have an even worse influence on vital and functional outcome than generalized epilepsy. Myoclonus may appear, like generalized seizures, as bilaterally synchronous myoclonic twitches [59] or, more frequently, as status epilepticus. Two variants are seen in VS patients: opsoclonus-myoclonus, defined as rapid chaotic movement of the eyes accompanied by myoclonus of the limbs and cerebellar signs [60]; and palatal myoclonus, defined as rhythmic contractions of the soft palate due to a lesion of the olivary nuclei in the medulla oblongata [61]. It is often discovered by the rhythmic "jumps" of the nasogastric tube, which rests on the palate. This disorder is sometimes accompanied by jerks of other muscled structures deriving from the same branchial arch – for example, the pharynx, larynx, tongue, face, orbicularis oris, and neck [62]. At times, it is triggered by sensory stimuli – even mild ones such as a gentle touch [63].

Ventricular Enlargement

Post-traumatic hydrocephalus or ventricular enlargement is considered a frequent complication or sequela of severe brain injury. The reported incidence varies widely, from 0.7% to 62% [64–70]. In VS specifically, studies note incidences of 37% [3] and 51% [2]. The dilatation may be widespread, involving the whole ventricular system, or may be limited mainly to the lateral ventricles (central atrophy) or cortical sulci (cortical atrophy). According to Kaliski et al. [3], the reported range of ventricular dilatation depends on the method used to determine ventricular size.

Post-traumatic ventricular dilatation may be due to wasting of the white matter (ex vacuo hydrocephalus), adhesions of the meninges and circulatory impairment of the cerebrospinal fluid (obstructive hydrocephalus), or malabsorption of the cerebrospinal fluid (normal-pressure hydrocephalus) [25]. Radiologically, empty images of the porencephalic type may be seen when they communicate with cerebrospinal fluid (CSF) passages [26]. It is particularly important to determine whether the ventricular enlargement is due to cerebral atrophy (ex vacuo) or to a communicating hydrocephalus, because there is no treatment for the former, whereas the latter requires ventricular shunting (see Chapter 6). In patients in VS, communicating hydrocephalus cannot be recognized clinically, as the classic diagnostic triad of dementia, incontinence, and gait disturbances is absent. The decision on whether to perform shunt procedures is based on the clinical course (i. e., arrest or regression in the clinical course), and on progressive enlargement of the ventricles, with ballooning of the third ventricle, without clear, dominant brain atrophy or massive loss of brain tissue.

Undernutrition

Severe brain trauma induces several metabolic changes leading to severe weight loss, often in the order of 50% of the previous weight. In VS, cachexia is frequent [26,71–73], with an incidence of 20% to 48% [2,22]. The weight loss is due to the elevated energy expenditures and increased catabolism characteristic of the acute phase of severe brain injury. This abnormality may continue for several months, into the stage of VS. In addition to the effects of neuroendocrine and autonomic alterations, the increased cardiac output, hyperventilation, fever, restlessness, posturing, seizures, and infections impose a metabolic burden [1]. Patients with abnormal posturing reactivity have the highest consumption of energy. When no nutritional support is provided, there is a large protein and caloric deficit and depletion of fat stores. This, in turn, leads to loss of immunocompetence, depression of defense mechanisms against infection [74], and hindrance of internal homeostasis, injury repair, and wound healing, and ultimately to a state of marasmus and cachexia. Calorie and protein supplementation, in the order of 40–60 cal/kg/day, drastically reduces mortality [75].

Water and Electrolyte Balance

Conditions of depletion or excess of water and electrolytes may appear separately, but a mixed syndrome is more common. Water constitutes approximately 60% of the total body weight, with two-thirds being intracellular and the rest consisting of plasma and interstitial fluids. Potassium is the predominant intracellular cation, and sodium the predominant extracellular cation; organic acids are the major intracellular anion, and chloride the major extracellular anion. In VS, there may be alterations in serum potassium, calcium and phosphorus concentrations, but more frequent and relevant are sodium disturbances – both hypernatremia and hyponatremia.

Hyponatremia and Hypernatremia

Hyponatremia has been related to permanent brain damage [76,77]. Among the syndromes involved are inappropriate antidiuretic hormone secretion (IADHS) syndrome and water intoxication [78]; the latter is usually iatrogenic. IADHS has been reported in 8.2% [79] and 12.3% [4] of brain-damaged patients. Dilutional hyponatremia may be caused by drugs such as thiazides, mannitol, barbiturates, and carbamazepine [80,81]. Endocrinological dysfunctions such as Addison's disease have also been implicated, but an acute etiologic diagnosis requires an evaluation of the extracellular fluid as well. In an unpublished work, Sazbon [82] suggested that for the clinical diagnosis of hyponatremia and hypo-osmolarity, the biceps should be pinched firmly between thumb and forefinger and quickly released; in affected patients, a thick, distinct band of muscle will be noted, which lasts for a few seconds. Signs of dehydration may be seen in cases of reduced extracellular fluid.

Hypernatremia is also often iatrogenic. It results from inadequate water replacement in the presence of an excess of water-to-sodium loss. The most representative syndrome is diabetes insipidus, due to lack of pituitary antidiuretic hormone secretion. Causes include exaggerated diuresis provoked by high protein tube feeding, gross sodium intake, or excessive water loss due to profuse sweating or diarrhea. There may also be water loss through the respiratory tract in patients who have undergone tracheostomy, and increased insensible water loss during periods of fever.

Hypokalemia and Hyperkalemia

Hypokalemia is more frequent than hyperkalemia. It can be due to gastrointestinal losses, large therapeutic use of laxatives, decreased dietary potassium intake, and loss of potassium in sweat. Other causes are corticosteroids or diuretics, or a hormonal imbalance. In vegetative patients, hypokalemia leads to muscular weakness, which may in turn lead to respiratory failure, paralytic ileus, and cardiac arrhythmia.

Hyperkalemia is associated with acidosis, renal failure, oliguric states, administration of potassium-sparing diuretics or exaggerated potassium supply. The most serious side effect is cardiac toxicity.

Other

Calcium, magnesium, and phosphorus disorders are seldom seen in VS. True hypocalcemia, when it occurs, is related to a reduction in protein-bound calcium due to hypoalbuminemia. It is asymptomatic, since membrane excitability is produced by the ionized fraction, which is unaltered. Hypomagnesemia is related to prolonged parenteral nutrition in combination with gastrointestinal losses or inadequate intake. Clinical manifestations are weakness, neuromuscular hyperexcitability, tremor, and changes in the electrocardiography (ECG) findings. Hypophosphatemia may be the result of the use of large amounts of aluminum hydroxide antacid, or may be part of the nutritional recovery syndrome.

Hematological Alterations

Diffuse intravascular coagulation (DIC) occurs as a consequence of a major intravascular activation of the coagulation cascade. In severe forms of brain injury, thromboplastin is released into the blood circulation from the injured zones [6,83–86], activating the extrinsic pathway of the clotting cascade. The actual incidence of DIC in VS is unknown, but it is likely very infrequent relative to its high frequency in the acute period of injury. Perpetuation of the syndrome has been reported in rare cases [87]. In spite of the decreased number of platelets, low level of fibrinogen, and abnormal values of plasma split products, clinical manifestations are extremely rare.

Anemia in VS is most often the "anemia of chronic or inflammatory diseases." It may also be due to dietary deficiencies of iron, vitamin B_{12}, or folic acid, or to drug sensitivity hemolysis in cases of glucose-6-phosphate dehydrogenase (G6PD). Although a mild degree of gastrointestinal bleeding is very frequent in VS, it is rarely the cause of anemia.

Hormonal Disorders

Hypothalamic – pituitary dysfunction may be manifested clinically as hypothyroidism, hypoadrenalism, hypopituitarism, diabetes insipidus, or IADHS. Hypopituitarism and diabetes insipidus are well recognized hormonal complications of the acute stage of head injury. In rare cases, they evolve into serious, life-threatening conditions; in others, minor degrees of hypothalamic – pituitary dysfunction may be present without clear, related symptomatology, especially in the presence of severe unconsciousness that may mask the clinical signs [88–100]. In VS, symptoms may begin a few hours after trauma or only days, months or years later. These include persistent low body temperature, low pulse and blood pressure, hypoglycemia, hyponatremia, and changes in diuresis volume. Slightly diminished levels of cortisol, testosterone, luteinizing hormone, follicle-stimulating hormone, triiodothyronine (T_3), thyroxine, and thyroid-stimulating hormone have been reported [5]. Sack et al. [101] suggested that a lack of reciprocity between T_3 and rT_3 may follow defective deiodination in both the alpha and beta rings of thyroxine. Precocious puberty, with elevated levels of 17-ketosteroids, and hyperthyreosis are unusual [5].

Sazbon and Groswasser [4] reported a 12% incidence of clinical signs of posterior lobe dysfunction in a series of 130 vegetative patients, and Bakay and Wood [102] noted transient blood hypo-osmolarity secondary to IADHS in two-thirds of their comatose patients. Daniel and Treip [103] reported hemorrhaging in the posterior lobe in 45% of fatal brain injuries, and Kornblum and Fischer [94] in 62%. All the suggested mechanisms of injury involve denervation of the posterior hypothalamus. Kornblum and Fischer [94] noted that injury to the stalk may be fatal, whereas Porter and Miller [104] emphasized the role of traumatic elongation of the stalk. The hypophysis sits in the sella turcica at the base of the cranium and is well protected by its bony sheath [89]. Some authors have reported that the culprit lesion is confined to the hypothalamus [92–96,100]. However, Crompton [88], in an autopsy study, reported that lesions of the hypothalamus occur together with lesions of the pituitary gland, especially in young males, and that they are often associated with a temporoparietal impact. They consist of microhemorrhages due either to venous engorgement subsequent to increased cranial pressure, or directly to elevated intracranial pressure. Ischemic necrosis can occur anywhere in the hypothalamus – pituitary axis.

The relative immunity of the anterior lobe [5,89,98,102] may be explained by its high location and lack of participation in the hypothalamopituitary portal system [105].

Immunologic Disorders

Humoral deficits, neutrophil dysfunction, a defective reticuloendothelial system, and depressed cellular immune function have all been documented in severe brain injury [106–108]. Hoyt et al. [109] reported a decreased proliferative response of T-cells to mitogen stimulation, with unaffected B-cells [109]. Wollaj et al. [106] noted impaired humoral immunity in three of 11 patients in VS. Hemolytic activity of the classical pathway was depressed in association with low levels of C1q, C1r and C4. One patient also had very decreased levels of immunoglobulin G2 (IgG2) and IgG4, which substantially influenced the phagocytic arm. Neutrophils showed impaired killing activity secondary to the humoral defect. Chemotaxis, random migration, and superoxide release were normal.

Infections

Patients in VS are particularly susceptible to nosocomial infections. Risk factors include the use of indwelling catheters, endotracheal tubes or cannulas, and nasogastric tubes, undernutrition, diminished immunologic defenses, immobility, atelectasis, lack of normal cough reflex, and bedsores. Rates range from 34% to 46% [3,4,22,110]. The most common nosocomial infections are pneumonia, urinary tract infection, sinusitis, and pseudomembranous colitis; the most common culprit organisms are *Pseudomonas* and *Klebsiella*. Meningitis, subdural empyema, and brain abscess occur rarely (1–2% of cases) following evacuation of delayed hematoma, shunt procedures, or cerebrospinal fluid fistula [2,3,111]. They are usually caused by *Staphylococcus aureus*, *S. epidermidis*, *Escherichia coli*, *Klebsiella*, and *Acinetobacter*. Pyogenic arthritis is very rare [112].

Deep Vein Thrombosis

Deep vein thrombosis (DVT) is a frequent complication in severely brain-injured patients [113], with a reported incidence of 20–54% [113–115]. The most frequent location is the calf, followed by the intrapelvic and humeral or subclavian veins. There are no statistics on DVT in VS, although this patient group is characterized by several important risk factors: long duration of bed confinement, long-term immobility, and motor deficits; some patients have undergone neurological, abdominal, or orthopedic operations, or have leg injuries and Gram-negative sepsis. In addition, free fatty acid mobilization, which is a typical response to head injury to increase energy needs [116], has a known tendency to cause DVT due to hypercoagulation [117]. DVT and its complication of pulmonary embolism is detectable with ^{125}I fibrinogen scanning, venous Doppler ultrasonography, and impedance plethysmography.

Autonomic Disturbances

Autonomic disorders are another well-recognized acute complication of traumatic brain injury. Symptoms may persist for months, even into VS.

Fever

Fever (hyperpyrexia) is extremely common in VS. In addition to such known causes as infections, other etiologies need to be considered as well – for example, PNBF, DVT, and drug reaction. The latter is found in 3–5% of cases, and is often related to hypersensitivity reactions [118]. Hypopyrexia due to hypothalamic damage is rare [4,57]. The diagnosis of fever of central origin is made by exclusion when a comprehensive work-up fails to yield a detectable cause. The reported incidence ranges between 4% and 7% [118,119]. Central fever is due to hypothalamic dysfunction. Its mediation by prostaglandin is controversial, although treatment with prostaglandin blockers such as indomethacin has been found beneficial. The fever is resistant to antipyretic drugs, but responds quickly to external cooling.

Sweating

Generalized sweating was noted in 25% of cases in one Israeli series [4]. In the absence of fever or other detectable causes, sweating indicates a failure of the hypothalamic thermoregulatory system. However, the underlying cause of bouts of localized sweating in the face and neck, often associated with flushing [4,71,120,121], is unclear.

Dysautonomia

Some authors consider dysautonomia, or vegetative storm, to be a distinct clinical entity affecting patients with severe traumatic brain injury [122,123]. It is characterized by a simultaneous and paroxysmal increase in at least five of the following seven autonomic parameters [123]:

- Heart rate (tachycardia > 120 beats/min)
- Respiratory rate (tachypnea > 30 breaths/min)
- Muscle tone (increased)
- Posture (decerebrate or decorticate)
- Blood pressure (systolic blood pressure > 160 mmHg)
- Sweating (profuse)
- Temperature (increased or decreased)

Episodes may occur with varying frequencies and times, or at specific hours of the day. They usually

Table 4.1 Vegetative state (VS) with and without dysautonomic syndrome [122]

Characteristics	VS with dysautonomia	VS without dysautonomia
Patients (n)	26	44
Mean age (years)	28.3	29.3
Admission GCS	6.7	7.7
Days in ICU for VS patients	168.5	85.6
Syndrome duration (days)	151	–
Outcome		
Moderate disability	11.50%	38.60%
Severe disability	30.70%	25.00%
VS > 1 y	38.40%	20.40%
Death	19.20%	15.90%*

* GCS, Glasgow Coma Scale; ICU, intensive-care unit.

disappear within 4 months of the onset of unconsciousness. A diencephalic epileptic origin has been suggested.

In a study of 70 patients in VS, Baguley et al. [123] found dysautonomic syndrome in about 30% of cases. According to Milano and Leto [122], the final functional outcome in affected patients is worse than that in patients without this syndrome. Their findings are summarized in Table 4.1.

Dermatological Changes and Bedsores

Acne vulgaris, seborrheic dermatitis, folliculitis, flat keloid changes, contact dermatitis, and allergic rash have all been reported in VS [2,3]. Patients are also prone to decubitus ulcers due to immobility, maceration of the skin due to contact with urine and feces, local sweating, and undernutrition. These may be exacerbated by deficient nursing care. Common sites of bedsores are the sacrum and trochanter region, heels, and occipital skin. Secondary complications of bedsores include localized osteoporosis, osteomyelitis, or osteoarthritis. Bedsores, in turn, may be a source of sepsis.

Complications of Medications

Drugs used in the treatment of patients in VS include anticonvulsants, benzodiazepines, beta blockers, antibiotics, L-dopa, and bromocriptine, among others. Skin reactions, angioedema, urticaria, fever, hematological changes, blood dyscrasias, and hepatic and renal toxicity may occur immediately after drug administration or later, with succeeding doses [124].

Other

Sharpening of the distal part of the fingers, finger clubbing, hypocratic fingers, hyperpigmentation of the dorsal aspect of the interphalangeal and metacarpophalangeal joints, ulnar deviation of the hands, longitudinal striation of the nails, and loss of hair are frequent findings, but of secondary value.

Neurological Aspects

Giuliano Dolce and Leon Sazbon

The neurological picture of the vegetative state has been described by several authors, mostly during the 1960s. In his book *Das traumatische apallische Syndrom*, Gerstenbrand described a number of detailed characterizing neurological signs [125], and included descriptions published by earlier authors, mostly in German or French [126]. These reports share a common fault: they contain an almost endless list of symptoms (mostly providing completely redundant information), but define poorly their sequence in time and their category of importance – possibly because most patients did not survive long enough. This refined exercise in neurological semiotics was curtailed by the appearance of emergency care and reanimation units/departments, and then by the development of brain imaging techniques for diagnosis. A list of neurological signs is given on p. 33–35. In our experience, however, we have always favored a standard neurological examination alongside morphological and functional examinations and brain imaging. As a result, we feel entitled to reduce expectations and above all to recognize the importance of numerous signs in the diagnostic and prognostic clinical evaluation (see p. 32–33).

Neurological Examination

The purpose of the neurological examination is to estimate the degree and level of functional organization of the patient's nervous system, at least once every 2 weeks until signs of initial recuperation appear. The conscious interaction between the patient and the observer that is required in conventional neurological examinations is lacking in the vegetative state. The examination is therefore limited to observations of spontaneous activity, reflexes, and pathological phenomena involving primitive reflexes, which are quite numerous and various in this type of patient. The patient should be supine and undressed for this functional examination. In this section, each step of the neurological examination will be described in full detail in relation to the inspection and observation of complex activities, reflexes, and reactivity.

Posture

The alignment of the body and head and the positioning of the limbs are observed. Hyperextension to opisthotonos of the head and trunk are rare, whereas flexion of the head and upper body or lateral deviation of the head are observed more frequently. Each limb (or pair of limbs) can assume its own posture: the upper limbs are mostly flexed (decorticate posture) or hyperextended (decerebrate posture) [7,127]. When decerebration and decortication occur in association, it is possible to observe a limb or a whole side of the body in flexion while the other side is in extension. The lower limbs are mostly in hyperextension, but flexion of one or both limbs is not exceptional. Wrists and fingers are usually in flexion and pronation, while the feet generally assume plantar flexion and supination. None of these postural positions have particular prognostic value when considered individually, and they can revert completely within the first 3–4 months of the vegetative state. In contrast, tonic and postural disturbances may become permanent after this period, with associated deficits that make functional recuperation more difficult.

Spontaneous and Pathological Movements

It is necessary to observe and describe in detail all subtle, segmental movements, as well as the presence of pathological movements such as clonic and myoclonic tremors [128–130]. Spontaneous movements of flexion and extension of each and any of the four limbs or of single parts of a limb (such as the body rotation often observed in the first weeks or months) constitute a favorable sign for recovery of conscious activity. Conversely, the complete absence of spontaneous movement of the four limbs after the third or fourth month of vegetative state is a poor prognostic indication of a vegetative state progressing towards a recuperation of conscious activity (see p. 32–33).

Among the various forms of spontaneous pathological movement, decerebrate and decorticate crises are common in the early months, but revert completely or occur only rarely after the eighth to tenth weeks. Tremors, clonus, and myoclonic and dystonic crises are clinical expressions of specific neurological injury to the cortex and underlying subcortical structures of the brainstem and cerebellum and their pathways. They often appear early in the first weeks, with total or partial later remissions, and manifest differently in each individual depending on the location and type of damage incurred. These deficits have no particular value in the evaluation of the course of the vegetative state. They cannot stand in the way of the resumption of conscious activity, but may reduce, to a greater or lesser extent, the recovery of motor functions.

Passive Movements and Muscular Tone

Passive mobilization of limb segments and large and small joints allows the evaluation of the muscular tone and the identification of ossifications, periosteomas, and retractions of individual joints. These observations are particularly important in the vegetative state in order to help ascertain whether the absence of spontaneous movements results from paralysis or from mechanical impediments, such as the frequent blocked joints.

When limited to a single limb or limb segment, disturbances of the muscular tone such as flaccidity or spasticity may have different significance in relation to the general muscular tone as expressions of local function. They are therefore important for evaluating actual conditions, especially when marked by sudden or rapid changes. Marked hypertonia, with all limbs hyperextended, reflects functions at the mesencephalic level. Sudden progression to flaccidity of all limbs does not signify amelioration, but rather a regression to a bulbar level not exceeding the pons. In general, sudden changes occur in the early stages of vegetative state, or when the patient is still in coma, due to compression, wedging, or edema of the mesencephalic structures. Progression to diffuse flaccidity or to hypertonus is more common.

Disturbances of the muscular tone are quite frequent and constitute a serious obstacle to functional recovery as well as a considerable therapeutic task (see p. 76). All changes in muscular tone can revert, sometimes totally within the first 3 months, and are generally preceded by a recovery of conscious activities. After this period, a therapy-resistant widespread spasticity is generally observed, which may become a serious complication and a very unfavorable condition for the recovery of conscious mental activity, by limiting or impeding the resumption of movements that permit exploration of space.

Behavioral Responses

Following inspection, the examination of the patient begins with an attempt to establish communication, when and if possible. The patient is supine and with the eyes open. The gaze is empty and glassy, although wakeful; eye movements can be conjugated, but are not finalized to fixate or follow objects moving in the visual field. Patients do not answer to their name, nor can they respond to simple verbal commands or requests for imitation. This first part of the examination must be carried out from both sides of the patient.

Contact with the outer world, environment or people – even the closest relatives – is completely absent [4,131,132]. No significant "refusal" motor response, such as closure of the eyelids or opening of the jaws, nor any defense mechanisms are evident, with a resistance indicative of a lack of complex motility involving active cognition. A quantitative scale exploring different dimensions of the patient's communication is useful to monitor the patient's progress over time (see page 46). The use of the Glasgow Coma Scale in this condition may be inappropriate, as it matches the diagnostic and prognostic requirements of a different clinical entity – i.e., coma.

The "behavioral" examination of the patient in the vegetative state requires attention, dedication and experience in the observation and interpretation of every sign potentially conveying relevant information. Often, even apparently insignificant or nonspecific signs can provide useful information or indications of a certain degree of conscious activity. Opening of the mouth is not necessarily just a primitive, automatic action, but at times can be the only practicable way to express a need ("I am hungry, I am thirsty") or to communicate feelings such as "I am surprised, I don't agree, help me, I don't feel well," etc. It is therefore also necessary to consider the context in which certain actions occur before they are deemed to be automatic motor actions unrelated to cognitive function [133]. Each individual sign, once observed by the whole team and discussed on scheduled rounds, can then be assigned a certain value.

Ocular Motility

Ocular motility is examined with the patient's head being kept in axis. Closed eyelids must be opened by applying intense pain stimuli to the skin of the clavicular fossa, first on one side and then the other. When the eyelids remain closed, the presence of local lesions or impairment of the oculomotor nerve must be checked for. In some cases, the patient forces his or her eyes shut, but this is not an act of volition. The same applies to the blink reflex to menace, which is sometimes absent at a first observation and may appear at a later time without signifying any integrated higher brain functions (such as those implied in the recognition of danger).

Spontaneous or provoked eye movements make it possible to note the presence of conjugated eye movements. Impairment of cranial nerves III and VI, possibly caused by peripheral lesions resulting from fractures and compressions at the base of the skull or orbits, must be recognized: monocular and binocular (horizontal, vertical, rotary, bobbing or retractive) nystagmus can be observed to occur either spontaneously or in response to passive head movements [7,134,135]. The presence of a bilateral nystagmus, in any more or less persistent form, is to be interpreted as the functional expression of massive anatomical damage at the mesencephalic level. It is hardly susceptible to regression, due to the likely involvement of the longitudinal medial bundle and reticular formation or of the centers regulating vigilance – which gives nystagmus a negative character.

It is not possible to evaluate a deficit of the fourth cranial nerve actively.

Pupils are observed for isocoria/anisocoria and isocyclicity, monolateral or bilateral miosis or mydriasis, and direct and consensual reflexes to light [136]. Accommodation cannot be tested in the absence of collaboration. The ciliospinal reflex, elicited by intense, painful stimulation of the neck or upper trunk skin, induces mydriasis. This reflex is almost always observed in the vegetative state (consequently excluding a deficit of the sympathetic cerebral chain in this condition), but can be absent in patients with concomitant direct trauma of the neck [137]. When observed in response to strong emotional stimulation, such as a visit from a special person, mydriasis may indicate that the afferent paths of Budge stemming indirectly from the hippocampus are unaffected.

The corneal reflex – i.e., closure of eyelids in response to a light touch on the cornea – makes it possible to evaluate the anatomical integrity of the afferent (trigeminal) pathway and motor response, in relation to the facial nerve and bulbopontine loop [43]. It is important to observe whether the corneal stimulus induces a corneo-chin reflex, a pathological response ascribed to the liberation of a cortical inhibition reflex of bulbopontine structures. A corneomandibular reflex (through contraction of the ipsilateral pterygoid muscle) can also be elicited in response to corneal stimulation and expresses cortical inhibition over a wider portion of the brainstem and bulbomesencephalic loop. The latter two reflexes are often observed in the vegetative state and constitute a characteristic indication of functional disconnection between cortical control and the brainstem (inhibitory function).

Oral Reflexes and Automatism

The "bulldog", tactile-oral, oculo-oral, labiomental, and snout reflexes and the chewing, sucking or swallowing automatisms (either spontaneous or provoked by stimulation of the lips or oropharyngeal cavity) are almost pathognomic of both the post-traumatic and non – post-traumatic vegetative state and are, in any event, expressions of diffuse brain damage.

Reflexes and automatisms are expressions of the level of functional arrangement attained by the postlesional brain organization. The presence of some or all reflexes/automatisms takes on significance in the light of time of appearance, duration, and remission. From a pathophysiological point of view, the functional area or anatomical level able to elicit reflexes or automatic activity is important to evaluate. Only the oculo-oral reflex, although somewhat rare, expresses an enlargement of the functional area, including involvement of diencephalic structures, such as the lateral thalamic geniculate body, its connection with the mesencephalic roof, and the quadrigeminal bodies. The result is a functional integration of higher level in a sequence including the retina, thalamus, mesencephalic roof, motor nucleus of the fifth cranial nerve, and reticulospinal tract inducing also body flexion. This condition describes a notable enlargement of the reflexogenic area. Continuous mastication, like other motor automatisms, expresses an enlargement of the reflex area, involving the loss of a certain degree of selectivity, indicating a globalization and extension of the functional deficit. The cervical myotatic reflex, or head-retraction reflex, which is elicited by the percussion of the upper lip while the head is kept slightly flexed, also has an analogous meaning and must be recognized. The involved area is large and involves the bulb, pons, and cervical medulla. This reflex is rare, and when it occurs it is usually observed after 3–6 months of vegetative state. Another characteristic sign involving the musculature controlling mastication and closure of the mouth is the rabbit-snout phenomenon, which may be seen when the patient bites his or her lower lip – at times even biting off a piece of the lip [5]. This phenomenon always occurs after about 6 months and constitutes a late negative prognostic sign. After this period, the so-called half-moon pucker mouth can be seen, which is also a very negative prognostic sign.

Oculocephalic Reflex

The patient is supine, with the head in line with the trunk, and the head is quickly rotated laterally by the examiner (the reflex is elicited by movements of the head on the horizontal plane in patients in the vegetative state, due to the presence of a tracheal cannula limiting the head flexion). The eyes should follow the direction of the head. In the absence of the oculocephalic reflex observed in concomitance with brainstem lesions the eyes do not follow the direction of the head. The result is the so-called "doll's eye sign" [138].

Trunk and Limbs

The patient's control of the head and chest is indispensable to elaborate a treatment plan to be initiated in the early phase (see p. 97), and needs to be evaluated as soon as possible. The patient should be in a sitting position, with proper support (the erect posture is generally impossible). An additional and more elaborate evaluation of head and body control must be carried out with the patient prone or lying on either side. The patient should also be observed erect while supported by a special lifting or standing device (Fig. 4.**1** and 7.**4**), and the presence of automatic step mechanisms should be checked for; rehabilitation procedures can take advantage of this function to facilitate motility of the lower limbs.

Motility of the limbs should be favored after the assessment of reflexes and only after having excluded impediments in the joints. For this purpose, automatic movements of portions of limbs from a painful stimulus applied to the skin can be evoked.

4 Clinical Picture

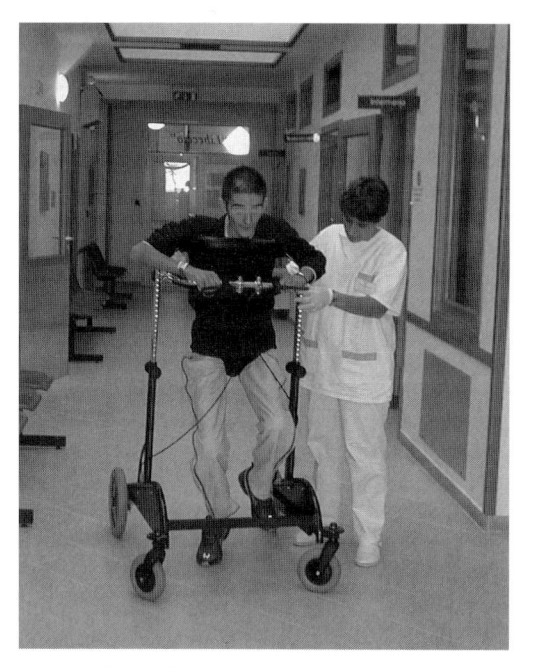

Fig. 4.1 The equipment used to position a patient in the vegetative state in an upright position, reducing the weight loading on the legs and feet and helping facilitate the motor scheme of walking

If present, these movements indicate that sensory functions are conserved to some degree.

Reflexes

Attenuated tendon reflexes are a functional correlate of compromised neuronal structures, without reflecting any functions peculiar to the vegetative state. Palm-chin and thumb-chin reflexes (physiological if observed until the third month of life) are always present in diffuse cerebropathies. At the beginning of vegetative state, the reflexogenic area can be enlarged to the extent that this reflex can be elicited by merely stroking the skin of the forearms and even the lateral parts of the trunk. This phenomenon expresses the functional liberation of structures of the brainstem and medulla from cortical control. This reflex can accompany head flexion and may be an indication of the level of functional organization of the cerebral structures.

Recovery of Conscious Activity

Recovery from the vegetative state occurs in different phases, notably: awakening with recovery of conscious activity, recuperation of functions through motor rehabilitation, readaptation based on the development of residual functions, and finally reintegration into family life and eventually into the working world.

These steps imply a neurological and psychological progression. During this entire period, the patient needs medical and social guidance in order to attain his or her objectives and must be assisted by a multidisciplinary team together with the family.

Patients usually progress from coma to the vegetative state while still in the emergency department. This progression is marked by two important steps – notably the patient's opening of the eyes with a watchful look (at first in response to painful stimuli, then spontaneously) and the subsequent appearance of sleep–wake cycles in long-term electroencephalography (EEG) recordings. Transient or pseudorhythmic EEG waveforms peculiar to slow-wave sleep are initially observed, together with spikes at the vertex and K complexes. The sleep patterns become progressively more organized and finally also include periods of rapid eye movement (REM) sleep. For most of the time, sleep cycles are short in duration and alternate with periods of wakefulness. Only after several weeks can longer periods of nocturnal sleep be observed (see p. 67).

The progression from the vegetative state to an adequate recovery of conscious functions, inappropriately described as "awakening" or "reawakening," is a pivotal moment in the patient's clinical progress. For such a progression to come about, functional organization must occur at levels of complexity comparable to those required for the progression from coma to vegetative state. The opening of the patient's eyes correlates functionally to a reestablished functional organization of the brain (or more precisely of the brain-stem structures), in which the nuclei of the cranial nerves regulating ocular globe and eyelid activity, as well as the part of the reticular formation in which the activating system originates, act together and simultaneously (arousal). It is therefore among these structures that a new functional organization allowing the resumption of conscious activity emerges. This is characterized by better control achieved by the brainstem structures partly substituting for the damaged cortex and by a higher degree of reciprocal interaction between these systems.

Clinically, this renewed organization of cerebral structures is expressed by a corresponding modification of neurological functions. The oral automatisms (such as chewing, sucking, swallowing) and pathological reflexes (such as the bulldog reflex or the oculo-oral and corneal-chin reflexes) disappear. Spontaneous mobility (if previously absent) reappears. A cardinal sign that anticipates the resumption of the most elementary conscious activities also appears-a conjugated "human" gaze following sources of visual stimulation (tracking) and oriented towards changes in the visual field induced by moving people or objects. This sign is an expression of functional integration at high levels of complexity, implying a recognition of form and significance of objects or people, and above all, indicating the complex motor activity required for spatial exploration. Thereafter, the ipsilateral and contralateral primitive motor systems resume function, together with the resumption of thalamocortical circuits through the pallidal system, in the absence of tectal reflexes. These neurological signs precede the resumption of conscious activity and are necessary prerequisites for this process to occur.

It is at this stage that the patient emerges from the vegetative state (awakening without awareness). The speed and quality of recuperation depend on the degree of residual functional plasticity. This factor is peculiar to each individual patient and linked to age, with the most extensive recuperation being observed in young patients 25–30 years old or younger. The recuperation of conscious functions presents very differently from case to case due to the involvement of many factors, the most relevant of which is undoubtedly the patient's own personality before the accident that led to the vegetative state.

Qualitative aspects, as well as the time necessary to stabilize functions, are diverse and do not always depend on small changes, but rather on individual curves of progress, without any correlation with the location and extension of the brain lesion. In all cases, the ability to execute simple commands is evident first, with the patient using an indifferent action (such as closing the eyes, opening of the mouth, or squeezing the hand) that can vouch for a certain function or response. The second level attained is defined as "reactive consciousness" [139], a term covering the state that lasts until the appearance of consciousness of the outer world. Then comes a phase defined by increasing interchange and interaction with the surroundings, which leads to recuperation of a certain degree of consciousness of the self.

The first stage ends when the patient is regularly able to follow simple commands such as closing the fist or eyes or opening the mouth in a predictable manner. This can last for weeks or months and does not make it possible to predict any progression into the next phase.

Gaze movements, unfinalized motor actions, yawning, chewing, and differentiated mimicry (expressing suffering or well-being) can arise and may be used to establish a primitive relationship with the patient and suggest a possible progression into successive phases. However, an established relationship with the outer world is not evident, nor is there by any means a capacity to recognize family members or familiar people. This is known as awakening without awareness.

A motor response, even if shaky, nevertheless stands as a very important initial event. Successive steps, bringing the patient toward recovery of the contents of consciousness, have been well defined by Cohadon [140] as follows:

Progressively, the catalogue of these brief responses expands. The patient does not spontaneously express any needs or desires, but seems to recognize concrete aspects of the outside world, progressively reacting to the presence of family members and members of the medical team. The first relational exchanges are built on this basis. The repertory of motor activity, even if limited, establishes a code: close your eyes to say yes, bend a finger to say no. These acts are limited to concrete, instantaneous situations to express acceptance or refusal. Progressively, it seems that the inner reconstruction of the present is possible and the first traces of memory begin, and in spite of emerging functional deficits in this period a global repertory of exchange grows. Data become installed about the present situation and about what preceded the trauma, while the bonds with family members and individuals in the medical team strengthen. Like an echo, it seems that a consciousness of self opens up.

While the time necessary to recover a higher level of integrated neurological performance (described earlier) is exhausted within 3–4 months, the time needed to recover behavioral performance in the sequence described above can be extremely variable and not synchronous. Very often, the patient seems extremely slow (sometimes 7 months or more) to achieve definite behavioral performance characteristic of emergence from the vegetative state. However, a careful and objective analysis may reveal that the first signs of communicability can often appear as early as the third month and then abate over time.

Recovery of consciousness is defined as the patient's ability to establish meaningful communicative contact with the environment by motor, visual, or verbal acts. Considerable experience is necessary to differentiate between reflex activity and meaningful responses. The *International Working Party Report on the Vegetative State* [141] suggested that a total lack of communication in patients in the vegetative state makes it impossible to determine whether they have an inner life, so that assessments need to be made on a behavioral basis. Furthermore, as the cognitive status fluctuates over time – even from minute to minute – the clinician has to perform frequent or continuous examinations, with a substantial investment of time. The report should highlight the role of family members in interpreting the first signs of recovery, especially in patients with severe motor limitations, because of their high sensitivity to changes in the patient and receptive interpretation of his or her behavioral patterns. Steady, long-term familiarity with the patient and his or her environment, knowledge of the patient's responses to visual or auditory stimuli, and interpersonal rapport with the patient are all important contributing factors. At the same time, however, physicians should be aware of the potential bias due to "wishful thinking" on the part of close relatives. The chances of recovery of patients in the vegetative state depend on three main factors: etiology, duration of unconsciousness, and age.

Prognostic Value of Neurological Signs

Giuliano Dolce and Leon Sazbon

The relevance of single neurological signs in predicting the outcome is discussed in the section on neurological examination. An assessment of the brain's degree of residual functional integration and the prediction of recovery are possible only through the neurological examination. By contrast, the neurophysiological parameters expressing higher brain function or the activation of sensory systems or subsystems (such as the EEG, somatosensory evoked potentials, event-related potentials, P300, contingent negative variation, mismatch negativity, etc.) do not provide reliable information to be used to predict the outcome; nor there is any consistent evidence of a correlation between these and the clinical course.

Quintieri and co-workers [142] have monitored the incidence and relevance of neurological signs every 2 weeks in a group of 70 patients in post-traumatic vegetative state. The prognostic relevance of each sign in relation to the outcome was estimated. No unique sign proved to be of any particular relevance. Changes over time in some neurological signs, such as their appearance or disappearance, are nevertheless important. A cluster of three signs (spontaneous mobility, oral automatism, eye tracking) has been identified, the temporal development of which has a remarkable prognostic value. A prediction of favorable outcome (with recovered neurological functions and awareness) proved legitimate when eye tracking and spontaneous mobility in at least one body segment were observed within 75 days of brain injury and oral automatisms had already disappeared. About one-third of the patients (32%) were discharged and returned home with restored ability to attend to the activities of daily life and with expectations of being able to resume work or education at levels comparable to those before the brain injury. A moderate to severe degree of disability persisted in about 30% of the patients in whom these signs had appeared late – i.e., more than 150 days after brain injury. Finally, it is possible to predict no recovery of conscious activities when no spontaneous motility or eye tracking are observed and oral automatisms are still present more than 200 days after trauma (Fig. 4.2). Under these conditions, a late recovery is only observed in excep-

Prognostic Value of Neurological Signs

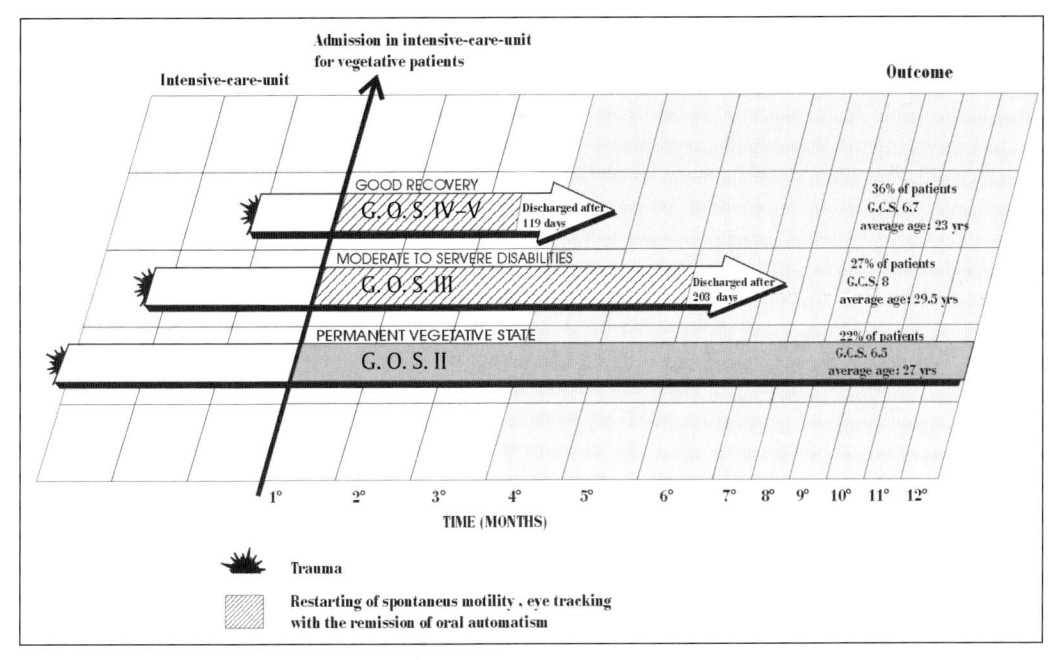

Fig. 4.2 Outcome of 100 patients in post-traumatic vegetative state, as estimated on the basis of three neurological signs (spontaneous movement, oral automatism, eye tracking). GCS: Glasgow Coma Scale

tional cases and never reaches above the minimally responding status. The so-called "late" neurological signs – i. e., those appearing only after 6 months from the beginning of vegetative state (such as rabbit-snout, half-moon pucker mouth and Klippel signs) – never disappear, and are a bad prognostic indication for the recovery of consciousness.

Basic Glossary and Definitions of Relevant Signs

- *Stereotyped movements.* These are involuntary, repetitive movements, with no finality or purpose, most often restricted to the buccal muscles in the form of chewing, swallowing or sucking.
- *Corneomandibular reflex.* Lateral movement of the jaw (as a result of the contracting external pterygoidal muscles) following stimulation of the ipsilateral cornea.
- *Snout reflex.* Sharp tapping of the middle of the upper lips induces exaggerated reflex contraction of the lips.
- *Flushing, excessive perspiration and drooling – emergency reactions.* A state that suddenly appears, usually after even minimal stimuli and on occasions without any detectable stimulus. It reflects vegetative unsteadiness, possibly due to inadequacy of the hypothalamic centers for thermal regulation.
- *Restlessness.* Psychomotor hyperactivity, including movements, vocalization and behavior.
- *Body position.*
  - *Decerebrate.* This is an opisthotonos position, with the upper limbs extended in adduction and hyperpronation and the lower limbs extended with plantar flexion of the feet. The extensor tonus is increased in all four limbs. The neurological damage responsible may be extensive subdural or intraventricular bleeding, usually localized in the midbrain structures.
  - *Decorticate.* In this condition, the patient's upper limbs are in adduction (with arms, palms and fingers in flexion), and the lower limbs are extended with plantar flexion of feet. The injury causing this is located in the internal capsule of the brain hemispheres and affects the corticospinal tracts.
  - *Normal position.* The position in which all four limbs and the head are straight.
  - *Paraplegia in flexion.* A position in which there are flexospasms of the lower limbs as a result of inhibition of the stretch reflex.

- *Fetal position.* A body attitude with limbs and neck in flexion, deriving its name from the similarity to the position of the fetus in the uterus.
- *Finger deformation.* A condition caused by periosteal ossification, bleeding inside the joints, erosion of cartilage, enlargement of periosteal soft tissues, thickening of skin, and increased perspiration of the hands and feet.
- *Epileptic fits.* These can appear as generalized tonic – clonic, partial, or focal seizures. Generalized fits start with a shout, a fall, and tonic spasms, followed by clonic convulsions of the limbs. Sometimes there are autonomous disturbances such as lack of control of body functions.
- *Abnormal movements.*
  - *Choreiform movements.* Rapid, sudden, involuntary movements without purpose or rhythm.
  - *Athetoid movements.* Slow, involuntary movements, reminiscent of those of a snake and more evident in the distal portions of the limbs.
  - *Tremor.* involuntary contraction of opposing groups of muscles, causing rhythmic or alternating movement of a joint or group of joints.
  - *Sketchy movements.* Uncoordinated defensive movements occurring as a result of a painful stimulus. They can cause skewing of the neck and body, or flexing of the neck.
  - *Slow-motion movements.* Very slow movements, similar to those of the characters in a movie in slow motion, which appear as a delayed reaction of the four limbs, trunk, and head to a painful stimulus.
  - *Balled-up movements.* Pelvicrural contraction resulting in an involuntary movement in flexion of the hips.
- *Clubbing.* A condition created as a result of enlargement of the tissue between the nail and the bone. This leads to a floating nail and changes the angle between the phalanx and the nail, apparently caused by a lack of oxygen (hypoxia).
- *Doll's eyes phenomenon.* The passive sudden movement of the patient's head in one direction causes the eyes to move in the opposite direction; alternatively, when the head is suddenly moved backward, the eyelids open.
- *Lateral conjugate deviation of the eyes.* Both eyes turn to the same side at a constant angle.
- *Skew deviation.* One eye moves upwards and the other downward, an indication of damage located between the nuclei of the pons and related pathways.
- *Blink reflex.* Blinking (closing) of the eyes in response to the sudden approach of an object. This reflex indicates an undamaged reticular ascending system in the pons.
- *Light reflex.* Contraction of the pupil when light falls on the retina; this indicates unaffected cranial nerves II and III.
- *Ciliospinal reflex.* Dilatation of the pupils on a painful stimulus, usually pinching of the neck area. This usually indicates integrity of the neck sympathetic system.
- *Corneal reflex.* Blinking when the cornea or conjunctiva are lightly touched – e.g., with a cotton patch. This reflex disappears if cranial nerves V or VII or nuclei in the pons have been damaged.
- *Klippel sign.* The thumb is continuously kept between the second and third fingers.
- *Orienting reaction and eye tracking.* When the patient turns his/her head or eyes in the direction of a sudden, loud noise. This indicates integrity of the thalamic structures and reticular ascending system.
- *Normal eye movement.* This occurs when there is integrity of the innervation of the external eye muscles. In this condition, the eyes look straight forwards in the resting condition.
- *Spontaneous eye movements.* When the oculomotor function of the brainstem is unaffected; may or may not be parallel, vertical or horizontal.
- *Eye movements in response to an order.* These indicate the patient's ability to follow verbal orders. Opening the eyes in response to a verbal order indicates that verbal stimulus of any kind causes opening of the eyes.
- *Finger following.* This is the movement of the patient's eyes following an examining finger in eight directions.
- *Movement of the limbs in response to painful stimuli.* Indicates residual function of thalamus, mesencephalon (and the connection between these structures), as well as of certain parts of the rhinencephalon. In a local response to a painful stimulus, a limb movement attempts to localize or remove it. An arm crossing the body midline or rising above the shoulder in the direction of the painful stimuli on the trunk, arm or skull is a pertinent example. More primitive movements are, for instance, the retraction of a limb or stretching it in an attempt to avoid the pain induced by a nociceptive stimulus.

- *Spontaneous vocalization.* In the vegetative state, groans or snores deprived of any specific significance are common.
- *Mimicry.* Spontaneous or imitative changes in facial expression resulting from a painful stimulus are absent in most patients in the vegetative state.
- *Sucking reflex.* Sucking of any object presented close enough to the mouth.
- *Cornea – chin reflex.* Turning leftwards of the chin if the cornea of the right eye is touched, and vice versa.
- *Lip – chin reflex.* A reflex similar to the Marinesco–Radovici reflex, in which stimulation of the lips results in the contraction of the chin.
- *Myotatic cervical reflex.* Straightening of the head in response to tapping on the face midline.
- *Marinescu – Radovici reflex.* Contraction of the muscles of the chin in response to stimulation of the thumb. The phenomenon indicates damage to the corticobulbar tract in a variety of brain diseases, including dementia, lateral amyotrophic sclerosis, and others.
- *Grasping reflex.* Closing the hand in response to any stimulus to the palm.
- *Retractory nystagmus.* Erratic, spontaneous backward movements of the eyeball in the orbit, as caused by the simultaneous contraction of the six muscles regulating extrinsic eye movements, and implying damage to the mesencephalon.
- *Opening the mouth.* The ability of patients in the vegetative state to open their mouths and receive food and drink.
- *Tactile oral stimulation.* Tactile stimulation around the mouth causes the mouth to open in an attempt to catch or bite the stimulating object.
- *Magnetic phenomenon.* When there is tactile stimulation around the mouth and the patient is unable to catch the stimulus, he/she is drawn after it.
- *Bulldog reflex.* In response to an object inserted into the mouth, the patient closes his or her teeth on it and does not allow it to be removed.
- *Optic – oral stimulation.* A phenomenon occurring when patients are shown an object and open the mouth or move the lips to search for it.
- *Exploration of the blanket and scratching.* Automatic movements performed by patients in the vegetative state, with the hands exploring the blanket (apparently searching) or scratching the body. In the most advanced stages of the syndrome, these movements are directed towards the genitals and in men may cause an erection.
- *Onanism.* Auto-eroticism (as defined by Shtekel). This is sexual self-satisfaction in which a man or woman use their hands or an object.

Differential Diagnosis

Erich Schmutzhard

Introduction

Although it is diffuse brain injury – such as severe traumatic brain injury, hypoxia/anoxia of the brain, rarely intracranial hemorrhage, or infection/inflammation – that more often leads to a vegetative state to be diagnosed by clinical and neurological examination or neuroimaging (particularly magnetic resonance imaging) and electrophysiological methods [143], focal neurological diseases may also result in a neurological syndrome which, in the hands of inexperienced physicians, may be mistaken for a vegetative state.

Both in children and adults, the accuracy of the diagnosis of a vegetative state – particularly if persistent – is not very good [144,145]. Misdiagnosis of the vegetative state includes akinetic mutism, locked-in syndrome and, in rare instances, a paramedian diencephalic syndrome (hypersomnia) [146]. These three clear-cut clinical entities in most instances show an easily distinguishable set of neurological signs and symptoms, but are liable to be misdiagnosed as vegetative state.

In the vegetative state, and particularly in the persistent vegetative state, as the consequence of a severe intracranial disease initially leading to coma, the patient is not comatose but completely unresponsive [147]. In these three clinical entities, the initial signs and symptoms may be a profound disturbance of vigilance/consciousness, i.e. coma; however, in all three the term "coma" is never applicable in a consistent way, and the patients regain full consciousness and at least partial responsiveness within days after the acute onset of disease.

The three diseases – locked-in syndrome, akinetic mutism and paramedian diencephalic syndrome – will be described here by definition, pathological basis/etiology, neurological signs and symptoms, prognosis, and specific differential diagnostics. Since there are specific causal treatments only for the acute phases (e. g., thrombolysis in basilar artery occlusion, external cerebrospinal fluid drainage in acute hydrocephalus, etc.), the therapeutic aspects of these three diseases will only be dealt with very briefly.

Locked-in Syndrome

Definition

Locked-in syndrome is defined by a complete de-efferentation at the level of the ventral pons. The patients are fully awake, alert, and are aware not only of their abnormal situation but also, and to a full extent, of their surroundings [148,149].

Pathology/Etiology

A bilateral lesion located in the ventral pons leads to a supranuclear interruption of the corticospinal and corticobulbar tracts. In the case of the full-blown picture of locked-in syndrome, the ascending fibers of the pontine/mesencephalic tegmentum are fully preserved, including the Dejerine bundle within the tectum of the mesencephalon. The unaffected tectum, projecting onto the oculomotor nuclei, therefore allows a fully preserved vertical eye movement [150].

In the vast majority (80–90%) of patients with a locked-in syndrome, the condition is caused by ischemia in the middle part of the basilar artery (Fig. 4.3) [146,148,149]. In addition to ischemia, pontine hemorrhage, infection and inflammation within the ventral pontine area, traumatic lesions, tumors located in the ventral pons, and pontine myelinolysis are further although infrequent causes of this disease entity [151–153].

Neurological Signs and Symptoms

Table 4.2 lists all the relevant neurological criteria for establishing a diagnosis of locked-in syndrome [146,149,150]. In the initial phase, the penumbra of the pontine ischemic lesion frequently leads, along with the de-efferentation, also to impairment of the afferent tracts, producing the more complex neurological picture of a pontine lesion, including impairment of consciousness (even coma). This impairment of consciousness usually improves within hours, or at the maximum within a few days. Prolonged impairment of consciousness is only very rarely seen in lesions located within the ventral pons.

As shown in Table 4.2, the dominant feature of the locked-in syndrome is spastic tetraplegia, with a bilateral extensor Babinski sign. Initially, signs of decortication are present. The destruction of the ventral pontine nuclei leads to impairment of swallowing and phonation, and the patient is therefore mute/mutistic. The destruction of the nuclei of the abducent nerves impairs both voluntary and reflex horizontal eye movements. The corneal reflex is interrupted due to the destruction of parts of the trigeminal nerves. In most instances, the sensory system is intact, with painful stimuli leading to extensor synergisms. Respiration is in most instances intact, but in the initial phase it is often at least partly impaired. The patient's cognitive capacities are fully intact. It is the vertical eye movements that allow the patients to communicate with their surroundings.

Electroencephalography shows a normal alpha-rhythm, which can be blocked by eye opening. Rarely, mild non-specific alterations of the electrical background activity are observed. While the sen-

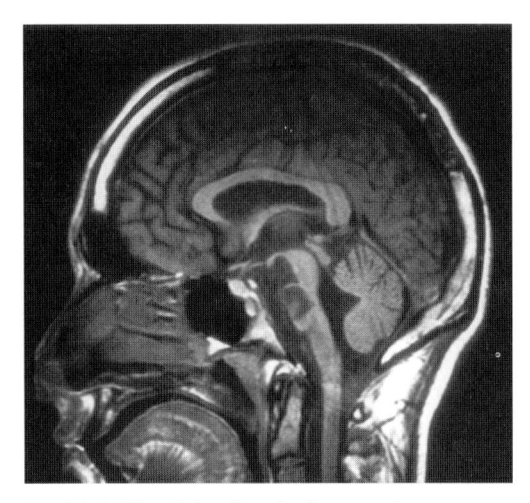

Fig. 4.3 A T1-weighted sagittal magnetic resonance image, showing ventral pontine ischemia in a patient with prolonged locked-in syndrome

Table 4.2 Clinical characteristics of locked-in syndrome

Self-awareness	Present
Sleep – wake rhythm	Intact
Motor function	Tetraplegia, pseudobulbar paralysis, vertical eye movement possible (incl. closure of the eyes)
Sensation of pain	Present
Respiration	(Occasionally) initially impaired, throughout the course of the disease normal
EEG activity	Normal or minimally abnormal
Neuroimaging	Ventral pontine lesion (Fig. 4.3)
Cerebral metabolism	Normal (in most instances)
Prognosis quo ad rehabilitationem	Recovery improbable (depending on the etiology), persistent tetraplegia, prolonged survival possible

sory evoked potentials and the early acoustic evoked potentials (as well as visually evoked potentials) do not usually show any abnormalities, the motor evoked potentials are partly or fully impaired, depending on the degree of the focal lesion [154]. The cerebral metabolism does not show any abnormalities.

Differential Diagnosis

The most important diagnostic aspect is recognition of the syndrome itself. Any form of coma can create diagnostic difficulties, as can progressive lesions of the peripheral nervous system such as Guillain–Barré inflammatory polyradiculoneuropathy, myasthenic crises, poliomyelitis, or polyneuropathy [146,149].

Therapy

The specific treatment needs to be organized in relation to the event causing the locked-in syndrome. In case of thrombosis of the basilar artery, local thrombolysis (in the acute stage) and/or full heparinization are the specific treatment modalities. As in all other tetraplegic patients who show additional impairment of various functions of the brainstem, early tracheostomy/tracheotomy and percutaneous endoscopic gastrostomy (PEG) need to be performed in order to allow the best possible management of respiration and nutrition. Early tracheostomy/tracheotomy also prevents potentially life-threatening aspiration pneumonia.

Prognosis

A transient locked-in syndrome is observed rarely and up to two-thirds of these patients died of acute pulmonary complications [155]. However, with early intensive care, including early tracheostomy/tracheotomy, the life-threatening pulmonary complications can be overcome and a high rate of survival can be achieved. If there are no or only few signs of recovery within the first week, further recovery seems unlikely despite the best efforts at rehabilitation. The major factor affecting the prognosis is the etiology of the locked-in syndrome. Whereas little recovery is to be expected beyond the first week after the onset of signs and symptoms in patients with an ischemic lesion, in other patients – e. g., those with brainstem encephalitis, pontine myelinolysis, etc. – at least partial recovery has been observed much more frequently, and even much later [156].

Although survival for more than 20 years has been described in single case reports of patients with a full-blown locked-in syndrome, the overall life expectancy is reduced. In one study, five patients requested full-scale medical care in case of life-threatening complications (including intravenous administration of antibiotics), despite the extreme reduction in the quality of their life [156].

In the age of electronic communications, all forms of high-tech communication can and must be incorporated into the rehabilitative program, allowing the patient to participate actively and communicate with the surroundings at least to some extent.

4 Clinical Picture

Akinetic Mutism

Definition

Akinetic mutism is defined as a condition in which the patient is without spontaneous movement (or at least shows very few, slow movements) and mutistic – i.e., not actively communicating [146,157,158]. However, the patient is able to fix the gaze on individuals and communicate with them. The immobility is not explained by a severe lesion of the peripheral or central motor systems.

Pathology/Etiology

Bilateral lesions of the corpus striatum, globus pallidus, lesions of the dorsomedial or ventrolateral thalamus, and paramedian lesions of the mesencephalic reticular formation or of the posterior diencephalon and the mesencephalon are usually found in akinetic mutism. Most frequently, however, extensive lesions of both frontal lobes are found (Fig. 4.4) [157–160]. These lesions can be caused either directly (frontal contusions, bilateral anterior cerebral artery infarction, bilateral intracranial/frontal hemorrhages, abscesses, etc.), or indirectly by compression of these structures by acute hydrocephalus or, at very advanced stages, by normal-pressure hydrocephalus [161–165]. Both the dopaminergic and noradrenergic systems seem to be involved, since pharmacological treatment has been shown to improve the signs and symptoms of akinetic mutism [161].

Neurological Signs and Symptoms

The patient appears to be alert, is easy to wake up and does not show any spontaneous, voluntary, or reflex movements. No, or very little movement is observed even on commands or in response to painful stimuli. However, spontaneous fixation of the gaze is observed regularly, always without head movement. Verbal communication is extremely limited. Overall, the general impression is that of a complete lack of impulse and spontaneity. Table 4.3 lists the most important clinical features of akinetic mutism [146,157,158].

Differential Diagnosis

In contrast to the locked-in syndrome, the caudal brainstem reflexes are usually intact. The fixation of the gaze allows objectivization of horizontal eye movements. This is the best possible method of distinguishing between akinetic mutism and the persistent vegetative state and locked-in syndrome. In addition, optokinetic nystagmus can be elicited. The major diagnostic problems are with psychiatric diseases such as catatonia and depressive stupor [157,158].

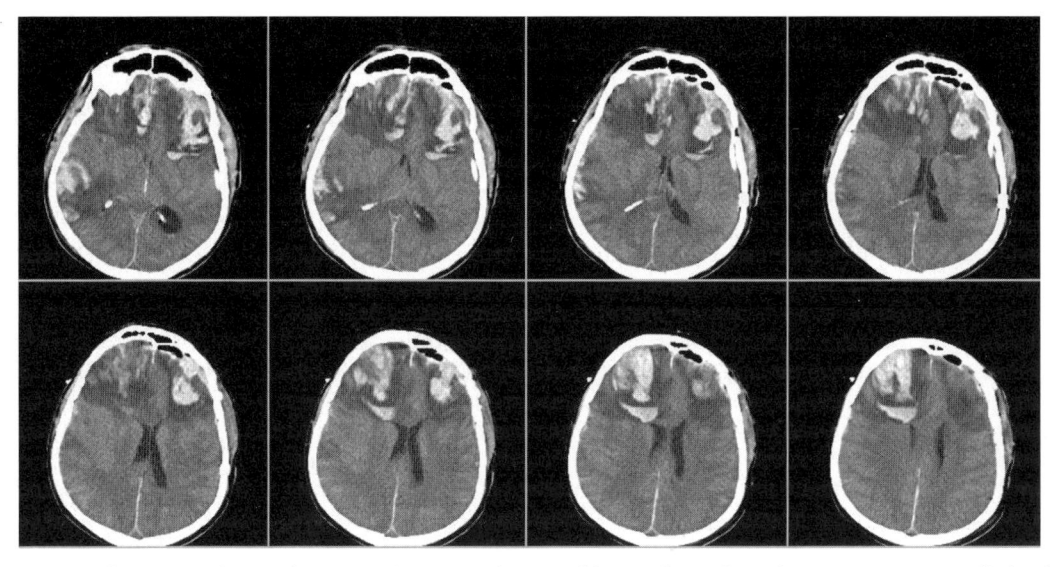

Fig. 4.4a–h A series of coronal computed tomography scans in the acute phase in a patient with severe bilateral hemorrhagic frontal contusions, eventually leading to akinetic mutism

Table 4.3 Clinical characteristics of akinetic mutism

Sleep – wake rhythm	Intact
Motor functions	Grossly reduced/absent
Pain sensation	Present
Respiration	Present
EEG activity	Unspecific slowing
Neuroimaging	Hydrocephalus or severe bilateral frontal lesions (Fig. 4.4)
Cerebral metabolism	Not known
Prognosis quo ad rehabilitationem	Depending on the etiology of the syndrome

Therapy

The initial treatment has to concentrate on the etiology, including evacuation of contusional hemorrhages, abscesses, etc. The earlier hydrocephalus is controlled by implanting a shunt system or by external cerebrospinal fluid drainage, the better are the chances of full recovery [157,158].

Prognosis

Depending on etiology, akinetic mutism may be fully reversible. However, full recovery appears to be highly unlikely in cases of contusional destruction of both frontal lobes or ischemic lesions after vasospasm in a patient with an anterior communicating artery aneurysm, whereas timely neurosurgical treatment of hydrocephalus may lead to impressive improvement in the clinical status. If the hydrocephalus has been present for a long time (e. g., normal-pressure hydrocephalus), a prolonged period of observation after neurosurgical correction (i. e., implantation of a shunt system) has to be allowed in order to achieve the best possible prognostic evaluation [146,157,158,161–163].

Paramedian Diencephalic Syndrome (Hypersomnia)

Definition

Hypersomnia represents a state of increased need of sleep. The patient with this syndrome is able to communicate, but only for short periods. The pa-

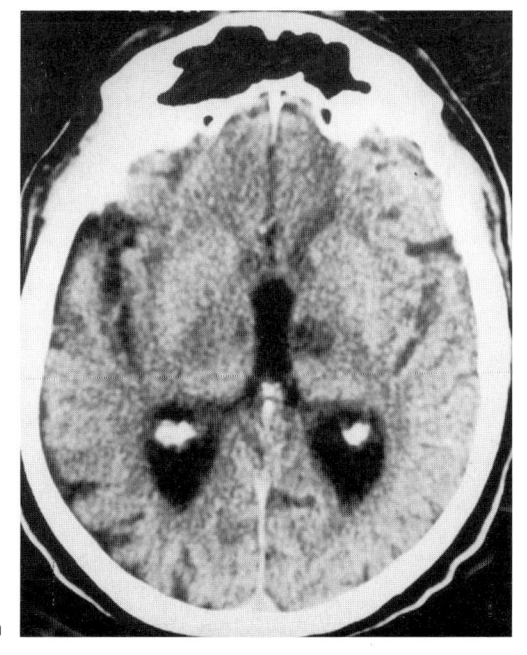

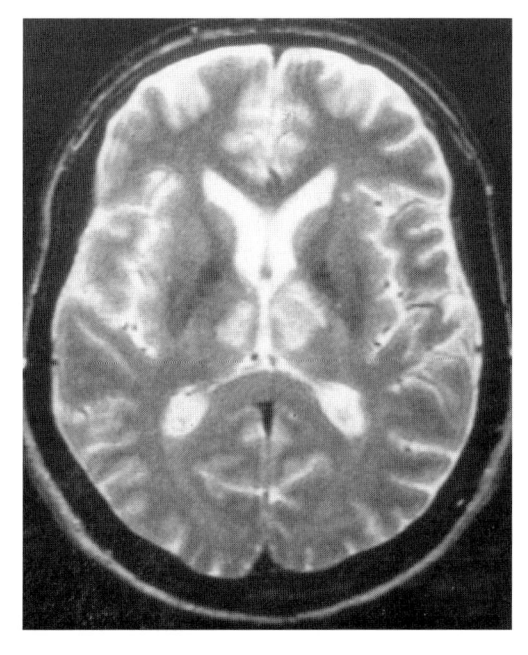

Fig. 4.5 Cerebral computed tomogram scan (**a**) and T2-weighted magnetic resonance image (**b**), showing a bilateral paramedian ischemic infarction in a patient with a transitory embolic occlusion of the basilar tip

tient is asleep for most of the time but can be awakened at any time [146,166]. Hypersomnia is due to an acute or subacute phase of disease, and it is not known to have irreversible neurological sequelae.

Pathology/Etiology

The neurological entity of hypersomnia is caused by bilateral lesions of the paramedian thalamus. Most cases are due to ischemic infarctions (Fig. 4.5); tumors or hemorrhages in this area, or within the third ventricle and tegmental mesencephalon, rarely cause hypersomnia [166–168]. The hypersomnia and insufficient arousal are caused by damage to the dopaminergic and noradrenergic fibers that ascend from the reticular formation to the thalamus. On electroencephalography, these patients have normal circadian rhythm and sleep architecture during the night. However, during the long phases in which they sleep throughout the day patients rarely reach stage two or deeper sleep stages (usually only stage one sleep during the day) [146].

Neurological Signs and Symptoms

The patients are in a fairly constant sleep-like condition, arousable for short periods. Throughout these short periods, they are attentive and aware, but in most instances this does not reach the normal level of being fully awake. Fairly normal communication is possible during these short waking phases, , but the patient tends to fall asleep easily even while talking or carrying out other activities. There is often amnesia, which may persist. In most cases, hypersomnia is the initial clinical diagnosis, and the patient is initially comatose only in rare cases. If this is the case, the transition from coma into hypersomnia is almost undetectable, and the diagnosis of hypersomnia is delayed. Hypersomnia usually lasts for several weeks, very rarely exceeding a period of 2 months [166,169].

This neurological condition is even more confusing if hypersomnia is accompanied by other mesencephalic signs and symptoms such as visuomotor disturbances, in particular blepharoptosis [146,166,167]. In such patients, only electrophysiological examinations (e. g., electroencephalography) can help to distinguish between those with hypersomnia plus blepharoptosis and those who are comatose. Table 4.4 lists the most important clinical aspects of paramedian diencephalic syndrome (hypersomnia) [146,166].

Differential Diagnosis

From a clinical viewpoint, it is difficult to distinguish between patients with hypersomnia plus visuomotor lesion (blepharoptosis) and patients in coma, but electroencephalography allows a decision. Since patients with hypersomnia usually have normal function of the pons and medulla oblongata, differentiating this from locked-in syndrome should not be difficult. Even in cases of visuomotor disturbance, patients with hypersomnia can be identified, since blepharoptosis and vertical ocular paresis do not usually exist in locked-in syndrome [146]. Spontaneous and adequate movements (to external stimuli such as pain, etc.) allow differentiation from akinetic mutism. A patient with hypersomnia is usually able to communicate actively, even speak and understand, although a simultaneous memory disturbance may impede the latter.

Therapy

Diagnosis (as early as possible) of basilar tip occlusion with subsequent ischemia, which is in most cases the cause of hypersomnia, may allow appropriate therapy with local thrombolysis and/or heparinization. Prevention of concomitant complications (e. g., aspiration pneumonia, malnutrition, etc.) is part of the initial therapy, and is often necessary for several weeks.

Prognosis

Hypersomnia usually persists for weeks or months. In most instances, impairment of memory

Table 4.4 Clinical characteristics of hypersomnia (paramedian diencephalic syndrome)

Self-awareness	Present
Sleep – wake rhythm	Hypersomnia
Motor functions	Present (occasionally reduced)
Pain sensation	Present
Respiration	Present
EEG activity	Sleep pattern
Neuroimaging	Bilateral paramedian thalamic lesions (Fig. 4.5)
Cerebral metabolism	Not known
Prognosis quo ad rehabilitationem	Frequently persistent amnesia

persists and, if associated with impaired attention, is termed "thalamic dementia." In other instances, apathy and psychomotor retardation and/or slowing may persist. There have been reports describing hypersomnia persisting for more than 1 year [166,167,170].

Prognosis and Outcome

Leon Sazbon and Giuliano Dolce

As described in detail in the section on clinical signs (p. 26), the vegetative State (VS) is characterized by unawareness of the self and of environment, absence of response to any type of stimulus, absence of communicative functions, and presence of wake–sleep cycles with preservation of autonomic functions and brainstem reflexes. The patient's total lack of communication with the external world makes it particularly difficult to assess the prognosis in vegetative state. However, the outcome is of paramount importance not only to the patient (whose survival, well-being and quality of life are directly affected), but also to the family, physician, and community. The family will need to cope with the cognitive, motor, and communications sequelae of the disorder, and the physician will be involved in the ongoing evaluation of the nature, intensity, and efficacy of treatment. The community shares in the economic burden of hospitalization, rehabilitation, medication, and compensation, where appropriate [171].

In this section, the outcome of VS is evaluated in relation to three aspects: survival, recovery of consciousness, and recovery of function (including vocational activities).

Survival

The survival of patients in VS is threatened by many factors and complications, both in the acute stage after injury (hypotension, hyperglycemia, risks of prolonged mechanical ventilation, unreactive pupils, etc.) [4,171,172] and in later stages, after autonomic stability has been achieved (see the section on complications, p. 18). Specific causes of death include, among others, infections, systemic failure, sudden death of unknown cause, and respiratory failure [22,173–176].

Table 4.5 summarizes several reports in the literature investigating mortality among patients in vegetative state. The cumulative rate in the different series is about 30% at the end of the first year after injury.

Strauss et al. [177] examined the records of 1021 patients in VS and noted that "during the first 10 years after onset, mortality declined by an estimated 8% per year. Thus, the chance of dying in the next year for a patient who has been in VS for 7 years is only 60%." Mortality did not correlate significantly with the patient's sex, residence (home, nursing home, hospital), occurrence of seizures, or associated medical conditions. Patients who were ventilator-dependent or fed via gastrostomy tube had a higher mortality rate, especially if they were very young or very old (see the section on complications, p. 18).

A remarkable study of the natural history of VS was published by a Japanese team, who followed 38 patients in traumatic VS, drawn from a heterogeneous group of 110 affected patients [22,178]. They found that 26% of patients died during the first year of the study, 42% by the end of the second year, and 55% by the end of the third year; the cumulative mortality by the end of the five-year follow-up period was 66%. However, these findings are difficult to compare with those of other series, as the patients were included at different time points after the onset of VS.

Studies on survival have yielded some controversial findings. Reported mean survival in patients of all ages was 15.5 months (SD 22) in the series reported by Sazbon and Groswasser [173] and 21.9 months in the series published by Rosin [179]. Higashi et al. [22] reported 33.0 months (SD 25.8), Minderhoud and Braakman [176] 4.4 years, and Tresch et al. [110] (all nursing home residents) 3.3 years (SD 0.5). In infants and children, estimates range from 4.1 (SD 0.7) to 7.4 (SD 1.8) years, depending on the specific age group [180]. The longest surviving patients in the Israeli sample reported by Sazbon and Groswasser [173] lived 10 years after sustaining injury. However, a number of authors have reported survival times of 10–20 years [22,25,43,180]. We suggest that these discrepancies are due to the fact that most of the reported series and case stud-

Table 4.5 Cumulative mortality (%) in patients in the vegetative state

First author (ref.)	Patients (n)	3 months (%)	6 months (%)	9 months (%)	1 year (%)	2 years (%)	3 years (%)	5 years (%)	7 years (%)	10 years (%)
Sazbon [173]	134	6.7	18.6	27.6	32.1	39.5	40.3	43.3	45.5	46.3
Brackman [175]	140	30	40	51						
Multi-Society Task Force [174]										
Adults	434	15	24	33						
Children	106	4	9	9						
Bricolo [43]	135				30					
Minderhoud [176]	53						47	76		

ies were published in the 1980s. Since then, the approach of medical professionals to patients with VS has changed considerably, and many patients today are managed in intensive-care units in major hospitals with continuous monitoring. In addition, the great majority of the studies have reported the median survival time, but not the life expectancy [181]. The median survival time reflects the point at which half the patients would have died, whereas the life expectancy is the arithmetic mean of the survival times [177]. Another question that has not yet been resolved is the number of patients who die due to withdrawal of supportive care.

The underlying condition also plays a role in survival. Comparisons of trauma and nontrauma (i. e., medical) patients in VS have shown a higher mortality rate and shorter survival time in the latter [5,22,174,182–185].

Recovery of Consciousness

Recovery of consciousness is defined as the ability of the patient to establish meaningful communicative contact with the environment by motor, visual or verbal acts [71,182]. Considerable experience is necessary to differentiate between reflex activity and meaningful responses. *The International Working Party Report on the Vegetative State* [141] suggested that the total lack of communication in VS patients excludes the possibility of determining whether they have an inner life, so assessments need to be made on a behavioral basis. In addition, as the cognitive status fluctuates over time, even from minute to minute, the clinician has to perform frequent or continuous examinations, with a great investment of time. The report highlights the role of family members in interpreting the first signs of recovery, especially in patients with severe motor limitations, because of their high sensitivity to changes in the patient and receptive interpretation of his or her behavioral patterns. Steady, long-term familiarity with the patient and his or her home environment, knowledge of the patient's responses to visual or auditory stimuli, and interpersonal rapport with the patient are all highly contributory [174]. At the same time, however, physicians should be aware of the bias of "wishful thinking" on the part of close relatives.

The chances of recovery of patients in VS depend on three factors: etiology, duration of unconsciousness, and age.

Etiology. Patients with a traumatic etiology have a greater chance of recovery than patients with a nontraumatic etiology, for the following reasons:
- The usually younger mean age of trauma patients compared to patients with anoxic ischemia.
- The prior existence in the medical group of cardiovascular, respiratory, or renal diseases or metabolic disorders that contribute to or prolong the VS.
- Differences in pathology: ischemia and anoxia cause cortical damage, laminar necrosis and diffuse demyelination, whereas trauma tends to cause diffuse axonal injury due to shearing forc-

es and microhemorrhages, with relative sparing of the cerebral cortex. In addition, anoxia due to an associated chest lesion, hypersecretions of the bronchial tree, or a state of shock is a more or less regular finding, with an undoubtedly bad influence on the final outcome [173,187]. Bricolo et al. [43] also emphasized the negative influence on recovery of alcohol use before injury and the presence of premorbid epilepsy or metabolic disorders.

Duration of unconsciousness. The duration of unconsciousness can serve as an important indicator of the severity of brain damage [175,186]. Table 4.6 shows the rates of recovery in patients in VS in relation to the duration of unconsciousness. The longer the unconscious state lasts, the poorer are the chances of recovering awareness and cortical function. Most of the patients who recover consciousness do so within the first 6 months of the onset of VS, especially in the first 4 months. Thereafter, the rate of recovery decreases to 7–11% in adults and 17–22% in children. Najenson et al. [11] reported a recovery rate of consciousness of 66% after 1 year in 15 patients in VS, and Bricolo et al. [43] reported a rate of 61% in 134 patients.

Age. The third important factor in the prognosis of VS is age. Many authors have noted that children have a better outcome than adults [22,174, 175,188,189–193]. However, older children apparently fare better than younger ones. Heindl and Laub [37] followed 82 affected children and adolescents for 19 months and found that 73% of the children younger than 6 years regained consciousness, compared to 89% of those older than 6 years. These findings were supported by the study by Mahoney et al. [44], who reported that children less than 2 years old have a worse prognosis, and the study by Jennett [194], who noted a poorer outcome in children less than 5 years of age. This may be due to the greater susceptibility of the immature and less myelinated brain to the damage induced by shearing forces and its lesser ability to autoregulate vascular perfusion [44].

In adults, studies in Israel [195] and America [174] have shown that patients over the age of 40 have a smaller chance of clinical improvement than younger ones. However, the reported rate of recovery in adults varies widely, probably owing to the different criteria used to define both VS and recovery of awareness from VS. For example, Sazbon and Groswasser [4] excluded patients with an inconsistent minimal response (see p. 110), but Bricolo et al. [43] did not; indeed, about half of the patients in the latter sample fell into this category.

Late Recovery

VS is considered to be permanent if consciousness is not regained within 1 year, with a 0.1% error, according to the Council on Scientific Affairs of the American Medical Association [192], and a 1.6% error according to the Multi-Society Task Force on PVS [174]. Nevertheless, there have been a few reports of patients recovering after 2 years or even later. For example, Higashi et al. [22] described five patients, and Levin et al. [187] reported on six of

Table 4.6 Rate of recovery of consciousness in patients in the vegetative state (% of total patients)

First author (ref).	Patients (n)	3 months (%)	6 months (%)	9 months (%)	12 months (%)	> 1 year (%)
Levin [187]	84	–	41	–	51	56
Kriel [188] (children)	40	20	55	67	72	77
Heindl [37] (children)	82	34	63	79	80	84
Sazbon [186]	134	43	49	52	54	–
Braakman [175]	140	25	38	–	42	–
Multi-Society Task Force						
Adults	434	33	46	–	52	54
Children	106	24	51	–	62	–

84 patients, who were found to be no longer vegetative between the first and third year of follow-up. Childs and Mercer [196] reported on an 18-year-old woman in VS of traumatic origin who experienced late recovery after 18 months, and the series published by Kriel et al. [188] included two patients who recovered during the second year. Arts et al. [197] published a case of a young woman who regained consciousness after 30 months. In addition, there have been several case reports of recovery from VS of nontraumatic etiology at 17–36 months after onset [22,198,199]. One particularly unusual case, observed by Tanhehco and Kaplan [200], involved a 25-year-old woman after head trauma, residing in a nursing home, who began to respond after 6 years. However, the authors provided no details on the patient's state during those years.

Owing to the legal and ethical implications of these cases, many clinicians are advocating that the term "permanent," with its negative and definitive connotations, should be replaced with the term "persistent" – a simple description of a continuous state over time.

Recovery of Function

The Multi-Society Task Force [174] described the recovery of function in patients in VS as the ability of the patient to communicate with the environment, perform adaptive tasks, perform tasks involving mobility, engage in self-care behaviors, and participate in recreational or vocational activities. The report states that: "Recovery of consciousness may occur without functional recovery, but functional recovery cannot occur without recovery of consciousness" [174]. Repeated examinations are necessary in order to evaluate the consistency and degree of signs of recovery.

Good recovery of function following brain damage apparently depends on the duration of unconsciousness and the extent of the deficit [43,44,201,202]. The greater the deficit, the worse the outcome. This is one of the largest problems in the rehabilitation of this patient group. One team in Israel has focused specifically on functional outcome in patients in VS for more than one month [4,203]. In the latter study, the authors followed 72 patients for 1 year after the onset of VS. By the end of the study period, half were independent in activities of daily life and 20% were partially dependent. The deficits in acquisition of information and in locomotion after 1 year were as follows: auditory deficits 16%, visual field defects 18%, ocular motility palsy 27%, motor deficits 66%, and ataxia 15% [195].

Cognitive and behavioral deficits of various degrees were the most common sequelae of central nervous system damage (93% and 32%, respectively). Cognitive disorders included memory deficits, problems of intellectual processing, praxis, gnosis, and problems of orientation. Almost 39% of the patients retained some aphasia and 55% retained dysphasia. Some patients were unaware of their disability, or suffered from apathy or lack of self-control as part of the frontal lobe syndrome; these had a poor rehabilitative, vocational, and social outcome. Locomotor dependence of various degrees was found in 66% of the patients and could be traced to two origins: skeletal trauma, such as fractures of the limbs and spine, and central nervous system trauma, causing paralysis and lack of coordination. In a comparison of children and adults, the Multi-Society Task Force [174] noted that at 1 year, 35% of the children had severe disability, 16% had moderate disability, and 11% had made a good recovery; the corresponding rates for the adult group were 28%, 17%, and 7%. In the series reported by Bricolo et al. [43], persistent severe disability was found in 31% of the patients (44% of survivors after 2 months), moderate recovery in 18% (25% of survivors), and good recovery in 13% (19% of survivors). Rates of severe and good to moderate recovery in the series reported by Braakman et al. [175] were 26% and 10%, respectively. Heindl and Laub [37] reported that at 19 months after onset, 19% of their 82 patients (all children or adolescents after trauma) became independent in activities of daily life. Of the six patients who regained consciousness after more than 1 year, none reached the level of independent living. Similarly, four of the six children followed by Kriel et al. [188] who recovered after 6 months achieved only limited language ability, although they were able to express wants and needs. The remaining two children recovered in the second year. One reached the level of the first four children, and the other achieved social responsiveness, but no language at all. Najenson and Groswasser [204] found that dysphasic patients have a poorer vocational outcome than nondysphasic ones.

Most patients who recover functional ability will eventually be able to live with their families, take part in community activities, and enjoy a reasonably good quality of life. Only a minority will be able to compete for jobs in the open market [4]. In the study by the Israeli group [195], despite the residual deficits, 72% of the patients returned home, 68% became independent or partially dependent in activities of daily life, and 60% found employment. The patients who recovered earlier had a better functional performance (Table 4.7).

In general, reasonable mental recovery cannot be expected if the coma lasts more than 2–4 months. In the study by Sazbon and Groswasser [203], 94% of the patients who recovered consciousness in the first 2 months after the onset of VS returned home, in comparison with 40% of those who recovered after 3 months. All patients who recovered after 6 months were referred to a nursing home facility. This series included 12 children younger than 12 years old. Only one of them recovered an age-adequate ability to learn (equivalent to return to work in adults); four returned to school but are now receiving education in a protected environment (equivalent to vocational training or sheltered workshop in adults); and seven were unable to learn (equivalent to inability to work in adults). Overall, five of the 12 children (42%) had a good functional recovery, compared to almost 60% of the adults.

The literature includes a few cases of late recovery of function. Najenson et al. [11] claimed that considerable improvement in communicative functions is possible even if the first manifestations of recovery appear as late as 5–7 months after the onset of the VS. They suggested that there is no one unique rhythm of recuperation and that each patient regains functional abilities at his or her own pace. The pattern of recovery, however, is predictable, starting with visual and auditory comprehension, followed by oral expression. Phonation returns slowly and incompletely, and patients tend to remain with evident dysphonia, rhinolalia or monotonous and harsh speech for a long time after recovery of consciousness [11].

Other studies in the literature support the possibility of perceptible mental recovery in patients in VS even after a long period. Bricolo et al. [43] described two patients who were able to execute commands after 6 months, and Arts et al. [197] reported on an unexpected improvement in awareness in a young girl after 2.5 years; she was able to comprehend and communicate and establish interpersonal relationships. In a 5-year follow-up study of 110 patients in VS, Higashi et al. [178] found five who showed a late recovery. Finally, Rosin [179] presented four patients who improved after 6 months, although all continue to have a severe disability and none was discharged home.

Table 4.7 Functional outcome relative to the duration of the vegetative state (% of recovered patients) [203]

	Duration of vegetative state				
	31–60 days	61–90 days	91–180 days	< 180 days	Total
Locomotion					
Full or aided	89%	75%	30%	0%	72%
Wheelchair	11%	25%	70%	100%	28%
ADL independence					
Full or partial	87%	40%	30%	0%	68%
Dependent	13%	65%	70%	100%	32%
Residence					
Home	94%	77%	40%	0%	76%
Institution	6%	23%	60%	100%	24%
Work					
Gainful or sheltered employment	82%	55%	20%	0%	62%
Unemployable	18%	45%	80%	100%	38%

ADL: activities of daily living.
Reproduced with permission from Taylor & Francis Limited http//www.tandf.co.uK. Brain Injury 5: 3–8, 1991.

These cases are all exceptions to the rule. The majority of researchers agree that if awareness is recovered after 6 months of VS, the chances of an acceptable functional outcome are practically negligible.

Assessment of the Vegetative State

Cecilia Koren, Mali Gil, Leon Sazbon

The successful evaluation of patients with severe brain injury who are unresponsive or minimally responsive remains one of the primary goals of professionals [205,206]. As noted by the *International Working Party Report on the Vegetative State* [141], the patients' lack of any means of communication makes it impossible for the clinician to determine the presence of an inner life (see p. 15). Therefore, the assessment has to be based on behavioral patterns. The constant fluctuation in the cognitive status over time, even from minute to minute, warrants frequent examinations, with a considerable investment of time. The report also emphasizes that the relatives, because of their high perceptiveness and receptivity to the patient's body language, play an important role in interpreting the first signs of cognitive recovery, especially in patients with severe motor limitations. However, in these cases, the physician must take the factor of "wishful thinking" into account.

The ideal assessment tool would be sufficiently sensitive to minimal subclinical changes to enable the clinician to determine not only the degree of disability, but also the possible rate of recovery, and to decrease or alter the course of the basic neurological deficit. For diagnosing the development and assessing the prognosis of the condition, the instrument must document the patient's state at each stage of the condition, highlighting behavioral deficiencies and abilities, thereby minimizing the time needed for treatment planning. The treatment course should be outlined in a user-friendly format for easy understanding by lay staff members and the patient's family. Grossman and Hagel [207] reported that "Some scales are more relevant for employment immediately or soon after injury, whereas others may be better applied to examine the long-term consequences of the brain injury. In both cases, the tests most commonly used represent compromises between reliable, comprehensive diagnostic and prognosis assessment, on the one hand, and the clinical necessity for quickly and easily administered instruments, on the other."

The *International Working Party Report on the Vegetative State* [141] divided assessments into two main types:
- Those that evaluate specific aspects of behavior according to predetermined criteria. These assessments have protocols that include the application of specific stimuli to elicit behavior.
- Techniques such as time sampling of spontaneous behavior, structured intervals with healthcare staff and/or relatives, and the ad-hoc recording of observations.

The report recommends nominal scales rather than ordinal ones. It also stresses the importance of recording accurate dates, the names of the persons providing information, clinically relevant factors, optimal channels of response for an individual patient, and reaction times.

Minimally responsive state (MRS) is a transitory or permanent stage of emergence from vegetative state. In the last two decades, professional groups worldwide have attempted to formulate a comprehensive and functional assessment tool for the evaluation and follow-up of patients in MRS. Zasler et al. [208] recommended the following scales for use in the "low-level patient with brain injury":
- The Glasgow Coma Scale (GCS) [209]
- The Rancho Los Amigos Levels of Cognitive Functioning Scale (LCFS) [210]
- The Disability Rating Scale (DRS) [211]
- The Western Neuro-Sensory Stimulation Profile (WNSSP) [212]
- The Coma/Near-Coma Scale (C/NC) [213]
- The Coma Recovery Scale (CRS) [214]
- The Sensory Stimulation Assessment Measure (SSAM) [215].

Since then, other assessments have been added, including:
- Prognostic Model of Emerging from VS [216]
- The Coma Exit Chart (CEC) [217]
- The Sensory Modality Assessment and Rehabilitation Technique (SMART) [218,219]
- The Preliminary Neuropsychological Battery (PNB) [205]
- The Loewenstein Communication Scale for the Minimally Responsive Patient (LCS)[220]

The application of so many different tools has produced an array of nonuniform data that are quite difficult to compare. Some are limited in efficacy to unconscious patients, because they consist of clinical indicators that may not retain prognostic utility beyond the acute period, such as corneal reflexes, pupillary reactivity, oculomotor responses, and spontaneous eye opening. These include the GCS, DRS, C/NC and LCFS (levels I, II). Some are insensitive to subtle neurological changes over time (WNSSP, LCFS levels II to VIII, and LCS).

This chapter will review some of these instruments.

The Glasgow Coma Scale (Table 4.8)

This GCS [209] is used worldwide and is very good for rapid, basic differentiation of coma/noncoma states and predicting survival. The GCS scores motor responsiveness, eye opening and verbal performance.

A score of 8 points or more is indicative of a noncoma state. The maximum score is 15. The GCS has proven universally useful for tracking emergence from coma, but its applicability in post-coma (MRS, VS) patients who are not yet ready for a more formal cognitive assessment is restricted by its ceiling effect [221].

The Rancho Los Amigos Levels of Cognitive Functioning Scale (Table 4.9)

The LCFS [210] measures outcome in terms of "general responsiveness" [222], and is able to distinguish among different levels of reactibility (see below), from comatose (I–II) to basic behavioral functioning (III–VIII). The scale is easy and quick to administer, but the passage between certain levels is sometimes unclear (III–VI) or crude (VII–VIII).

Table 4.8 The Glasgow Coma Scale

Eye opening	1	Nil
	2	To pain
	3	To speech
	4	Spontaneous
Verbal response	1	None
	2	Incomprehensible sounds
	3	Inappropriate words
	4	Confused conversation
	5	Oriented
Best motor response	1	None
	2	Extensor response
	3	Abnormal flexion
	4	Withdraws
	5	Localizes
	6	Obeys

Reproduced with permission from Prof. B. Jennett. Jennett B, Teasdale G, *Management of head injuries*. Philadelphia: Davis, 1981: 78.

Table 4.9 The Rancho Los Amigos Levels of Cognitive Functioning Scale

Level	Response
I	No response
II	General response
III	Localized response
IV	Confusion and restlessness
V	Confusion; inconsistent and incorrect responses
VI	Confusion; consistent, correct responses
VII	Correct automatic responses
VIII	Correct

Reproduced with permission from Dept. los Amigos Research Institute. Rancho los Amigos National Rehabilitation Center.

The Disability Rating Scale

The DRS [211] is used to identify those patients who are most likely to benefit from intensive therapy; emphasis is placed on community reentry. It covers eight dimensions of functioning: arousability; verbalization; motor responsiveness and cognitive ability for self-care activities; feeding; toileting; grooming; overall level of dependence on others and psychological adaptability; and employability. Each dimension is ranked by level of disability: 0, no gross disability; 1, mild; 2–3, partial; 4–6, moderate; 7–11, moderately severe; 12–16, severe; 17–21, extremely severe; 22–24, vegetative state; 25–29, extreme vegetative state; 30, death. Rating is based on information gathered from direct observation and personal contacts with the patient, or from interviews with the nursing staff (for feeding, toileting, grooming). Patients are evaluated at three time points over 1 year (6, 12, and 24 months). Since the feeding, toileting and grooming categories correlate very highly with the verbal category ($r = 0.90$, 0.86, and 0.89, respectively), the DRS provides a short global description that can be easily interpreted by carers. Interrater and test-retest reliability levels are good [221].

Novak et al. [206] pointed out that the "window surrounding the time intervals may be extremely large," so the information about the pace of recovery may be inconsistent.

The Western Neuro-Sensory Stimulation Profile

The WNSSP [212] was formulated to evaluate function and trace outcome in patients at higher levels of performance (II–V in the LCFS). It contains 33 items divided into six cognitive/communicative subscales: arousal/attention (wakefulness, eye contact); auditory comprehension (following one-step spoken commands); visual comprehension (following one-step written commands); visual tracking (horizontal/vertical tracking); object manipulation (use of familiar objects); and expressive communication (yes/no responses, vocal/nonvocal communication). Responses to sound, speech, smell, and touch are also examined. Scoring is based not only on the type of stimulation (general or specific), but also on the latency of the reaction and the need for cueing. Each subscale has a different score range; the auditory comprehension and visual comprehension subscales contribute almost half the points towards the total. Total scores range from 0 to 113.

The administration of the WNSSP may be slow and complicated, because the analyses of the response patterns are more sophisticated than in earlier tests.

The Coma/Near Coma Scale

The 11-item C/NC scale [213] is an extension of the DRS, described above, with a very narrow range of testing, making it sensitive to small clinical changes in patients with severe brain injuries functioning at levels characteristic of VS (i.e., DRS scores of 21–29). It scores five levels of performance for the severity of sensory, perceptual, and primitive response deficits, as follows: level 1, no coma; 2, near coma; 3, moderate coma; 4, marked coma; 5, extreme coma. (Note the wrong use of the word "coma" when evaluating VS.) There is a good correlation between the C/NC and multisensory evoked potentials [223].

The Coma Recovery Scale (Table 4.10)

The CRS [214] consists of 35 items, each of which assesses the absence or presence (scoring 0, 1) of a specific physical sign representative of the integ-

Table 4.10 The Coma Recovery Scale

Area	Items (n)	Lowest item	Highest item
Arousal and attention	6	Eyes open to pain	Attends for 15 min
Auditory	5	Blinks to noise	Replicates command
Visual	7	Blinks to threat	Tracks bilaterally without cues
Motor	7	Abnormal extension	Automatic response to familiar object or task
Oromotor	2	Spontaneous swallow	Assisted or independent feeding
Communication	6	Incomprehensible vocalization	Functional use of communication system
Initiative	2	Initiates behavior when distressed	Initiated behavior to environmental cue

Reproduced with permission from W. B. Saunders Co. Arch. Phys. Med. Rehabil 72: 897–901; 1991

rity of brain function at four levels: generalized, localized, emergent, and cognitively mediated responsiveness. The lowest ranking items within each category assess reflexive responses; the highest items, cortically based abilities. Table 4.**10** shows a sample of the items included in each area.

The approximate administration time is 30 minutes. The authors report high levels of concurrence between this scale and the GCS and DRS [214]. Interrater reliability is good. Ng et al. [224] evaluated one patient over 9 months using four measures – the GCS, Functional Independence Measure (FIM), CRS, and DRS. They found that the CRS was the one best able to detect subtle changes and fluctuations in neurobehavioral status.

The Sensory Stimulation Assessment Measure

The SSAM was formulated by Rader and Ellis [215] on the basis of their pioneering use of sensory stimulation as a treatment tool in unresponsive patients. Using a measure of responsiveness, the SSAM follows reactions to an array of stimuli in patients at different levels of MRS. Patients are reassessed at several predetermined time points in order to monitor the optimum effects of stimulatory treatment for all five senses. The instrument also takes into account the effect of family visits, prior education, age, time since injury, neurological status, amount of interpersonal contact (low/high), and the patient's position (upright/supine) during treatments.

Although no significant differences in behavioral changes were observed among the patients treated, the introduction of sensory stimulation has been followed by the development of a range of related methods for the treatment of this population [171,209,218,222,225,226]. The results are still not clear-cut, and further research is needed.

Prognostic Model of Emergence from Vegetative States

The prognostic model [216] is used with patients who have emerged from coma and are in a state of prolonged unconsciousness (at least 30 days). It provides a prognosis regarding recovery of consciousness rather than survival. Its eight easily evaluated parameters have been found to be significantly associated with failure to recover [216]. Six of them are already observable in the acute phase of coma – i. e., in the first week after trauma: fever of central origin, diffuse body sweating, disturbances in antidiuretic hormone secretion (all of these being manifestations of hypothalamic damage), failure of motor reactivity, respiratory disturbances, and multiple nonneurological injuries. The other two parameters are epilepsy and hydrocephalus, which become evident at a later phase, after 1 month. The first three parameters are all manifestations of hypothalamic damage. Studies have shown that they do not contribute significantly to the prediction of outcome, because the set of the five other factors reaches a probability level of 98 %.

The prognostic indicators and outcome were fitted to two logistic models. The first was designed to predict recovery of consciousness in the first week after onset, if the patient (still in comatose state) survived and remained in VS. This model included

Table 4.11 Model 1: estimated probabilities of the recovery of awareness for combinations of the significant early predictor variables [216]

		Extraneural trauma	
Ventilatory disturbances	Motor reactivity	Absent	Present
Absent	Decortication	0.94	0.85
	Decerebration	0.90	0.75
	Flaccidity	0.30	0.13
Present	Decortication	0.86	0.68
	Decerebration	0.72	0.53
	Flaccidity	0.14	0.06

Reproduced from *J Neurol Neurosurg Psychiatry* 1991; 54: 149–52, with permission from the BMJ Publishing Group.

Table 4.12 Model 2: estimated probabilities of recovery of awareness for combinations of significant predictor variables [216]

Hydrocephalus	Ventilatory disturbances	Motor reactivity	None	Epilepsy Early	Late
Absent	Absent	Decortication	0.93	0.86	0.78
		Decerebration	0.86	0.74	0.82
		Flaccidity	0.59	0.39	0.57
Absent	Present	Decortication	0.89	0.78	0.67
		Decerebration	0.77	0.61	0.47
		Flaccidity	0.44	0.26	0.17
Present	Absent	Decortication	0.75	0.58	0.44
		Decerebration	0.57	0.38	0.26
		Flaccidity	0.24	0.13	0.08
Present	Present	Decortication	0.63	0.44	0.31
		Decerebration	0.43	0.26	0.16
		Flaccidity	0.15	0.07	0.04

Reproduced from J *Neurol Neurosurg Psychiatry* 1991; 54: 149–52, with permission from the BMJ Publishing Group.

only three early parameters as categorical predictors. The second model evaluated higher brain function 30 days after onset, and included the two late variables (hydrocephalus status and epilepsy) in addition to the two early ones. The estimated probabilities of recovery for combinations of the significant predictor variables are shown in Tables 4.11 and 4.12.

The Coma Exit Chart

The CEC [217] is based on three sources: the medical interview, the clinical examination, and the postexamination discussion. Information obtained from the medical staff and, particularly, the patients' relatives is considered essential to the assessment, because they spend considerable time with the patient and are very familiar with his or her body language and facial expressions. The data are divided into three classes: 1, facial expressions; 2, sensory functions (visual, auditory, tactile); and 3, motor abilities (eye opening, head control, arm and hand control, leg control, vocalization). Responses are defined as "unconfirmed" if seen only once by a single person, or "confirmed" if seen by several people on different occasions. Once responses are confirmed, they are further classified as "variable" or "constant." The chart is organized in such a way as to allow several assessments over time.

Table 4.13 shows an example of the way in which information is gathered.

The results of the medical interrogation are compared with the findings by direct observation and discussed among the multidisciplinary team. All the stages assessed are presented in order and in detail. It is important to reach general agreement on observations that are seen as positive, and to leave other matters open for future clarification.

In general, the assessment is simple and enables the team to gather accurate and relevant information on the patient's conscious state. However, some caution is advised [217]. Firstly, patients may "close in" if they feel threatened in any manner, or they may have "low" days for various reasons. In these cases, the examination should be postponed. The time of day at which the assessment takes place is also important and should be noted. Secondly, there may be a lag between the presentation of the stimulus and patient's response. Physicians must be sure to take their time, and they must be

Table 4.13 The Coma Exit Chart: emotional facial expression

	Anxiety/fear	Anger	Pleasure	Sadness	Disgust	Surprise
Appropriate/constant						
Appropriate/not constant						
Inappropriate						
Nil						

Reproduced with permission from Taylor and Francis Limited http//www.tandf.co.uK. Brain Injury 10: 615–624, 1996.

gentle for the assessment to be correct. The patient should always be warned before being touched. Third, the relatives may feel that their findings are not been taken seriously, and they may become reluctant to provide information, or even hostile. Physicians and members of the staff must demonstrate an open and receptive approach.

The Sensory Modality Assessment and Rehabilitation Technique

The SMART [218,219] was developed as a quantitative scientific and methodological tool for the incontrovertible diagnosis of the vegetative patient. It is an expanded form of Freeman's Coma Exit Chart [217], assessing function on the basis of a hierarchical categorization derived from the parameters of the GCS and expanded to include all behavioral responses observed during sensory stimulation. The tool includes seven subscales: responses to visual, tactile, auditory, olfactory and gustatory stimuli, level of wakefulness, and functional motor and communicative abilities. The response to each modality is ranked on a five-point scale: 1, no response; 2, reflexive response; 3, withdrawal response; 4, localization response; 5, differentiating response. Scores from sensory modality components can be converted to levels on the LCFS. [210]

The SMART also provides qualitative information that is comparable across sensory modalities and can identify evidence of awareness.

The SMART may provide a good indication of the patient's best functional response, as it does not rely only on the patient's physical ability to respond to stimuli. Patients need to demonstrate only one consistent response in order to receive the maximum score of 60. The scale is also more sensitive than the WNSSP in detecting cognitive functions [227]. It can apparently also identify the initial point of awareness and subtle shifts in function. The only limitation of the SMART is that it is a therapeutic tool designed for patient follow-up and therefore cannot be administered at the bedside.

The Preliminary Neuropsychological Battery

The PNB [205] is a psychometric tool for the cognitive evaluation of patients who are unable to give verbal or complex motor answers. It uses a set of nonsymbolic (section 1) and symbolic (section 2) verification tasks, divided into five stages each. The nonsymbolic section tests comparisons of size, shape, number of spots, color and quasi-lateral shapes. The symbolic section tests the correspondence of capital/small letters, drawings/words, colors/names of colors, and digits/names of digits, and judgment of the correctness of calculations. The PNB is short, reliable, easy to administer, and suitable for patients with severe motor and/or speech restrictions; it also seems to be very sensitive to the identification of attentional deficits [205]. However, it does not sufficiently differentiate between different types of cognitive impairment. Furthermore, the presence of certain language deficits (e.g., aphasia) could impair the patient's performance, especially on the symbolic part of the test.

Loewenstein Communication Scale for the Minimally Responsive Patient (Table 4.14)

A review of the different evaluation tools developed worldwide reveals that they all test the same areas of minimal function and regaining of consciousness. As these areas are not yet well defined, the use of "wide-ranging" assessments tends to yield unclear results.

Table 4.14 Loewenstein Communication Scale for the minimally responsive patient

Motility	• Responsiveness
	• Head/eye control
	• Extremity control
	• Speech/swallowing mechanisms
	• Mimicry
Respiration	• Assisted respiration
	• Spontaneous respiration
	• Respiration for voice production
	• Respiration for speech production
	• Coordination for speech
Visual responsiveness	• Gaze
	• Blink reflex
	• Environmental stimulation
	• Tracking
	• Matching tasks
Auditory comprehension	• Response to noise
	• Response to voice
	• One-step commands
	• Object recognition
	• Two-step commands
Communication	
Verbal	• Use of speech articulators
	• Basic speech
	• Articulation
	• Rhythm/fluency
	• Message quality
Alternative	• Need for outside assistance
	• Use of body parts
	• Initiative
	• Speed
	• Message quality

Reproduced with permission from Taylor & Francis Limited, http//www.tandf.co.uK. In press with Brain Injury, 2002.

Reflexes of cortical liberation are generally accepted as expressions of the earliest stages of ontogenetic development or phylogenetic regression. In all vertebrate embryos, the perioral area is the first to respond to exteroceptive stimuli. The same type of reflex activity can also be seen in patients in VS, and in elderly people and patients with presenile dementia due to bilateral, diffuse and severe central nervous system lesions. This anatomic area is also directly related to the development of acquired, cognitive, swallow, and speech functions. Thus, the study of the development of this specific neuroanatomic system may throw light on the rate of improvement in VS patients, and may even be of prognostic value [228].

The recently developed LCS [220] consists of five hierarchical functions, as shown in the table, divided into five parameters and rated in developmental order on a five-point scale by level of difficulty: 0, nonfunctional response; 1, minimally functional; 2, partly functional; 3, usually functional; 4, functional. The maximum score for each function is 20; the maximum score for the total quantitative communication profile is 100. A total score of at least 50 successfully distinguishes VS patients who have the potential for further treatment; it is therefore predictive of communication (cognitive ability) [211].

This scale has the advantage over other assessment scales of evaluating both oral and alternative communication possibilities. It can be easily and quickly administered even by untrained professionals, and interrater agreement is good. The tool can assist clinicians in formulating targeted treatment plans and provides good back-up information for patients' families.

As a final note, it should be emphasized that the function and rehabilitation potential of patients who have advanced from the minimally responsive or vegetative state should be evaluated with different tools from the ones presented here. These are beyond the scope of this book.

References

1. Kaufman HH, Timberlake G, Voelker J, et al. Medical complications of head injury. Contemporary Clin Neurol 1993; 77: 43–60.
2. Sazbon L, Groswasser Z. Medical complications and mortality of patients in the postcomatose unawareness (PC-U) state. Acta Neurochirur 1991; 112: 110–2.

3. Kaliski Z, Morrison DP, Meyers CA, et al. Medical problems encountered during rehabilitation of patients with head injury. Arch Phys Med Rehabil 1985; 66: 25–9.
4. Sazbon L, Groswasser Z. Outcome in 134 patients with prolonged post-traumatic unawareness, 1: parameters determining late recovery of consciousness. J Neurosurg 1990; 72: 75–80.
5. Sazbon L. Prolonged coma. Prog Clin Neurosci 1985; 2: 65–81.
6. Kirland LL, Wilson GL. Extracranial effects of acute brain injury. Prob Crit Care 1991; 5: 292–306.
7. Plum F, Posner JB. Diagnosis of stupor and coma, 3rd ed. Philadelphia: Davis, 1982.
8. Gildenberg PL, Frost EAM. Respiratory care in head trauma. In: Becker DP, Povlishock JT, editors. Central nervous system trauma: status report. Bethesda, MD: National Institutes of Health, 1985: 161–176.
9. Frost EA. Effects of positive end-expiratory pressure on intracranial pressure in brain-injured patients. J Neurosurg 1979; 50: 768–72.
10. Eisenberg HM, Levin HS. Outcome after head injury: general considerations and neurobehavioral recovery. In: Becker DP, Povlishock JT, editors. Central nervous system trauma: status report. Bethesda, MD: National Institutes of Health, 1985: 271–302.
11. Najenson T, Sazbon L, Fiselzon J, et al. Recovery of communicative functions after prolonged traumatic coma. Scand J Rehabil Med 1978; 10: 15–21.
12. Becker E, Sazbon L, Najenson T. Gastrointestinal hemorrhage in long lasting traumatic coma. Scand J Rehabil Med 1978; 10: 23–6.
13. Krimchansky B, Sazbon L, Heller L, et al. Bladder tone in patients in post-traumatic vegetative state. Brain Inj 1999; 13: 899–903.
14. Coleman Gross J. Bladder dysfunction after stroke. Urol Nursing 1992; 12: 55–63.
15. Abramson AS, Roussan M, Feibel A. Pathophysiology of the neurogenic bladder. Bull NY Acad Med 1983; 19: 775–85.
16. Sazbon L. Prolonged coma. Prog Clin Neurosci 1985; 2: 65–81.
17. Monath C, Weil JP, Sibilly A, et al. Fibrogastroscopie gastrique systématique chez les traumatisés craniens graves. Semin Hosp Paris 1975; 51: 1281–4.
18. Sazbon L. [Personal communication.]
19. Aiges HW, Daum F, Olson M, et al. Effects of phenobarbital and diphenylhydantoin on liver function and morphology. J Pediatr 1980; 97: 22–6.
20. Mayer N. Functional management of spasticity after head injury. J Neurol Rehabil 1991; 5: S1–S4.
21. Awaad Y. Spasticity. In: Gilman S, editor. Neurobase on CD. 4th ed. San Diego, CA: Arbor, 1998.
22. Higashi H, Sakata Y, Hatano M, et al. Epidemiological studies on patients with a persistent vegetative state. J Neurol Neurosurg Psychiatry 1977; 40: 876–85.
23. Filloux FM. Neuropathophysiology of movement disorders in cerebral palsy. J Child Neurol 1996; 11 (Suppl 1): S5–12.
24. Young RR. Spasticity: a review. Neurology 1994; 44 (Suppl 9): S12–20.
25. Jennett B, Teasdale G. Management of head injuries. Philadelphia: Davis, 1981.
26. Bricolo A. Prolonged post-traumatic coma. In: Vinken P, Bruyn GW, editors. Handbook of clinical neurology. Amsterdam: North-Holland, 1976: 699–755.
27. Graham DI, Adams JH, Genarelli T. Pathology of brain damage in head injury. In: Cooper PR, editor. Head injury. Baltimore: William & Wilkins, 1993: 91–114.
28. Feldman S. Prolonged coma: outcome and prognosis. Unpublished monograph, Tel Aviv University, Israel, 1985.
29. Mielants H, Vanhove E, de Neels J, et al. Clinical survey of and pathogenic approach to para-articular ossification in long-term coma. Acta Orthop Scand 1975; 46: 196–8.
30. Sazbon L, Najenson T, Tartakovsky M, Becker E, Grosswasser Z. Widespread periarticular new-bone formation in long-term comatose patients. J Bone Joint Surg Br 1981; 63-B(1): 120–5.
31. Melamed E, Keren O, Robinson D, et al. Extraskeletal new bone formation after brain injury. Harefuah 2000; 139: 368–71.
32. Garland DE, Blum CE, Waters RL, et al. Periarticular ectopic ossification in head-injured adults. J Bone Joint Surg 1980; 62A: 1143–6.
33. Garland DE. A clinical perspective of common forms of acquired heterotopic ossification. Clin Orthop Rel Res 1991; 263: 13–27.
34. Mendelson L, Groswasser Z, Najenson T, et al. Periarticular new bone formation in patients suffering from severe head injuries. Scand J Rehabil Med 1975; 7: 141–5.
35. Sazbon L, Groswasser Z. Heterotopic bone formation involving wrist and fingers in brain-injured patients: a report of three cases. Brain Inj 1989; 3: 57–61.
36. Groswasser Z, Reider-Groswasser I. Heterotopic new bone formation in the cervical spine following head injury. J Neurosurg 1986; 64: 513–5.
37. Heindl UT, Laub MC. Outcome of persistent vegetative state following hypoxic or traumatic brain injury in children and adolescents. Neuropediatrics 1996; 27: 94–100.

38. Sazbon L, Sack J, Najenson T. Growth hormone and periarticular new bone formation: a causal relationship? Scand J Rehabil Med 1982; 15: 43-6.
39. Hauser WA, Rich SS, Annegers JF, et al. Seizure recurrence after a first unprovoked seizure: an extended follow-up. Neurology 1990; 40: 1163-70.
40. Scheuer ML, Pedley TA. The evaluation and treatment of seizures. N Engl J Med 1990; 323: 1468-74.
41. Yablon SA. Post-traumatic seizures. Arch Phys Med Rehabil 1993; 74: 983-1001.
42. Black P, Sheppard RH, Walker AE. Outcome of head trauma: age and post-traumatic seizures. In: Outcome of severe damage to the central nervous system, Symposium 34. Amsterdam: Ciba Elsevier, 1975: 215-77.
43. Bricolo A, Turazzi S, Feriotti G. Prolonged post-traumatic unconsciousness. J Neurosurg 1980; 52: 625-34.
44. Mahoney WJ, D'Souza BJ, Haller JA, et al. Long-term outcome in children with severe head trauma and prolonged coma. Pediatrics 1983; 71: 756-62.
45. Snyder BD, Hauser WA, Loewenson RB, et al. Neurologic prognosis after cardiopulmonary arrest, 3: seizure activity. Neurology 1980; 30: 1292-7.
46. Annegers JF, Grabow JD, Groover RV, et al. Seizures after head trauma: a population study. Neurology 1980; 30: 683-9.
47. Salazar AM, Jabbari B, Vance SC, et al. Epilepsy after penetrating head injury, 1: clinical correlates. Neurology 1985; 35: 1406-14.
48. Ascroft PB. Traumatic epilepsy after gunshot wounds of the head. Br Med J 1941; 1: 739-44.
49. Phillips G. Traumatic epilepsy after closed head injury. J Neurol Neurochir Psychiatry 1954; 17: 1-10.
50. Walker AE, Erculei F. Post-traumatic epilepsy 15 years later. Epilepsia 1970; 11: 17-26.
51. Jennett B. Epilepsy after non-missile head injury. Chicago: Heineman, 1975.
52. Neufeld M, Korczyn A. Post-traumatic epilepsy. Harefuah 1986; 110: 353-5.
53. Caveness WF, Liss HR. Incidence of post-traumatic epilepsy. Epilepsia 1961; 2: 123-9.
54. Wilberger JE. Emergency care and initial evaluation. In: Cooper PR, editor. Head injury. Baltimore: William & Wilkins, 1993: 27-42.
55. Jennett B, Miller JD, Braakman R. Epilepsy after nonmissile depressed fracture. J Neurosurg 1974; 41: 208-16.
56. Caveness WF, Meirowsky AM, Rish BL, et al. The nature of post-traumatic epilepsy. J Neurosurg 1979; 50: 545-53.
57. Edwards RH, Simon RP. Coma. In: Joynt RB, editor. Clinical neurology, vol 2. Philadelphia: Lippincott, 1989: 1-51.
58. Johnston B, Sheshia SS. Prediction of outcome in nontraumatic coma in childhood. Acta Neurol Scand 1984; 69: 417-27.
59. Young GB, Gilbert JJ, Zochodne DW. The significance of myoclonic status epilepticus in postanoxic coma. Neurology 1990; 40: 1843-8.
60. Tuchman RF, Alvarez LA, Kantrowitz AB, et al. Opsoclonus–myoclonus syndrome: correlation of radiographic and pathological observations. Neuroradiology 1989; 31: 250-2.
61. Lapresle J. Rhythmic palatal myoclonus and the dentate–olivary pathway. J Neurol 1979; 220: 223-30.
62. Shuttleworth EC, Voto S, Sahar D. Palatal myoclonus in Behçet's disease. Arch Intern Med 1985; 145: 949-50.
63. Van Cot AC, Blatt I, Brenner R. Stimulus-sensitive seizures in postanoxic coma. Epilepsia 1996; 37: 868- 74.
64. Gotthard T, Oder W. Outcome after shunt implantation in severe head injury with post-traumatic hydrocephalus. Brain Inj 2000; 14: 345-54.
65. Bontke CF, Zasler ND, Boake C. Rehabilitation of the head-injured patient. In: Narayan RK, Wilberger JE, Povlishock JT, editors. Neurotrauma. New York: McGraw-Hill, 1996: 841-58.
66. Gudeman KS, Kishore PR, Becker DP. Computed tomography in the evaluation of incidence and significance of post-traumatic hydrocephalus. Radiology 1981; 141: 397-402.
67. Herrmann HD. Neurotraumatologie. Weinheim, Germany: Medizin VCH, 1991: 185-6.
68. Kishore PR, Lipper MH, Miller JD. Post-traumatic hydrocephalus in patients with severe head injury. Neuroradiology 1978; 16: 261-5.
69. Kampfl A, Franz G, Aichner F, et al. The persistent vegetative state after closed head injury: clinical and magnetic resonance imaging findings in 42 patients. J Neurosurg 1989; 88: 809-16.
70. Guyot LL, Michael DB. Post-traumatic hydrocephalus. Neurol Res 2000; 22: 25-8.
71. Najenson T, Sazbon L, Mainz T, et al. Rehabilitation of the long lasting comatose traumatic brain injured patients. Proceedings of the first Convegno Internazionale Associazione Rihabilitazione Comatosi. Milan. 1983; 109-24.
72. Sazbon L, Becker E, Costeff H, et al. Développement fétale normale chez une femme en coma traumatique prolongé. J Readap Med 1984; 4: 133-5.
73. Binder H, Getstenbrand F. Post-traumatic vegetative syndrome. In: Vinken P, Bruyn GW,

editors. Handbook of clinical neurology. Amsterdam: North-Holland, 1976: 575–98.
74. Gadisseau PH. Nutrition and CNS trauma. In: Becker DP, Povlishock JT, editors. Central nervous system trauma: status report. Bethesda, MD: National Institutes of Health, 1985; 207–16.
75. Turner WW. Nutritional considerations in the patient with disabling brain disease. Neurosurgery 1985; 16: 707–13.
76. Arieff AI. Hyponatremia, convulsions, respiratory arrest, and permanent brain damage after elective surgery in healthy women. N Engl J Med 1986; 314: 1529–35.
77. Sterns RH, Riggs JE, Schoshet SSJ. Osmotic demyelination syndrome following correction of hyponatremia. N Engl J Med 1986; 314: 1535–42.
78. Braunwald R, Iselbachern KJ, Petersdorf RG, Wilson JD, Martin JB, Fauci AS, editors. Harrison's principles of internal medicine. 11th ed., vol 2. New York: McGraw-Hill, 1987.
79. Doczi T, Tarjanyi J, Huszka E, et al. Syndrome of inappropriate secretion of antidiuretic hormone after subarachnoid hemorrhage. Neurosurgery 1981; 10: 685–8.
80. Berkow R, Fletcher AJ, editors. The Merck manual of diagnosis and therapy. Rahway, NJ: Merck Sharp & Dohme Research Laboratories, 1987.
81. Chesnut RM, Marshall LF, Bower Marshall S. Medical complications of the head injured patient. In: Cooper PR, editor. Head injury. Baltimore: William & Wilkins, 1993: 225–246.
82. Sazbon L. [Personal communication.]
83. Clark JA, Finelli RE, Netsky MG. Disseminated intravascular coagulation following cranial trauma. J Neurosurg 1980; 52: 266–9.
84. Auer L. Disturbances of the coagulatory system in patients with severe cerebral trauma, 1. Acta Neurochir 1978; 43: 51–9.
85. Auer LM, Ott E. Disturbances of the coagulatory system in patients with severe cerebral trauma, 2. Acta Neurochir 1979; 49: 219–26.
86. Kaufman HH, Mattson JC. Coagulopathy in head injury. In: Becker DP, Povlishock JT, editors. Central nervous system trauma: status report. Bethesda, MD: National Institutes of Health, 1985: 187–206.
87. Barmada MA, Moossy J, Shuman RM. Cerebral infarcts with arterial occlusion in neonates. Ann Neurol 1979; 6: 495–502.
88. Crompton MR. Hypothalamic and pituitary lesions. In: Vinken PJ, Bruyn GW, editors. Handbook of clinical neurology, Vol. 23. Amsterdam: North-Holland, 1975: 465–470.
89. Klingbeil GE, Cline P. Anterior hypopituitarism: a consequence of head injury. Arch Phys Med Rehabil 1985; 66: 44–6.
90. Altman R, Pruzanski W. Post-traumatic hypopituitarism: anterior pituitary insufficiency following skull fracture. Ann Intern Med 1961; 55: 149–54.
91. Escamilla RF, Lisser H. Simmond's disease (hypophyseal cachexia). J Clin Endocrinol 1942; 2: 65–96.
92. Jambart S, Turpin G, De Genes JL. Panhypopituitarism secondary to head trauma; evidence for hypothalamic origin of deficit. Acta Endocrinol 1980; 93: 264–70.
93. Jambart S, Turpin G, De Genes JL. Acquired post-traumatic and idiopathic hypothalamic panhypopituitarism. Nouv Presse Médicale 1981; 70: 975–8.
94. Kornblum RN, Fischer RS. Pituitary lesions in craniocerebral injuries. Arch Pathol 1969; 88: 242–8.
95. Miller WL, Kaplan SL, Grumbach MM. Child abuse as a cause of post-traumatic hypopituitarism. N Engl J Med 1980; 302: 724–8.
96. Sheehan HL. Post-partum necrosis of the anterior pituitary. J Pathol Bact 1937; 45: 189–214.
97. Simmonds M. Über embolische Prozesse in der Hypophysis. Virchow's Arch 1914; 217: 226–39.
98. Rudman D, Fleischer AS, Kutner MH, et al. Suprahypophyseal hypogonadism and hypothyroidism during prolonged coma after head injury. J Clin Endocrinol Metab 1977; 45: 747–54.
99. Sack J, Sazbon L, Lunenfeld B, et al. Hypothalamic pituitary functions in patients with prolonged coma. J Clin Endocrinol Metab 1983; 56: 635–8.
100. Valenta LJ, De Feo DR. Post-traumatic hypopituitarism due to hypothalamic lesion. Ann J Med 1980; 68: 614–7.
101. Sack J, Sazbon L, Melamed S, et al. Low serum T3 and rT3 concentrations in patients with prolonged coma. Isr J Med Sci 1980; 16: 402–3.
102. Bakay RAE, Wood JH. Pathophysiology of cerebrospinal fluid in trauma. In: Becker DP, Povlishock TT, editors. Central nervous system trauma: status report. Bethesda, MD: National Institutes of Health, 1985: 89–122.
103. Daniel PM, Treip CS. Quoted in Crompton MR. Hypothalamic and pituitary lesions. In: Vinken PJ, Bruyn GW, editors. Handbook of clinical neurology, Vol. 23. Amsterdam: North-Holland, 1975: 465–470.
104. Porter RJ, Miller RA. Diabetes insipidus following closed head injury. J Neurol Neurosurg Psychiatry 1948; 11: 258–62.
105. Halimi PH, Sigal R, Doyon D, et al. Post-traumtic diabetes insipidus: MR demonstration of pituitary stalk rupture. J Comput Assist Tomogr 1988; 12: 135–7.

106. Wollaj B, Sazbon L, Gavrieli R, et al. Some aspects of the humoral and neutrophil functions in post-comatose unawareness patients. Brain Inj 1993; 7: 401–10.
107. Wollaj B, Coates TD, Hugli TI. Plasma lactoferrin reflects granulocyte activation via complement in burn patients. J Lab Clin Med 1984; 103: 284–93.
108. Donovan AJ. The effect of surgery on reticuloendothelial system. Arch Surg 1967; 94: 247–50.
109. Hoyt DB, Oskan AN, Hansbrough JF, et al. Head injury: an immunologic deficit in T-cell activation. J Trauma 1990; 30: 759–66.
110. Tresch DD, Sims FH, Duthie EH, et al. Clinical characteristics of patients in the persistent vegetative state. Arch Intern Med 1991; 151: 930–2.
111. Landesman S, Cooper PR. Infectious complications of head injury. In: Cooper PR, editor. Head injury. Baltimore: William & Wilkins, 1993: 503–524.
112. Sazbon L. [Personal communication.]
113. Kaufman HH, Satterwhite T, McConnell BJ, et al. Deep vein thrombosis and pulmonary embolism in head injured patients. Angiology 1983; 34: 627–38.
114. Anon. Prevention of venous thrombosis and pulmonary embolism: NIH consensus development. JAMA 1986; 256: 744–9.
115. Geerts W, Code K, Jay R, et al. Prospective study of venous thromboembolism after major trauma. N Engl J Med 1994; 331: 1601–4.
116. Warner WA. Release of free fatty acid following trauma. J Trauma 1969; 9: 692–9.
117. Attar S, Boyd D, Layhe D, et al. Alterations in coagulation and fibrinolytic mechanisms in acute trauma. J Trauma 1969; 9: 939–65.
118. Clinchot DM, Otis S, Colachis SC. Incidence of fever in the rehabilitation phase following brain injury. Am J Phys Med Rehabil 1997; 76: 323–7.
119. Childers MK, Rupright J, Smith DW. Post-traumatic hypernatermia in acute brain injury rehabilitation. Brain Inj 1996; 8: 335–43.
120. Lance JW, Drummond PD, Gandevia SC, et al. Harlequin syndrome: the sudden onset of unilateral flushing and sweating. J Neurol Neurosurg Psychiatry 1988; 51: 635–42.
121. Morrison DA, Bibby K, Woodruff G. The "harlequin" sign and congenital Horner's syndrome. J Neurol Neurosurg Psychiatry 1997; 61: 626–8.
122. Milano M, Leto C. The dysautonomic syndrome. Poster. 4th Congress of Brain Injury, Turin, Italy, September 2001.
123. Baguley IJ, Nicholls JI, Feldminham KL, et al. Dysautonomia after traumatic brain injury: a forgotten syndrome. J Neurol Neurosurg Psychiatry 1999; 67: 39–43.
124. Beringer PM, Middleton RK. Anaphylaxis and drug allergies. In: Young LY, Koda-Kimble MA, editors. Applied therapeutics: the clinical use of drugs. Vancouver: Applied Therapeutics, 1995: 1–21.
125. Gerstenbrand F. Das traumatische apallische Syndrom. Heidelberg: Springer, 1967.
126. Bricolo A, Dolce G. Evoluzioni cliniche del coma posttraumatico grave. Minerva Neurochir 1969; 13: 61–8.
127. Bricolo A. Decerebrate rigidity in acure head injury. J Neurosurg 1977; 47: 680–98.
128. Bricolo A. Prolonged post-traumatic coma. In: Vinken PJ, Bruyn GW, editors. Handbook of clinical neurology. Vol. 24, Amsterdam: North-Holland, 1975: 699–755.
129. Bottinelli MD, Bogarz J. Estupor hypertonico posttraumatico. Acta Neurol Latinoam 1962; 8: 102–20.
130. Adams RD. Tremor, chorea, athetosis, ataxia, and other abnormalities of movement and posture. In: Thorn GW, Adams RD, Braunwald R, Iselbachern KJ, Petersdorf RG, editors. Harrison's Principles of Internal Medicine, 8th ed. Tokyo: McGraw-Hill Kogakusha, 1980: 87–93.
131. Multi-Society Task Force on PVS. Medical aspects of the persistent vegetative state, 1. N Engl J Med 1994: 330: 1499–508.
132. Jennett B, Plum F. Vegetative state after brain damage: a syndrome in search of a name. Lancet 1972; i : 734–7.
133. Cohadon F, Richer E. Etats végétatives posttraumatique. Neurochirurgia 1993; 12: 269–80.
134. Bates D, Caronna JJ, Cartlidge NE, et al. A prospective study of nontraumatic coma: methods and results in 310 patients. Ann Neurol 1977; 2: 211–20.
135. Singh BM, Strobos RJ. Retraction nystagmus elicited by bilateral simultaneous cold caloric stimulation. Ann Neurol 1980; 8: 79.
136. Chusid JG. Reflexes. In: Chusid JG. Correlative neuroanatomy and functional neurology. Los Altos, CA: Lange, 1976: 206–210.
137. Chusid JG. Reflexes. In: Chusid JG. Correlative neuroanatomy and functional neurology. Los Altos, CA: Lange, 1976: 206–210.
138. Plum F, Posner JB. Occular Movements. In: Plum F, editor. Diagnosis of stupor and coma. 3rd ed. Philadelphia: Davis, 1980: 47–53.
139. Cohadon F. Phase d'éveil et de reprise de conscience. In: Cohadon F, editor. Le traumatisé cranien. Paris: Arnette, 1998: 205–7.
140. Cohadon F. Sortir du coma. Paris: Jacob, 2000.
141. Andrews K, Beaumont JG, Danze F, et al. International Working Party report on the vegetative state. London: Royal Hospital for Neurodisability, 1996 (http://www.comarecovery.org/pvs.htm).

142. Quintieri M, Serra S, Pileggi A, Dolce G. The neurological test and outcome of patients in a post traumatic vegetative state [abstract]. In: Abstracts of Fourth World Congress on Brain Injury, Turin, Italy, 4–9 May 2001. Alexandria, VA: International Brain Injury Assocation, 2001: 382.
143. Andrews K. The vegetative state: clinical diagnosis. Postgrad Med J 1999; 75: 321–4.
144. Andrews K, Murphy L, Munday R, et al. Misdiagnosis of the vegetative state: retrospective study in a rehabilitation unit. Br Med J 1996; 313: 5–6.
145. Childs NL, Mercer WN, Childs HW. Accuracy of diagnosis of persistent vegetative state. Neurology 1993, 43: 1465–7.
146. Weber JR, Einhäupl KM. Neurologische Defektsyndrome. In: Stöhr M, Brand T, Einhäupl KM, editors. Neurologische Syndrome in der Intensivmedizin. 2nd ed. Stuttgart: Kohlhammer, 1998: 111–9.
147. Zeman A. Consciousness. Brain 2001; 124: 1263–89.
148. Firsching R. Moral dilemmas of tetraplegia: the locked-in syndrome, the persistent vegetative state and brain death. Spinal Cord 1998; 36: 741–3.
149. Santosh C. Locked-in syndrome. J Neurol Neurosurg Psychiatry 2001; 71 (Suppl 1): 12.
150. Virgile RS. Locked-in syndrome: case and literature review. Clin Neurol Neurosurg 1984; 86: 275–9.
151. Hirabayashi H. Pontine bleeding showing locked-in syndrome over 5 years. No To Shinkei 1988; 50: 476–7.
152. Odabasi Z, Kutukcu Y, Gokcil Z, et al. Traumatic basilar artery dissection causing locked-in syndrome. Minim Invasive Neurosurg 1988; 41: 46–8.
153. Pirzada NA, Ali II. Central pontine myelinolysis. Mayo Clin Proc 2001; 76: 559–62.
154. Cincotta M, Tozzi F, Zaccara G, et al. Motor imagery in a locked-in patients: evidence from transcranial magnetic stimulation. Ital J Neurol Sci 1999; 20: 37–41.
155. Haig AJ, Katz RT, Sahgal V. Mortality and complications of the locked-in syndrome. Arch Phys Med Rehabil 1987; 68: 24–7.
156. Katz RT, Haig AJ, Clark BB, et al. Long-term survival, prognosis, and life-care planning for 29 patients with chronic locked-in syndrome. Arch Phys Med Rehabil 1992; 73: 403–8.
157. Ackermann H, Ziegler W. Akinetischer Mutismus. Literatur-Übersicht. Fortschr Neurol Psychiatr 1995; 63: 59–67.
158. Altshuler L, Cummings J, Mills M. Mutism: review, differential diagnosis, and report of 22 cases. Am J Psychiatry 1986; 143: 1409–14.
159. Minagar A, David NJ. Bilateral infarction in the territory of the anterior cerebral artery. Neurology 1999; 52: 886–8.
160. Nemeth G, Hegedus K, Molnar L. Akinetic mutism associated with bicingular lesions: clinicopathological and functional anatomical correlates. Eur Arch Psychiatry Neurol Sci 1988; 237: 218–22.
161. Aidi S, Elalaoui-Faris M, Benabdeljlil M, et al. Akinetic mutism and progressive supranuclear palsy-like syndrome after the shunt of an obstructive hydrocephalus: successful treatment with bromocriptine: 2 cases. Rev Neurol 2000; 156: 380–3.
162. Cairns H, Oldfield RC, Pennybacks JS. Akinetic mutism with an epidermoid cyst of the third ventricle. Brain 1941; 64: 273–290.
163. Messert B, Henke TK, Langheim W. Syndrome of akinetic mutism associated with obstructive hydrocephalus. Neurology 1966; 16: 635–49.
164. Nicolai J, van Putten MJ, Tavy DL. BIPLEDs in akinetic mutism caused by bilateral anterior cerebral artery infarction. Clin Neurophysiol 2001; 112: 1726–8.
165. Oomman A, Madhusudhanan M. A case of unpaired anterior cerebral artery occlusion producing akinetic mutism. Neurol India 1999; 47: 157–8.
166. Bassetti C, Mathis J, Gugger M, et al. Hypersomnia following paramedian thalamic stroke: a report of 12 patients. Ann Neurol 1996; 39: 471–80.
167. Biller J, Sand J, Corbet J, et al. Syndrome of the paramedian thalamic arteries: clinical and neuroimaging correlation. J Clin Neuroopthalmol 1985; 5: 217–23.
168. Dromerick AW, Meschia JF, Kumar A, et al. Simultaneous bilateral thalamic hemorrhages following the administration of intravenous tissue plasminogen activator. Arch Phys Med Rehabil 1997; 78: 92–4.
169. Krolak-Salmon P, Croisile B, Houzard C, et al. Total recovery after bilateral paramedian thalamic infarct. Eur Neurol 2000; 44: 216–8.
170. Leathem JM, Martin GT. Cognitive deficits due to asymmetrical bilateral lesions. Brain Inj 2001; 15: 455–62.
171. Giacino JT, Zasler ND. Outcome after severe traumatic brain injury: coma, vegetative state and the minimally responsive state. J Head Trauma Rehabil 1995; 10: 40–56.
172. Jennett B, Teasdale G, Braakman R, et al. Predicting outcome in individual patients after severe head injury. Lancet 1976; i: 1031–4.
173. Sazbon L, Groswasser Z. Medical complications and mortality of patients in the postcomatose unawareness (PC-U) state. Acta Neurochir 1991; 112: 110–2.

174. The Multi-Society Task Force on PVS. Medical aspects of the persistent vegetative state, 2. N Engl J Med 1994; 330: 1572–9.
175. Braakman R, Jennett B, Minderhoud M. Prognosis of the post-traumatic vegetative state. Acta Neurochir 1988; 95: 49–52.
176. Minderhoud JM, Braackman R. Het vegeterende bestaan. Ned Tijdschr Geneeskd 1985; 129: 2385–8.
177. Strauss DJ, Shavelle RM, Ashwal S. Life expectancy and median survival time in the permanent vegetative state. Pediatr Neurol 1999; 21: 626–31.
178. Higashi H, Hatano M, Abiko S, et al. Five-year follow-up study of patients with persistent vegetative state. J Neurol Neurosurg Psychiatry 1981; 44: 552–4.
179. Rosin AJ. Very prolonged unresponsive state following brain injury. Scand J Rehabil Med 1978; 10: 33–8.
180. Ashwal S, Bale JF, Coulter DL et al. The persistent vegetative state in children: report of the Child Neurology Society Ethics Committee. Ann Neurol 1992; 32: 570–6.
181. Eyman RK, Strauss DJ, Grossman HJ. Survival of children with severe development disability. In: Rosenbloom L, editor. Baillière's Clinical Pediatrics. Diagnosis and Management of neurological disabilities in childhood. London: Baillière Tindall, 1996; 543–56.
182. Sazbon L, Zagreba F, Ronen J, et al. Course and outcome of patients in vegetative state of nontraumatic aetiology. J Neurol Neurosurg Psychiatry 1993; 56: 407–9.
183. Sacco RL, Van Gool R, Mohr JP, et al. Nontraumatic coma: Glasgow Coma Scale and coma etiology as predictors of two week outcome. Arch Neurol 1990; 47: 1181–4.
184. Shats V, Kozakov S, Sazbon L. Vegetative state (postcoma unawareness): a review. J Irish Coll Phys Surg 1996; 24: 87–90.
185. Kallert TW. Das "Apallischen syndrom." Zu Notwendigkeit und Konsequenzen einer Begriffserklärung. Fortschr Neurol Psychiatr 1994; 62: 241–55.
186. Sazbon L, Costeff H, Groswasser Z. Epidemiological findings in traumatic post-comatose unawareness. Brain Inj 1992; 6: 359–62.
187. Levin HS, Saydjari C, Eisenberg HM, et al. Vegetative state after closed-head injury: a Traumatic Coma Data Bank report. Arch Neurol 1991; 46: 580–5.
188. Kriel RL, Krach LE, Jones-Saete C. Outcome of children with prolonged unconsciousness and vegetative states. Pediatr Neurol 1993; 9: 362–8.
189. Johnston RB, Mellits DE. Pediatric coma: prognosis and outcome. Dev Med Child Neurol 1980; 22: 3–12.
190. Bruce DA, Schut L, Bruno L, et al. Outcome following severe head injuries in children. J Neurosurg 1978; 48: 679–88.
191. Ashwal S. The persistent vegetative state in children. Adv Pediatr 1994; 41: 195–209.
192. Council on Scientific Affairs and Council on Ethical and Judicial Affairs. Persistent vegetative state and the decision to withdraw or withhold life support. JAMA 1990; 263: 426–30.
193. Lang DA, Teasdale GM, MacPherson P, et al. Diffuse brain swelling after head injury: more often malignant in adults than children? J Neurosurg 1994; 80: 675–80.
194. Jennett B. Head injuries in children. Dev Med Child Neurol 1972; 14: 137–46.
195. Groswasser Z, Sazbon L. Outcome of 134 patients with prolonged post-traumatic unawareness, 2: functional outcome of 72 patients recovering consciousness. J Neurosurg 1990; 72: 81–4.
196. Childs NL, Mercer WN. Brief report: late improvement in consciousness after post-traumatic vegetative state. N Engl J Med 1996; 334: 24–5.
197. Arts WFM, Van Dongen HR, Van Hof-Van Duin J, et al. Unexpected improvement after prolonged post-traumatic vegetative state. J Neurol Neurosurg Psychiatry 1985; 48: 1300–3.
198. Rosenberg GA, Johnson SF, Brenner RP. Recovery of cognition after prolonged vegetative state. Ann Neurol 1977; 2: 167–8.
199. Snyder BD, Cranford RE, Rubens AB, et al. Delayed recovery from post anoxic persistent vegetative state [abstract]. Ann Neurol 1983; 14: 152.
200. Tanhehco J, Kaplan PE. Physical and surgical examination of patient after 6-year coma. Arch Phys Med Rehabil 1982; 63: 36–7.
201. Levin HS. Outcome after head injury, 2: neurobehavioural recovery. In: Becker DP, Povlishock JT, editors. Central system nervous trauma: status report. Bethesda, MD: National Institutes of Health, 1985: 281–302.
202. Vigouroux PR, Bauraud C, Choux M, et al. Etat actuel des aspects séquellaires graves dans les traumatismes craniens de l'adult, 4: incidence des lesions associées. Neurochirurgie 1972; 18 (Suppl 2): 123–36.
203. Sazbon L, Groswasser Z. Time-related sequelae of TBI in patients with prolonged postcomatose unawareness (PC-U) state. Brain Inj 1991; 5: 3–8.
204. Najenson T, Groswasser Z, Mendelson L, et al. Rehabilitation outcome of brain damaged patients after severe head injury. Intern Rehabil 1980; 2: 17–22.
205. Cossa FM, Fabiani M, Farinato A, et al. The Preliminary Neuropsychological Battery: an instrument to grade the cognitive level of

minimally responsive patients. Brain Inj 1999; 13: 583–92.
206. Novack TA, Alderson AL, Bush BA, et al. Cognitive and functional recovery at 6 and 12 months post-TBI. Brain Inj 2000; 14: 987–96.
207. Grossman P, Hagel K. Post-traumatic apallic syndrome following head injury, 1: clinical characteristics. Disabil Rehabil 1996; 18: 1–20.
208. Zasler ND, Kreutzer JS, Taylor D. Coma stimulation and coma recovery. Neurorehabilitation 1991; 1: 33–40.
209. Teasdale G, Jennett B. Assessment of coma and impaired consciousness: a practical scale. Lancet 1974; ii: 81–3.
210. Hagen C, Malkmus D, Durham P. Levels of cognitive functioning. Rehabilitation of the head injury adult: Comprehensive physical management. Downey, CA: Professional Staff Association of Rancho Los Amigos Hospital, Inc., 1979.
211. Rappaport M, Hall KM, Hopkins HK, et al. Disability Rating Scale for severe head trauma patients: coma to community. Arch Phys Med Rehabil 1982; 63: 118–23.
212. Ansell BJ, Keenan JE. The Western Neurosensory Stimulation Profile: a tool for assessing slow-to-recover head injured patients. Arch Phys Med Rehabil 1989; 70: 104–8.
213. Rappaport M, Herrero-Backe C, Rappaport ML, et al. Head injury outcome: up to ten years later. Arch Phys Med Rehabil 1989; 70: 885–92.
214. Giacino JT, Kezmarsky MA, DeLuca J, et al. Monitoring rate of recovery to predict outcome in minimally responsive patients. Arch Phys Med Rehabil 1991;72: 897– 901.
215. Rader MA, Ellis DW. The Sensory Stimulation Assessment Measure (SSAM): a tool for early evaluation of severely brain injured patients. Brain Inj 1994; 8: 309–21.
216. Sazbon L, Fucks C, Costeff H. Prognosis for recovery from prolonged post-traumatic unawareness: logistic analysis. J Neurol Neurosurg Psychiatry 1991; 54: 149–52.
217. Freeman EA. The Coma Exit Chart: assessing the patient in prolonged coma and the vegetative state. Brain Inj 1996; 10: 615–24.
218. Gill-Thwaites H. The Sensory Modality Assessment Technique: a tool for assessment and treatment of patients with severe brain injury in a vegetative state. Brain Inj 1997; 11: 723–34.
219. Gill-Thwaites H, Munday R. The Sensory Modality Assessment and Rehabilitation Technique (SMART): a comprehensive and integrated assessment and treatment protocol for the vegetative state and minimally conscious patient. Neuropsychol Rehabil 1999; 9: 305–20.
220. Borer-Alafi N, Gill M, Sazbon L, Korn C. The Loewenstein Communication Scale for the minimally responsive patient. Brain Inj 2002; (In print). http//www.tandf.co.uK.
221. Gouvier WD, Blanton PD, LaPorte KK, et al. Reliability and validity of the Disability Rating Scale and the levels of the Cognitive Functioning Scale in monitoring recovery from severe head injury. Arch Phys Med Rehabil 1987; 68: 94–7.
222. Wilson SL, MacMillan TM. A review of the evidence for the effectiveness of sensory stimulation treatment for coma and vegetative states. Neuropsychol Rehabil 1993; 3: 149–60.
223. Rappaport M, Dougherty AM, Kelting DL. Evaluation of coma and vegetative states. Arch Phys Med Rehabil 1992; 73: 628–34.
224. Ng WK, Nakase-Thompson R, Yablon SA, et al. Conceptual dilemmas in evaluating individuals with severely impaired consciousness. Brain Inj 2001; 15: 639–43.
225. Rader MA, Alston JB, Ellis DW. Sensory stimulation of severely brain injured patients. Brain Inj 1989; 3: 141–7.
226. Wilson SL, Powell GE, Elliot K, et al. Sensory stimulation in prolonged coma: four single case studies. Brain Inj 1991; 5: 393–400.
227. Wilson SL, Gill-Thwaites H. Early indication of emergence from vegetative state derived from assessment with the SMART: a preliminary report. Brain Inj 2000; 14: 319–31.

5 Ancillary Examination

Laboratory Findings

Leon Sazbon

Although some laboratory parameters have prognostic significance in acute head injury, they are of minimal or no value for evaluating the vegetative state (VS). In patients in VS, laboratory tests are used mainly as a prophylactic screen to detect and follow up complications.

In acute coma, stress-induced acute hyperglycemia, which is often accompanied by impaired oxidative metabolism, leads to high serum lactate values and metabolic acidosis [1,2]. These alterations are of short duration and not generally seen in VS. If they persist, they may be predictive of irreversible VS [2].

Hypoglycemia, serum or urine electrolyte imbalance, leukocytosis, and accelerated sedimentation rate are all frequent findings related to multiple complications.

The development of periarticular bone formation may increase alkaline phosphatase levels [3]. Occult blood in feces or gastric juice is almost always present, with gastric acidity and normal pH [4]. Hypoproteinuria and inversion albuminoglobulins are linked to nutrition or hepatic disorders (see p. 19, 22).

Changes in hormone profile are described in the section on medical complications in Chapter 4 (see p. 23).

The first stage of acute injury is associated with enzymatic changes in serum or cerebrospinal fluid, or both: creatine phosphokinase (CPK) and its isoenzymes, mainly CPK1 of the brain type in the brain (also known as CKBB); lactic dehydrogenase (LDH) and its isoenzymes; and glutamic oxalacetic transaminase (GOT) and pyruvates. Levels of all of these generally return to normal in the stage of VS [2,5–8].

Low cerebrospinal fluid cAMP was observed by Rudman et al. [9] and Sazbon [10]. A trend toward normalization of this parameter might indicate a good prognosis.

A certain degree of hypoxia, with Po_2 values of 60–80 mmHg in arterial blood, is the rule. Recovered patients show a marked diminution of forced vital capacity and both expiratory and inspiratory reserves [11]. This may be explained by paresis of the respiratory muscles (except the diaphragm), or the effect of possible bronchial aspiration, with subsequent inflammation of the pulmonary parenchyma by irritative acid gastric contents, alveolar collapse, microatelectasis, and interstitial sclerosis.

The increase in adrenocortical parameters – namely cortisol, norepinephrine, and catecholamines – which is characteristic of the first days after brain injury, regresses and then almost completely disappears in VS [5,12,13].

Pezzilli et al. [14] reported that hyperamylasemia and, less frequently, hyperlipidemia occur in the first phase of unconsciousness, but without proof of pancreatic involvement. These observations require further study.

A decrease in serum zinc concentrations, with loss of urinary zinc, is the rule in acute coma and is clearly correlated with the extent of brain damage. These parameters usually normalize within 2 weeks, although they have rarely been observed in VS [15,16]. The cause of the hypozincemia may be stress [17].

In the last few years, genetic factors such as the ε4 (epsilon 4) allele of apolipoprotein E have been found to have possible prognostic significance in post-traumatic coma and VS. Patients with this gene were likely to have a bad outcome [18–20].

Neuroimaging in the Vegetative State

Hans Hacker

The pathological conditions underlying the clinical picture in patients in the vegetative state are well known. Important information concerning the anatomical and pathological state of the brain [21,22], its functional, vascular, and chemical state, and regional cerebral blood flow, can be obtained using computed tomography (CT) [23], magnetic resonance imaging (MRI) [24,25], functional MRI, magnetic resonance angiography (MRA), MRI perfusion studies, magnetic resonance spectroscopy, and positron emission tomography (PET) [26]. In the usual clinical surroundings, many of these sophisticated techniques are not available. The absence of cooperation of patients in a vegetative state excludes complicated or long examinations without general anesthesia. It is also debatable how much of the information that can be obtained is relevant to the treatment or prognosis. At present, only a detailed anatomical diagnosis of brain lesions and vascular efficiency is indispensable. This is best obtained with MRI and MRA or, if these are not possible, with CT [27] contrast imaging.

The imaging findings at the time of examination, which may well be weeks after the injury, may conceal the extent and multiplicity of brain lesions in the immediate post-traumatic phase. For this reason, it is necessary to collect all previous examinations as well, although this is sometimes difficult to achieve. Reading and interpreting a series of older examinations, with a large number of films, and comparing them with the current examination is always a time-consuming and difficult task, but it is indispensable. Finally, a detailed description of the development of each of the different lesions over the previous few weeks should be presented.

Many types of traumatic brain lesion are demonstrated by imaging techniques:
- Compression by external hematomas: epidural; subdural, acute or chronic
- Brain swelling with internal shifting of parts of the brain, herniation, and compression of vessels
- Open or penetrating brain lesions
- Cortical lacerations
- Contusions
- Hemorrhages
- Subarachnoid bleeding
- Infarcts
- Shearing injuries
- Diffuse axonal injuries (DAIs)
- Vascular occlusions (neck or brain)
- Hydrocephalus: acute or low pressure
- Secondary lesions: thrombosis, infection

There is agreement among neuropathological and neuroradiological investigators that the most frequently found lesions in VS are:
- Diffuse axonal injuries (DAIs)
- Shearing injuries
- Extended cortical contusions

The most frequent locations for DAIs are:
- Corpus callosum and corona radiata
- Dorsolateral brain stem

Less frequent locations include:
- Bilateral thalamus
- Parahippocampal gyrus
- Ventral brain stem and medulla oblongata

The following grading of DAIs and shearing injuries is used:
- Grade 1: hemispheric white matter
- Grade 2: hemispheric white matter and corpus callosum
- Grade 3: hemispheric white matter, corpus callosum, and brain stem

A careful statistical study of lesions in 80 patients in post-traumatic vegetative state presented by Kampfl et al. showed that lesions in the corpus callosum and dorsolateral upper brainstem correlate with failure to recover [28,29]; this would correspond to grade 3. Most patients present with multiple locations of lesions with different pathologies. There have been no reports of patients with a single lesion or no lesions on MRI [30]. The main location observed in more than 40% of patients by Kampfl et al., are:
- Lobar white matter, mainly in the frontal and temporal lobes
- Cortical contusions
- Corpus callosum

62   5 Ancillary Examination

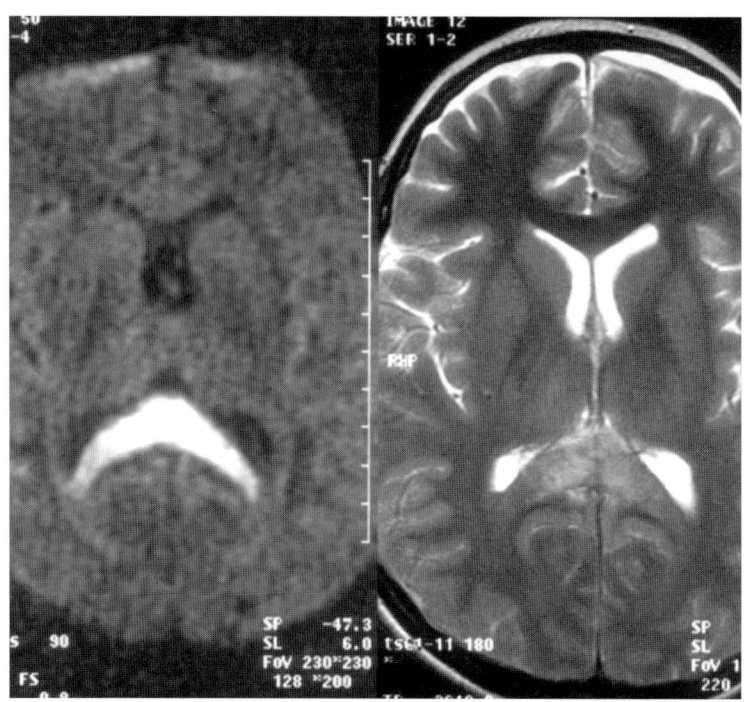

Fig. 5.1 Case 1: a 12-year-old child with coma following a fall from horseback. Magnetic resonance imaging (MRI), 2 days after the trauma.

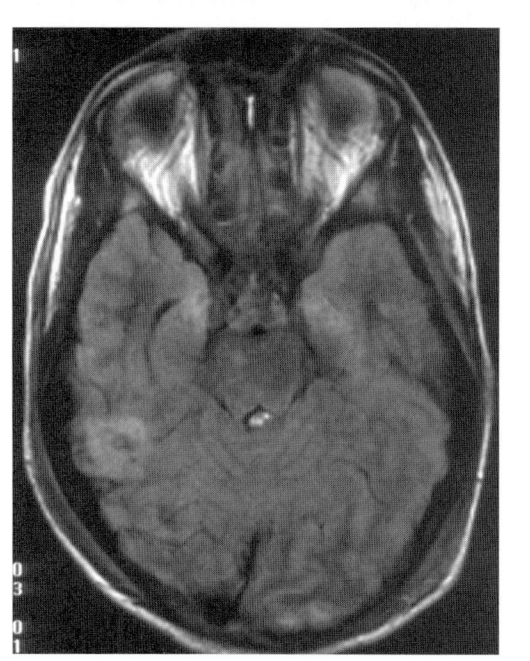

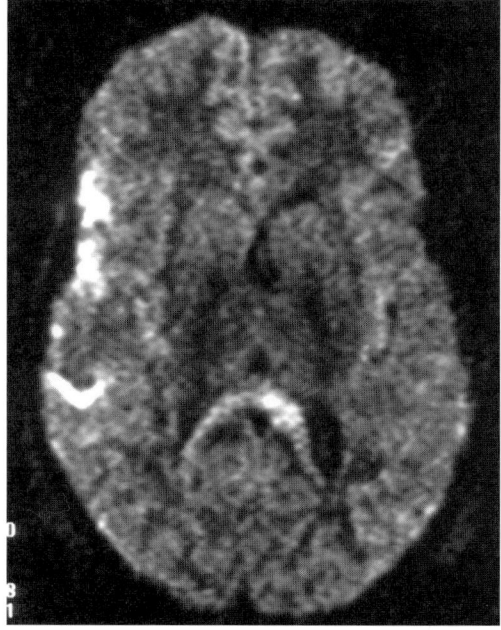

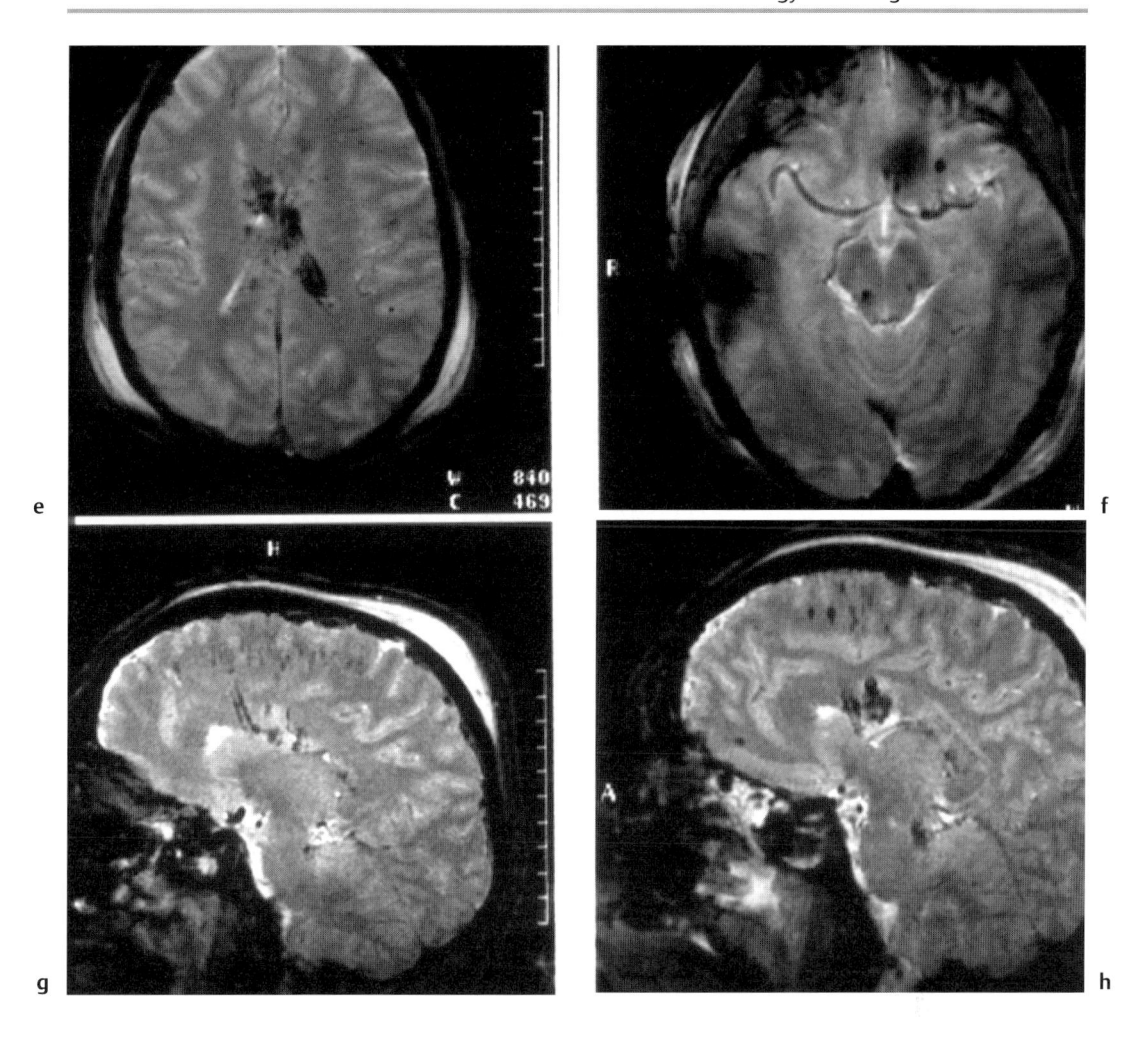

a Diffusion-weighted imaging (DWI).
b Spin-echo T2-weighted MRI, showing a lesion in the posterior corpus callosum, which is more clearly evident on the diffusion-weighted image.
c Fluid-attenuated inversion recovery (FLAIR). There are cortical and subcortical lesions in the right temporal lobe and in the medial parts of both temporal lobes-parahippocampal gyrus, right pons.

d DWI, with an axial section higher than in **c**. Lesions are seen in the right temporal lobe, right operculum, and right and left cingulum.
e–h Gadolinium-enhanced T2*-weighted MRI. There are lesions in the corpus callosum, multiple diffuse axonal injuries with subcortical microhemorrhage, in the corona radiata, and in the right lateral dorsal mesencephalon

64   5 Ancillary Examination

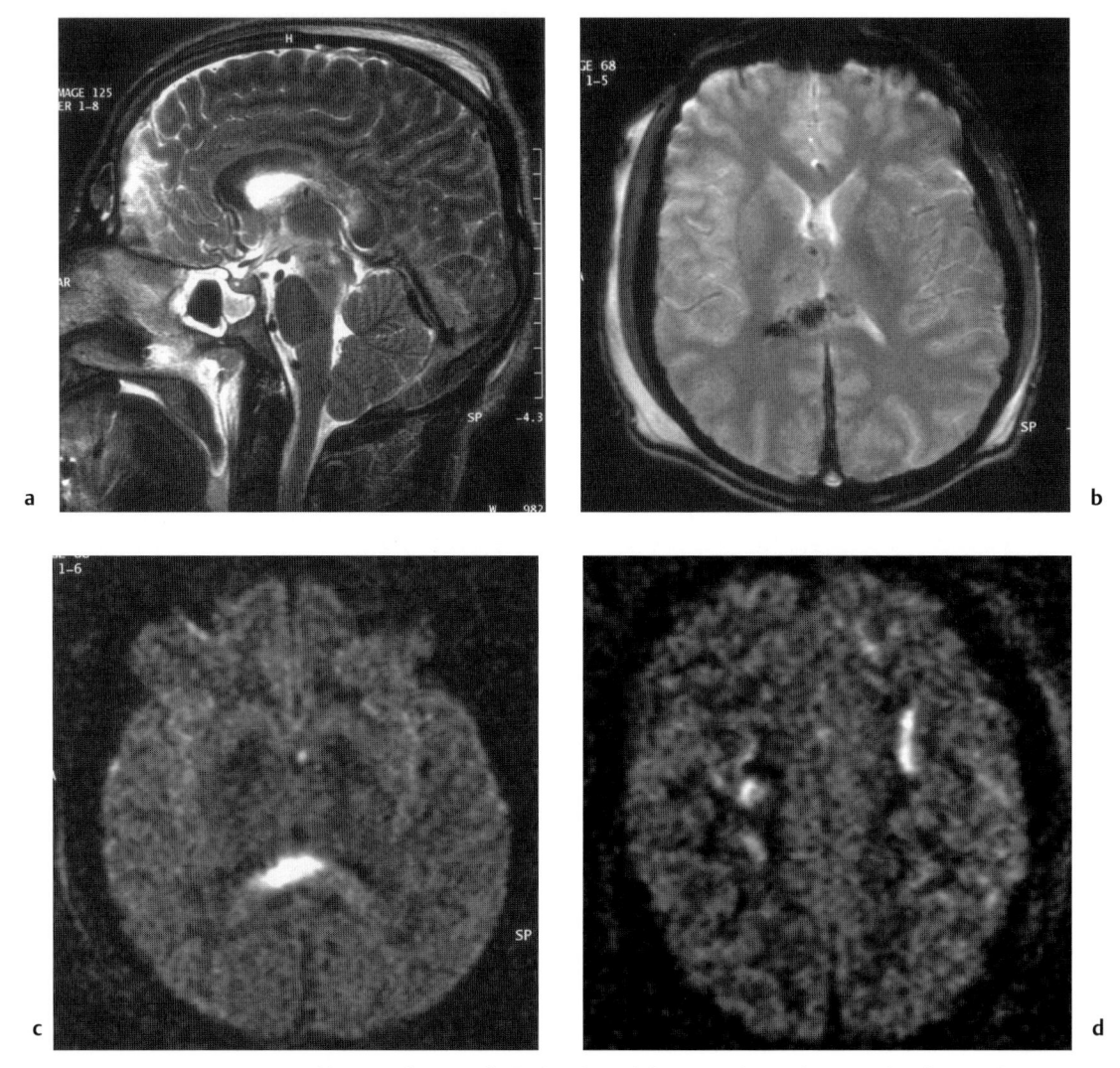

Fig. 5.2 Case 2: a 31-year-old man who initially had coma after a car accident, with a vegetative state after 6 weeks. Magnetic resonance imaging (MRI) 6 weeks after the trauma.
a Spin-echo T2-weighted MRI. Lesions include frontal cortical defects, destruction and atrophy of the posterior part of the corpus callosum, and diffuse axonal injury in the rostral mesencephalon.
b Gadolinium-enhanced T2-weighted MRI. There are frontal cortical contusions, hemosiderin in the right thalamus, and lesions in the basal ganglia and corpus callosum.
c Diffusion-weighted imaging (DWI). There is a lesion in the corpus callosum.
d DWI. Diffuse axonal injury in the centrum semiovale

- Thalamic and basal ganglia
- Parahippocampal region
- Dorsolateral brain stem
- Rostral ventral brain stem and medulla oblongata

Lesions interfering with the connection between central and cortical structures, in addition to partial interruptions of transcallosal connections, are likely to be at the origin of locking-out from perception and reaction to external stimuli. These lesions are best seen during the first few weeks. Lesions found in the basal ganglia, especially when bilateral, also contribute to loss of consciousness. If brain-stem lesions are visualized, an impaired arousal reaction is explained. Pathological MRI findings in two patients are shown in Figs. 5.**1** and 5.**2**.

Evidence in perfusion studies of a reduced regional cortical blood flow adds to the understanding of coma. It can also be assumed that a persistent flow rate below 20 mL/100 g/min provokes cortical atrophy. The value of spectroscopic magnetic resonance studies [31] is as yet unclear. In the future, spectroscopic imaging may allow the detection of regions in which there is no recovery. At present, CT studies in the acute stage and MRI in the postacute phase are the crucial examinations.

MRI examinations should include the following sequences:

- Spin-echo (SE) T1-weighted
- Proton density
- SE T2-weighted
- Gadolinium-enhanced (GE) T2*

These can be supplemented by the following techniques, if available:

- Fluid-attenuated inversion recovery (FLAIR)
- Diffusion-weighted imaging (DWI)

And, if vascular occlusion is suspected:

- Magnetic resonance angiography (MRA)

T2* images are sensitive for hemosiderin, and even after many weeks may indicate the presence of tiny shearing injuries. FLAIR and DWI are superior for demonstrating small and faint shifts in tissue water and of small foci of demyelination, allowing visualization of small DAIs.

Check-up examinations to assess the development of hydrocephalus can be carried out using CT, which should be performed every 3 months, or more frequently, during the first post-traumatic year.

Recent publications [32] on magnetic resonance spectrography in the mesencephalon have reported that reduced nuclear aspartic acid (NAA) appears to be predictive of a poor outcome. Confirmation of this finding by other groups must be awaited.

Acknowledgment

I am grateful Dr. S. Weidauer and Prof. Zanella at the Institute of Neuroradiology, University of Frankfurt, Germany, for kindly providing the clinical cases.

Neurophysiological Assessment of Brain Function in the Persistent Vegetative State

Alessandro Pincherle, Walter G. Sannita

The electrophysiological signals recorded by macroelectrodes from the surface of scalp (or, in selected instances, brain cortex) reflect spatially averaged postsynaptic potentials originating in large neuronal populations, notably ionic currents generated by membrane and volume-conducted through the extracellular media [34–36]. The functions of cerebral cortex are implicitly accepted to depend to a significant extent on the integrated activity of neuronal assemblies and circuitry. The hypothesis that collective signals recorded by macroelectrodes reflect with acceptable approximation the activity of these neural populations is therefore practicable. Experimental evidence and clinical observations converge in suggesting some functional correlation between neuronal mechanisms of, for example, sensory information processing, higher ("cognitive") performance, sleep–wakefulness cycle, vigilance, etc., and the electrophysiological signals generated in the activated neuronal assemblies. This correlation allows some extrapolation from single-unit/multi-unit cell recording to human data and privileged methods of investigation [37,38]

Electroencephalography

Spontaneous brain signals are recorded routinely for diagnostic purposes using electroencephalography (EEG) [39]. Under properly controlled experimental conditions (and with due approximation), the technique has also proved a reliable method in brain research, as it is noninvasive and can be applied repeatedly with minimal discomfort even in the absence of collaboration by the patient. Remarkably, the EEG is modulated by processes that also regulate vigilance [40]. These peculiarities make it a selective approach to the investigation of brain function or malfunctioning in intensive-care routine and, eventually, in research on the electrophysiological concomitants of vigilance and consciousness [41]. EEG transient or rhythmic patterns (e. g., triphasic complexes in hepatic encephalopathies, asymmetric or focal slow activities in supratentorial hemispheric lesions, diffuse EEG slowing, etc.) provide the clinician with indications of diagnostic relevance also in the absence of clinical signs [42]. Epileptic events without motor symptoms can be documented in comatose patients only by EEG recordings. The sleep phases are classified on the basis of EEG patterns (slow waves, spindles, sharp waves, K complex, etc.) that also provide information about the responsiveness of the thalamocortical system and its abnormalities. A variety of EEG patterns have been observed in patients in coma or vegetative state, including burst-suppression, bilateral periodic complexes, epileptic discharges, diffuse nonreactive alpha activity, spindle activity, and other abnormalities with or without pathological connotation.

Dolce and Kaemmerer [43] studied the EEG evolution from onset of coma to outcome in five patients. Three patients died, one recovered completely, and one only partially; the duration of coma was 2–5 weeks, with a subsequent vegetative state lasting 4–40 weeks. The EEG recordings showed slow (delta) waves with low amplitude and no detectable reactivity. During the evolution into a vegetative state, the EEG became progressively rhythmic in the 4–6 Hz frequency range and slightly reactive. In the late recordings, a 6–7 Hz activity was observed, with the delta activity (if present) restricted to the scalp locations over the lesional areas. The longitudinal EEG and clinical monitoring suggest that recovery of electrophysiological brain activities anticipates, even by months, the recovery of consciousness and motor function. In general, however, the information provided by the conventional EEG parameters is limited [44–46].

A number of studies have specifically focused on the EEG reactivity, which reflects to a relevant extent the anatomic/functional integrity of cortex, reticular brainstem formation, diffuse thalamocortical projecting systems, and extrathalamic pathways from subthalamic and hypothalamic regions [47,48]. According to early and recent reports [49–51], EEG reactivity (possibly in association with evidence of stimulus-evoked sensory responses) is a reliable long-term predictor of outcome after brain injury, with a reported 92% predictive accuracy of EEG reactivity (98% in combination with Tc or MRI brain scans), compared to 72% of the Glasgow Coma Scale [51]. Computer-assisted methods for EEG quantitative analysis have been applied extensively in the investigation of EEG reactivity patterns and have documented effects of sensory stimulation otherwise undetectable after conventional visual EEG inspection [e. g. 52–54]. Analyses of the coherence between EEG signals recorded from distinct areas of the scalp (a measure of correlation in the frequencies domain) were applied to describe changes in the functional relationship among brain cortical structures (either interacting or driven by a common regulating structure) in patients with closed head injuries [55]. Davey et al. [56] measured interhemispheric coherence in a patient in persistent vegetative state after stroke, with destruction of right basal ganglia and thalamus and atrophic cerebral cortex of the same side documented by MRI. Damage in the left hemisphere was restricted to part of the posterior areas. Notable interhemispheric asymmetry was observed, suggesting that subcortical structures (primarily the basal ganglia and thalamus) regulate, at least in part, the coherence among cortical/subcortical structures involved in the generation of EEG signals. It has been proposed that changes in coherence induced by thalamocortical activation may sustain integrative forebrain function, with damage to these structures conceivably being at the basis of the pathophysiology of vegetative state.

Sleep EEG

EEG patterns peculiar to functional correlates of physiological sleep (such as spindle activity) are observed in patients in coma, regardless of depth, and are indicated as an index of favorable prognosis in spite of their still undefined pathophysiology [57]. In general, the appearance of a sleep – wake cycle (no matter how rudimentary) is correlated to a better outcome and is a common observation in the transition from coma to a vegetative state (Fig. 5.**3**) [58,59]. Evans and Bartlett [60] studied a population of 138 patients with brain injury, subdivided into classes according to a number of EEG and polygraphic parameters (wakefulness, sleep-like patterns, normal, abnormal, or absent arousal, etc.) and found the absence of any arousal activity to be highly predictive of development into a persistent vegetative state. D'Aleo et al. [61] observed that progressive restoration of the sleep – wake cycle and increase of rapid eye movement (REM) sleep are associated with clinical recovery from the vegetative state. Also, Bricolo and co-workers [62] report a correlation between REM sleep, non-REM sleep, sleep-like patterns, diffuse nonreactive high-amplitude delta (0.5–6.0 Hz) activity, etc., in repeating sleep recordings and the clinical course in 22 long-term comatose patients after a brain injury. These studies agree in indicating some correlation between the occurrence, degree of organization, and progressive organization of sleep patterns in longitudinal recordings and the development of the comatose state. There is evidence [63,64] of functional interaction between REM sleep and processes of memory consolidation (specifically of perception traces), which are affected by selective REM-sleep deprivation [65]. In perspective, increased REM sleep in patients recovering from the vegetative state [66] is a possible correlate of recovery of the memory mechanisms necessary for conscious cognitive functions.

Recently, researchers from the Loewenstein Rehabilitation Center in Tel Aviv [67] observed an association between sleep-related erection episodes and REM sleep (95% of episodes) in a group of patients who recovered from vegetative state. This association was comparable with that in healthy controls, with no differences in the duration and characteristics of both events. Although preliminary, this observation suggests that hypothalamic mechanisms may be unaffected in the vegetative state. Following a comparable approach, spontaneous nystagmus was observed by electro-oculographic recording methods in six patients in the vegetative state during wakefulness, phase I and REM sleep, but never in phase II and slow-wave sleep [68]. Although not predictive of outcome, the presence itself of the rapid phase of nystagmus implies some integrity of the paramedian pontine reticular formation and frontal cortex [69].

Stimulus-Related Evoked Potentials

Cortical and precortical brain structures respond to adequate sensory inputs also through changes in the electrophysiological activities (evoked potentials), which are time-locked to stimulus onset, depend on the dynamics of activation of stimulus-specific central nervous system (CNS) pathways/structures, and reflect the mechanisms of sensory information processing. Visual, somatosensory and auditory stimulus-related potentials are used in clinical practice, as well as in animal and human research, following reliable methodological and interpretative standards [70].

Somatosensory Evoked Potentials

Somatosensory evoked potentials have been proposed as an acceptable predictor of output in early phases of coma [46,71,72], despite the differences existing between studies with regard, for example, to the study design, etiology of coma, age of patients, type of and time from brain injury (from coma to locked-in or apallic syndromes). The EEG and somatosensory evoked potentials were studied within 3 days of head injury in 100 patients [73] ranked according to their somatosensory responses (group 1, central conduction time within normal values bilaterally; group 2, central conduction time abnormally increased on one side; and group 3, cortical wave N20 undetectable on one side or both sides). The outcome was favorable in 90% of patients in group 1, 69% in group 2, and 6% in group 3, respectively. The EEG was not predictive, except in case of poor outcome for patients with isoelectric or severely abnormal EEG recordings. The prognostic values of EEG reactivity, somatosensory evoked potentials, and the Glasgow Coma Scale measured in the early days after coma onset were compared in 40 patients, 33 post-traumatic and seven post-anoxic [74]. The study reports a higher predictive value of the somatosensory evoked potentials (92%) compared to EEG reactivity (67%) and Glasgow Coma Scale (62%). The prediction of

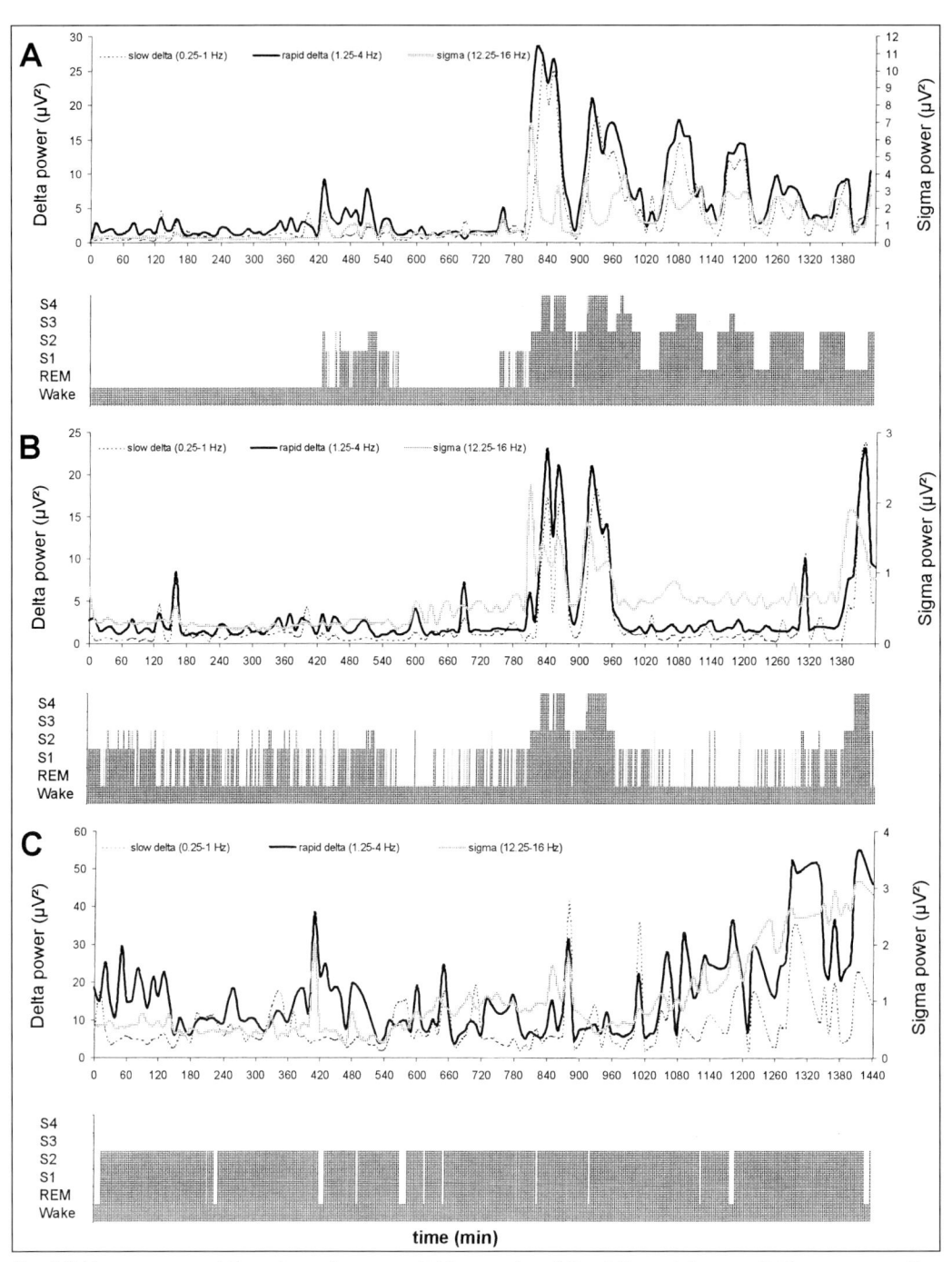

Fig. 5.3 Hypnogram and time dynamics over a 24-h period of quantitative electroencephalography (EEG) in the 0.2–4.0 Hz (delta) and 12.2–16.0 Hz (sigma) activities of a normal individual (**a**) and two patients in permanent vegetative state (**b, c**). A short and rudimentary sleep organization is evident in **b**, with two cycles of the delta and sigma activities corresponding to episodes of deep sleep; the occurrence of consecutive deep sleep and delta activity cycles that are peculiar to the normal sleep–wake function (as seen in **a**) is truncated. No organized sleep–waking cycle can be recognized in **c**

good outcome in post-traumatic patients with normal or borderline somatosensory evoked potentials, however, was not confirmed in post-anoxic patients, no matter how organized their somatosensory responses were. The latter observation suggests that etiology may play a role as a prognostic factor of outcome from coma and vegetative state, taking into account the several concomitant pathologies (such as brain edema or hydrocephalus) that may affect brain electrophysiology in the acute phases after brain injury. A study of the effects of brain injury and vegetative state on the somatosensory evoked potentials [75,76] did not detect any pattern common to all patients besides a normal response at Erb's recording position excluding peripheral nerve damage, and a prolonged central conduction time, conceivably due to diffuse subcortical axonal injury, which was also documented at the postmortem examinations [77,78]. Interestingly enough, progressive clinical improvement and reduction of the central conduction time were concomitant in one patient, suggesting that recovery of sensory processes may be essential in order to regain a conscious state. Concomitant improvement of the clinical condition and somatosensory evoked potentials was also recently reported by Claassen and Hansen [79].

Auditory Evoked Potentials

The brainstem evoked response to auditory stimulation is a compound potential generated within several structures of the brainstem auditory pathway [70]. In standard conditions, it is resistant to endogenous factors (e. g., ammonia, electrolytes, pH, Pco_2) and exogenous factors (e. g., neuroactive drugs) [71,80,81], and it may therefore also be useful in metabolic coma. Changes in the latencies and conduction times between waves, high variability, changes in amplitude, or loss of individual waves can occur in different phases of acute midbrain syndromes. Recovery can be related to clinical improvement [82–84]. The reliability of brainstem auditory responses as a prognostic index is questioned, but a combined study of brainstem and middle-latency auditory responses appears to improve the prediction of outcome [71,85–87]. Frank et al. [88] reported on five nontraumatic comatose children, whose brainstem responses in the absence of a response to stimulation of the median nerve (reflecting thalamocortical network activation) was predictive of a permanent vegetative state.

Rappaport et al. [89] compared brainstem and long-latency auditory evoked responses in 75 patients with long-term traumatic brain injury. Increased latencies of long-latency responses proved to correlate significantly with the clinical outcome, while the brain-stem responses did not.

Jones et al. [90] measured the long-latency auditory responses to synthesized musical tones in 22 post-comatose patients. The presence of a response to complex tone stimuli was associated with discriminative hearing, i.e. the ability to respond differentially to verbal commands. The behavioral and electrophysiological findings were in agreement in 18 patients, suggesting that this approach may be suitable when identifying patients with "perception" capabilities in the presence of severe communication or motor disabilities.

Recently, Laureys et al. [91], in a PET study on patients in permanent vegetative state, documented a cascade of functional disconnection along the auditory cortical pathway, from the primary auditory area to parietal associative and limbic areas. The primary auditory cortex was activated by appropriate stimulation, and a brain-stem response was recorded.

Visual Evoked Potentials

Visual evoked potential studies in unresponsive patients mostly investigate the cortical/precortical responses to luminance stimuli, as investigation of the contrast visual function is not practicable in subjects who are unable to attend to the stimulation paradigm properly. Adler [92] studied these responses in 40 comatose patients in intensive care and assessed their relationship to intraventricular pressure. The complexity of the response (estimated as the number of detectable wave components) decreased with increasing depth of coma. Increased pressure resulted in a considerable reduction in the response amplitude, which recovered to baseline values after reduction of pressure. Clinical application of visual evoked responses in comatose patients is limited in comparison with somatosensory and auditory responses, and prediction of the clinical outcome is poor [71]. On the other hand, damage to the visual system, ranging from reduced visual acuity to visual field loss or even to functional blindness, often occurs after head injury [93], and visual evoked responses have proved useful in monitoring the recovery of visual function after trauma [94].

Event-Related Potentials

The definition of event-related potentials refers to a class of transient, phasic potentials elicited in conjunction with perceptual, cognitive, or motor events and regarded as concomitants of higher ('cognitive") brain functions. Unlike the responses to sensory stimulation, event-related potentials neither reflect the physical properties of stimulus nor depend on sensory input with physiological relevance, but result from situational links such as the significant association or omission, convergence, interaction, or unpredictable occurrence of significant events. In this respect, event-related potentials are, within limits, specific to the cognitive function explored, while sharing the sensitivity of electrophysiological measures. In the conventional experimental paradigms, conscious collaboration is required. However, studies in psychiatric or demented patients and animals have been performed successfully. The resulting evidence suggests that several physiological mechanisms concur in the generation of event-related potentials and reflect partly undefined neural functions that contribute to conscious behavior, but can occur independently [95–97]. Contingent negative variation (CNV) and P300 are classic examples of this, in a rapidly evolving field.

The CNV [98,99] is in agreement with theoretical models of operant conditioning. A negative steady potential shift with positive monotonic and inverted-U correlation with attention and arousal, respectively, the CNV is evoked by a temporal association between (conditional and imperative) stimuli. A motor response to the imperative stimulus is a rule. However, steady-state potentials comparable in shape to the CNV recorded in conscious subjects were obtained from two patients in deep coma (one of whom developed the vegetative state) by increasing the number of paired stimuli (Fig. 5.**4**) [100]. This observation is consistent with experimental evidence that steady shifts in membrane potential occur in the cortex and subcortical structures during memory processes, at levels of complexity of the involved neuronal assemblies that are not compatible with conscious operations [101–105].

A late positive response to attended stimuli, usually referred to as "P300" based on polarity and latency, is recorded at appropriate scalp locations when stimuli in the same sensory modality, but with differing physical characteristics and frequency of occurrence, are presented and the subject is requested to attend the infrequent stimulus. The generators are unknown, but experimental evidence suggests interaction of cortical/subcortical structures such as the limbic system, thalamus, corpus callosum, and distributed cortical areas [106–113]. Tomberg and Desmedt [114] suggest that the P300 may reflect time-related inhibition (possibly due to subcortical activation) of the neuronal functional assemblies involved in the processing of attended stimuli. Kotchoubey et al. [115] reported observing P300 responses in 14 patients in the vegetative state and 19 patients who had recovered to the condition of minimal response. In all cases, conventional brain-stem acoustic responses made it possible to exclude significant impairment of the precortical auditory system. Three different acoustic stimulation paradigms were applied: two (target and nontarget) sinusoidal tones, two complex tones, and two vowels (an "O" in a female voice and an "I" in a male voice). In both groups of patients, the P300 response was observed more frequently when the complex paradigms were applied. Comparable results were obtained in patients in permanent vegetative state when verbal paradigms with affective-emotional connotations, eliciting a P300 (e. g., the patient's names compared to other names) were compared with the classic oddball paradigms [116]. Keren and co-workers [117] reported on 16 severely brain-injured patients, whose P300 and neuropsychological assessments were performed 1, 2, and 5 months after the trauma. At the beginning of follow-up, the P300 latencies were significantly longer in patients with lower Glasgow Coma Scale scores. A progressive reduction in the P300 latencies was observed in patients with low scores, with the differences from patients with high scores disappearing at a later time in parallel with improvements in cognitive performance as detected by neuropsychological tests. These observations suggest a possible clinical use of event-related potentials as an index of brain activity relating to the recovery from coma or vegetative state, as well as some participation of limbic structures (involved in the "emotional recognition" of human voice and names) in the generation of a P300 response in vegetative patients and, conceivably, in healthy subjects. However, a prediction of favorable outcome based on the observation of a P300 response is still speculative.

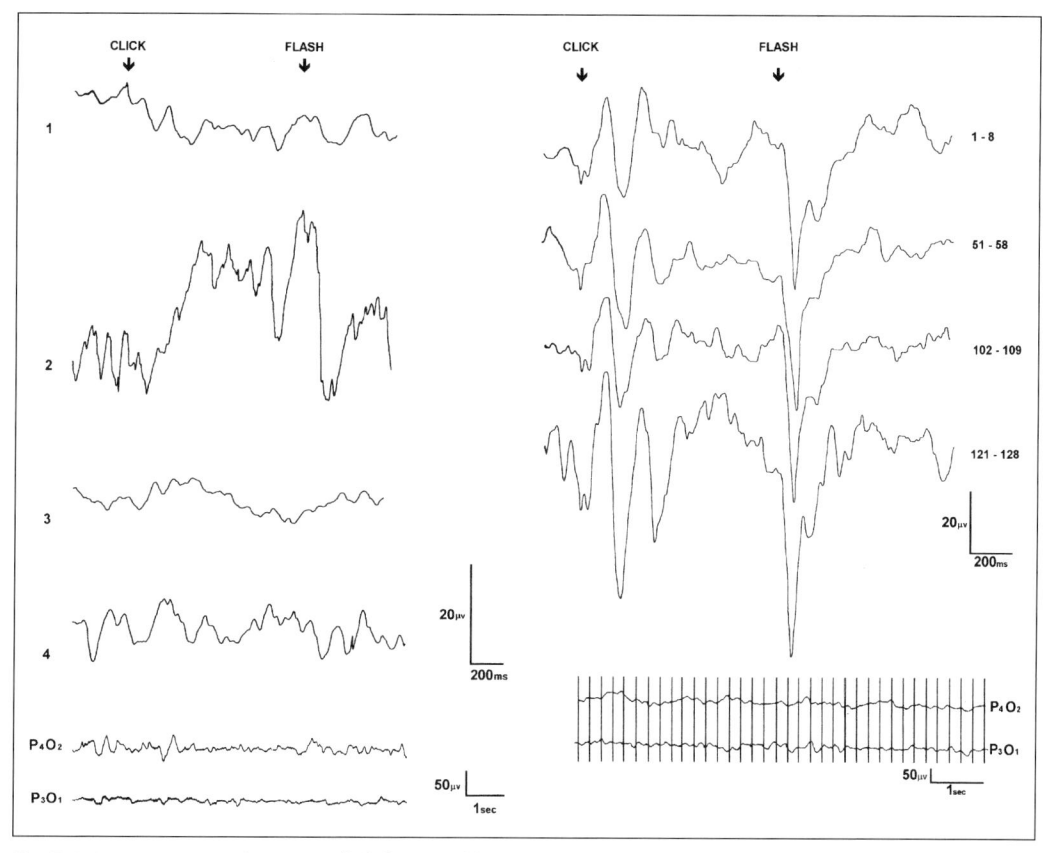

Fig. 5.4 A negative steady potential shift resembling contingent negative variation (CNV), recorded by conventional methods in two patients in deep coma (see the original report for details). On the left are shown: 1) the absence of response to a first standard sequence of eight paired stimuli (sufficient to evoke CNV in healthy subjects) and the averaged response to eight paired stimuli obtained after a long series of stimuli (about 150) as recorded from the vertex (2) and midparietal areas (3). On the right are shown the averaged responses to sequences of eight paired stimuli, with a CNV-like response appearing only after a long series of stimuli. (Reproduced from *Electroencephalography and Clinical Neurophysiology* [100], with permission from Elsevier Science)

Jennett and Plum [45] introduced the term "persistent vegetative state" to describe the condition of "wakefulness without awareness" following brain injuries. The cortical-subcortical structures involved in the regulation of vigilance also modulate cortical electrophysiology. An electrophysiological approach to the understanding of the mechanisms of coma and vegetative state therefore appeared conceptually and methodologically appropriate and was favored. However, research in this field did not expand and become systematic, as in other areas of clinical neurology (e.g., epilepsy, dementia, movement or vascular disorders, etc.), and the available information is often derived from case reports or studies in small groups of patients. Methodologies have often differed among studies, making meta-analyses impracticable, and prospective study designs are exceptional.

The approach nevertheless still appears promising, and it seems realistic to expect that more refined and controlled methodologies and research strategies may help predict the outcome and allow physicians to allocate resources. Remarkably, questions about the physiological concomitants of consciousness have expanded beyond the fields of philosophy and epistemology and are becoming key issues in today's neuroscience, as well as in neuroinformatics and in research on artificial intelligence and robotics. Improved and systematic neurophysiological investigations combined with up-to-date functional neuroimaging techniques – such as functional MRI (fMRI) and PET – as well as collaboration between neuroscientists and anesthesiologists, should be regarded as a sound approach to understanding CNS function, the mechanisms regulating vigilance and allowing conscious behavior, and the pathophysiology of the conditions of impaired consciousness that can follow brain injuries.

References

1. De Salles AAF, Muizelaar JP, Young HF. Hyperglycemia, cerebrospinal fluid lactic acidosis, and cerebral blood flow in severely head-injured patients. Neurosurgery 1987; 21: 45–50.
2. Zupping R, Magi M, Tikk A et al. Cerebral metabolic disorders during prolonged unconsciousness after severe head injury. Eur Neurol 1972; 9: 145–50.
3. Sazbon L, Solzi P, Berghaus N. Periarticular new bone formation in hemiplegic patients. Harefuah 1980; 99: 317–8.
4. Becker E, Sazbon L, Najenson T. Gastrointestinal haemorrhage in long lasting traumatic coma. Scand J Rehabil Med 1978; 10: 23–6.
5. Hamil RW, Woolf PD, McDonald JV, et al. Catecholamines predict outcome in traumatic brain injury. Ann Neurol 1987; 21: 438–43.
6. Hans P, Born JD, Albert A. Extrapolated creatine kinase-BB isoenzyme activity in assessment of initial brain damage after severe head injury. J Neurosurg 1987; 66: 714–7.
7. Rabow L, Dec Salles AAF, Becker DP, et al. CSF brain creatinine kinase levels and lactic acidosis in severe head injury. J Neurosurg 1986; 65: 625–9.
8. Bakay RAE, Ward AA. Enzymatic changes in serum and cerebrospinal fluid in neurological injury. J Neurosurg 1983; 58: 27–37.
9. Rudman D, Fleischer AS, Kutner MH, Raggio JF. Suprahypophyseal hypogonadism and hypothyroidism during prolonged coma after head injury. J Clin Endocrinol Metab 1977; 45: 747–54.
10. Sazbon L. Prolonged coma. Prog Clin Neurosci 1985; 2: 65–81.
11. Najenson T, Sazbon L, Fiselson J, et al. Recovery of communicative functions after prolonged traumatic coma. Scand J Rehabil Med 1978; 10: 15–21.
12. Woolf, PD, Hamill RW, Lee RA, et al. The predictive value of catecholamines in assessing outcome in traumatic brain injury. J Neurosurg 1987; 66: 875–82.
13. Woolf PD, Cox C, Kelly M, et al. The adrenocortical response to brain injury. Alcohol Clin Exp Res 1990; 14: 917–21.
14. Pezzili R, Billi P, Barakat B, et al. Serum pancreatic enzymes in patients with coma due to head injury or acute stroke. Int J Clin Lab Res 1997; 27: 244–6.
15. Sazbon L. [Personal communication].
16. Kapaki E, Segditsa J, Papageorgiou C. Zinc, copper and magnesium concentration in serum and CSF of patients with neurological disorders. Acta Neurol Scand 1989; 79: 373–8.
17. McClain CJ, Twyman DL, Ott LG, et al. Serum and urine zinc response in head- injured patients. J Neurosurg 1986; 64: 224–30.
18. Sorbi S, Nacmias B, Piacentini S, et al. ApoE as a prognostic factor for post-traumatic coma [letter]. Nature Med 1995; 1: 852.
19. Friedman G, Froom P, Sazbon L, et al. Apolipoprotein E e4 genotype predicts a poor outcome in survivors of traumatic brain injury. Neurology 1999; 52: 244–8.
20. Roses AD, Saunders A. Head injury, amyloid and Alzheimer disease. Nature Med 1995; 1: 603–4.
21. Adams JH. Brain damage in fatal nonmissile head injury in man. In: Vinken PJ, Bruyn GW, editors. Handbook of clinical neurology, vol 53. Amsterdam: North-Holland, 1990: 43.
22. Kinney HC, Samuels MA. Neuropathology of the persistent vegetative state: a review. J Neuropathol Exp Neurol 1994; 53: 548–58.
23. Zimmermann RA, Bilaniuk LT, Genneralli T. Computed tomography of shearing injuries of the cerebral white matter. Radiology 1978; 127: 393–6.
24. Vallasciani M, Gironelli L, Tulli D, Chiaramoni L, Salvolini U. Neuroradiological investigations in patients with persistent vegetative state. Rev Neuroradiol 2000; 13 (Suppl 2): 81.
25. Santoro G, Lanza PL. Traumi cranio-encefalici. [Personal communication].
26. Hijdra A, Zandbergen EG, de Haan RJ. PET scanning and neuronal loss in acute vegetative state. Lancet 2000; 355: 1826.
27. Reider-Groswasser I, Costeff H, Sazbon L, Groswasser Z. CT findings in persistent vegetative state following blunt traumatic brain injury. Brain Inj 1997;11: 865–70.
28. Kampfl A, Schmutzhard E, Franz G, et al. Prediction of recovery from post-traumatic vegetative state with cerebral magnetic resonance imaging. Lancet 1998;351: 1763–7.
29. Kampfl A, Franz G, Aichner F, et al. The persistent vegetative state after closed head injury: clinical and magnetic resonance imaging findings in 42 patients. J Neurosurg 1998; 88: 809–16.

30. Gieron MA, Korthals JK, Riggs CD. Diffuse axonal injury without direct head trauma and with delayed onset of coma. Pediatr Neurol 1998; 19: 382–4.
31. Ricci R, Barbarella G, Musi P, Boldrini P, Treviasn C, Basaglia N. Localized proton MR spectroscopy of brain metabolism changes in vegetative patients. Neuroradiology 1997; 39: 313–9.
32. Sinson G, Bagley LJ, Cecil KM, et al. Magnetization transfer imaging and proton MR spectroscopy in the evaluation of axonal injury: correlation with clinical outcome after traumatic brain injury. Am J Neuroradiol 2001; 22: 143–51.
34. Petsche H, Pockberger H, Rappelsberger P. On the search for the sources of the electroencephalogram. Neuroscience 1984; 11: 1–27.
35. Elul R. The genesis of the EEG. Int Rev Neurobiol 1971; 15: 227–72.
36. Speckmann EJ, Caspers H, editors. Origin of cerebral field potentials. Stuttgart: Thieme, 1979.
37. Pilgreen KL. Physiologic, medical and cognitive correlates of electroencephalography. In: Nunez P, editor. Neocortical dynamics and human EEG rhythms. New York: Oxford University Press, 1995: 195–248.
38. Steriade M. Corticothalamic resonance, states of vigilance and mentation Neuroscience 2000; 101: 243–76.
39. Niedermayer E, editor. Electroencephalography: basic principles, clinical applications and related fields. Baltimore: Williams and Wilkins, 1993.
40. Coenen AM. Neuronal phenomena associated with vigilance and consciousness: from cellular mechanisms to electroencephalographic patterns. Conscious Cogn 1998; 7: 42–53.
41. Celesia GG. EEG and coma: is there a prognostic role for EEG? Clin Neurophysiol 1999; 110: 203–4.
42. Plum F, Posner JB, editors. The diagnosis of stupor and coma. Philadelphia: FADC, 1980.
43. Dolce G, Kaemmerer E. Contributo anatomo clinico alla conoscenza della sindrome apallica. Sistema Nervoso 1967; 19: 12–23.
44. Lucking CH, Mullner E, Pateisky K, Gerstendbrand F. Electroencephalographic findings in apallic syndrome. In: Dalle Ore G, Gerstendbrand F, Lucking CH, Peters G, Peters UH, editors. The apallic syndrome. New York: Springer, 1977: 144–54.
45. Jennett B, Plum F. Persistent vegetative state after brain damage. Lancet 1972; i: 734–7.
46. Chatrian G, Bergamasco B, Bricolo A, Frost JD, Prior P. IFCN recommended standards for elctrophysiologic monitoring in comatose and other unresponsive states: report of an IFCN committee. Electroencephalogr Clin Neurophysiol 1996; 99: 103–23.
47. Steriade M, Buzsàki G. Parallel activation of thalamic and cortical neurons by brainstem and basal forebrain cholinergic systems. In: Steriade M, Biesold S, editors. Brain cholinergic systems. Oxford: Oxford University Press, 1990: 3.
48. Steriade M, Jones EG, Llinas RR, editors. Thalamic oscillations and signaling. New York: Wiley, 1990.
49. Chatrian G. Electroencephalographic patterns resembling those of sleep in certain comatose states after injuries to the head. Electroencephalogr Clin Neurophysiol 1963; 15: 272–80.
50. Courjon J, Naquet R. Value of the EEG in diagnosis and prognosis immediately after cranial trauma. Rev EEG Neurophysiol 1971; 1: 133–50.
51. Gutling E, Gosner A, Imhof HG, Landis T. EEG reactivity in the prognosis of severe head injury. Neurology 1995; 45: 915–8.
52. Ferrillo F, Rivano C, Rosadini G, Rossi GF, Turella C. EEG spectral analysis in coma. Electroencephalogr Clin Neurophysiol 1969; 27: 700.
53. Rosadini G, Ferrillo F. Automatic analysis of spontaneous EEG activity in the functional exploration of the human brain. In: Somjen GG, editor. Neurophysiology studied in man: proceedings of a symposium held in Paris at the Faculté des Sciences, 20–22 July 1971. Amsterdam: Excerpta Medica, 1972: 453–460.
54. Sannita WG, Rosadini G. Computerized EEG analysis in the management of comatose patients: an operational proposal. In: Lechner H, Aranibar A, editors. EEG and clinical neurophysiology. Amsterdam: Excepta Medica, 1980: 583–91.
55. Tatcher RW, Cantor DS, McAlaster R, Geisler F, Krause P. Comprehensive predictions of outcome in closed head injured patients: the development of prognostic equations. Ann NY Acad Sci 1991; 620: 82–101.
56. Davey M, Victor J, Schiff N. Power spectra and coherence in the EEG of a vegetative patient with severe asymmetric brain damage. Clin Neurophysiol 2000;111: 1949–54.
57. Kaplan PW, Genoud D, Ho TW, Jallon P. Clinical correlates and prognosis in early spindle coma. Clin Neurophysiol 2000; 111: 584–90.
58. Gerstenbrand F. Das traumatische apalliche syndrom. Vienna: Springer, 1967: 344.
59. Zeman A. Persistent vegetative state. Lancet 1997; 350: 795–9.
60. Evans BM, Bartlett JR. Prediction of outcome in severe head injury based on recognition of sleep related activity in the polygraphic electroencephalogram. J Neurol Neuros Psych 1995; 59: 17–25.

61. D'Aleo G, Saltuari L, Gerstenbrand F, Bramanti P. Sleep in the last remission stages of vegetative state of traumatic nature. Funct Neurol 1994; 9: 189–92.
62. Bricolo A, Gentilomo A, Rosadini G, Rossi F. Long lasting post-traumatic unconsciousness. Acta Neurol Scand 1968; 44: 512–32.
63. Crick F, Mitchinson G. The function of dream sleep. Nature 1983; 304: 111–4.
64. Kavanau JL. Memory, sleep and the evolution of mechanisms of synaptic efficacy maintenance. Neuroscience 1997; 79: 7–44.
65. Karni A, Tanne D, Rubenstain BS, Askenasy JJ, Sagi D. Dependence on REM sleep of overnight improvement of a perceptual skill. Science 1994; 265: 679–82.
66. D'Aleo G, Bramanti P, Silvestri R, Saltuari L, Gerstenbrand F, Di Perri R. Sleep spindles in the initial stages of the vegetative state. Ital J Neurol Sci 1994; 15: 347–51.
67. Oksenberg A, Arons E, Sazbon L, Mizrahi A, Radwan H. Sleep-related erections in vegetative state patients. Sleep 2000; 23: 953–7.
68. Gordon C, Oksenberg A. Spontaneous nystagmus across the sleep-wake cycle in vegetative state patients. Electroencephalogr Clin Neurophysiol 1993; 86: 132–7.
69. Leigh R, Zee D. The neurology of eye movements. Philadelphia: Davis, 1983.
70. Regan D. Human brain electrophysiology: evoked potentials and evoked magnetic fields in science and medicine. New York: Elsevier, 1989.
71. Greenberg RP, Mayer DJ, Becker DP, Miller JD. Evaluation of brain function in severe human head trauma with multimodality evoked potentials. J Neurosurg 1977; 47: 150–77.
72. Sleigh JW, Havill JH, Frith R, Kersel D, Marsh N, Ulyatt D. Somatosensory evoked potentials in severe traumatic brain injury: a blinded study. J Neurosurg 1999; 91: 577–80.
73. Hutchinson DO, Frith RW, Shaw NA, Judson JA, Cant BR. A comparison between electroencephalography and somatosensory evoked potentials for outcome prediction following severe head injury. Electroencephalogr Clin Neurophysiol 1991; 78: 228–33.
74. Piersanti P, Cesaretti C, Matà S, et al. Reattività EEG e potenziali evocati somatosensitivi. Confronto e possibili discordanze nella prognosi precoce del coma grave. In: Rossi B, Gabrielli L, Murri L, editors. Atti del VI Congresso della Società Italiana di Psicofisiologia, Pisa, Italy, 1996: 49–57.
75. Keren O, Groswasser Z, Sazbon L, Ring C. Somatosensory evoked potentials in prolonged post-comatose unawareness state following traumatic brain injury. Brain Inj 1991; 3: 233–40.
76. Keren O, Sazbon L, Groswasser Z, Shmuel M. Follow-up studies of somatosensory evoked potentials and auditory evoked potentials in patients with post-coma unawareness of traumatic brain injury. Brain Inj 1994; 8: 239–47.
77. Adams JH, Graham DI, Murray LS, Scott G. Diffuse axonal injury due to non-missile head injury in humans: analysis of 45 cases. Ann Neurol 1982; 27: 557–63.
78. Adams JH, Graham DI, Gennarelli TA, Maxwell WL. Diffuse axonal injury in non-missile head injury. J Neurol Neurosurg Psychiatry 1991; 54: 481–3.
79. Claassen J, Hansen HC. Early recovery after closed traumatic head injury: somatosensory evoked potentials and clinical findings. Crit Care Med 2001; 29: 494–502.
80. Sutton LN, Frewen T, Mausch R, Jaggi J, Bruce DA. The effect of deep barbiturate coma on multimodality evoked potentials. J Neurosurg 1982; 57: 178–85
81. Sannita WG. Stimulus-related evoked potentials: from basic science to clinical neuropharmacology. Electroencephalogr Clin Neurophysiol Suppl 1996; 46: 95–106.
82. Rumpl E, Prugger M, Gerstenbrand F, Brunnhuber W, Badry F, Hackl JM. Central somatosensory conduction time and acoustic brainstem transmission time in post-traumatic coma. J Clin Neurophysiol 1988; 3: 237–60.
83. Schwarz G, Litscher G, Rumpl E, Pfurtscheller G, Reimann R. Brainstem auditory evoked potentials in respiratory insufficiency following encephalitis. Int J Neurosci 1996; 84: 35–44.
84. Werner RA, Vanderzant CW. Multimodality evoked potentials testing in acute mild closed head injury. Arch Phys Med Rehabil 1991; 72: 31–4.
85. Litscher G. Middle latency auditory evoked potentials in intensive care patients and normal controls. Int J Neurosci 1995; 83: 253–67.
86. Sazbon L, Solzi P, Steinvil Y, Becker E. Blink reflex in patients in prolonged comatose state. Electromyogr Clin Neurophysiol 1988; 28: 151–8.
87. Hall JW, Mackey-Hargadine J, Allen SJ. Monitoring neurological status of comatose patients in the intensive care unit. In: Jacobson JT, editor. The auditory brainstem response. San Diego: College Hill Press, 1985: 253–83.
88. Frank M, Furgiuele T, Etheridge J. Predicting of chronic vegetative state in children using evoked potentials. Neurology 1985; 35: 931–4.
89. Rappaport M, Hemmerle AV, Rappaport ML. Short and long latency auditory evoked potentials in traumatic brain injury patients. Clin Electroencephalogr 1991; 22: 199–202.
90. Jones SJ, Vaz Pato M, Sprague L, Stokes M, Munday R, Haque N. Auditory evoked poten-

tials to spectro-temporal modulation of complex tones in normal subjects and patients with severe brain injury. Brain 2000; 123: 1007–16.
91. Laureys S, Faymonville ME, Degueldre C, et al. Auditory processing in the vegetative state. Brain 2000; 123: 1589–601.
92. Adler G, Bransi A, Prange HW. Neuro-monitoring using visual evoked potentials in comatose neurologic intensive care patients. EEG EMG Z Elektroenzephalogr Elektromyogr Verwandte Geb 1991; 22: 254–8.
93. Tierney DW. Visual dysfunction in closed head injury. J Am Optom Assoc 1988; 59: 614–22.
94. Freed S, Hellerstein LF. Visual electrodiagnostic findings in mild traumatic brain injury. Brain Inj 1997; 11: 25–36.
95. Johnson R, Rohrbaugh JW, Parasuraman R, editors. Currents trend in event-related potentials research. Electroencephalogr Clin Neurophysiol Suppl 1987; 40 [special issue].
96. Brunia CHM, Mulder G, Verbaten MN, editors. Event related brain research. Electroencephalogr Clin Neurophysiol Suppl 1991; 42 [special issue].
97. Naatanen R. Attention and brain function. Hillsdale, NJ: Erlbaum, 1992.
98. Walter WG, Cooper R, Aldridge VJ, McCallum WC, Winter AL. Contingency negative variation: an electric sign of sensori-motor association and expectancy in the human brain. Nature 1964; 203: 380–4.
99. Tecce JJ, Savignano-Bowman J, Cole JO. Drug effects on CNV and eyeblinks: the distraction arousal hypothesis. In: Lipton MA, DiMascio A, Killam KF, editors. Psychopharmacology: a generation of progress. New York: Raven Press, 1978: 745–58.
100. Dolce G, Sannita W. A CNV-like negative shift in deep coma. Electroencephalogr Clin Neurophysiol 1973; 34: 647–50.
101. John ER, Herrington RN, Sutton S. Effects of visual form on the evoked response. Science 1967; 155: 1439–42.
102. Horel JA, Vierck CJ Jr, Pribram KH, Spinelli DN, John ER, Ruchkin DS. Average evoked responses and learning. Science 1967; 158: 394–5.
103. Albright TD, Kandel ER, Posner MI. Cognitive neuroscience. Curr Opin Neurobiol 2000; 10: 612–24.
104. Spencer WA, Kandel ER. Cellular and integrative properties of the hippocampal pyramidal cell and the comparative electrophysiology of cortical neurons. Int J Neurol 1968; 6: 266–96.
105. Kandel ER, Hawkins RD. The biological basis of learning and individuality. Sci Am 1992; 267: 78–86.
106. Polich J, Squire LR. P300 from amnesic patients with bilateral hippocampal lesions. Electroencephalogr Clin Neurophysiol 1993; 86: 408–17.
107. Ji J, Porjesz B, Begleiter H, Chorlian D. P300: the similarities and differences in the scalp distribution of visual and auditory modality. Brain Topogr 1999; 11: 315–27.
108. Katayama J, Polich J. Auditory and visual P300 topography from a 3 stimulus paradigm. Clin Neurophysiol 1999; 110: 463–8.
109. Frodl-Bauch T, Bottlender R, Hegerl U. Neurochemical substrates and neuroanatomical generators of the event-related P300. Neuropsychobiology 1999; 40: 86–94.
110. Buchner H, Gobbele R, Waberski TD, Wagner M, Fuchs M. Evidence for independent thalamic and cortical sources involved in the generation of the visual 40 Hz response in humans. Neurosci Lett 1999; 269: 59–62.
111. Clark VP, Fannon S, Lai S, Benson R, Bauer L. Responses to rare visual target and distractor stimuli using event-related fMRI. J Neurophysiol 2000; 83: 3133–9.
112. Trinka E, Pfisterer G, Unterrainer J, et al. Multimodal event-related potential P3 after transient global amnesia. Eur J Neurol 2000; 7: 81–5.
113. Trinka E, Unterrainer J, Staffen W, Loscher NW, Ladurner G. Delayed visual P3 in unilateral thalamic stroke. Eur J Neurol 2000; 7: 517–22.
114. Tomberg C, Desmedt JE. Human perceptual processing: inhibition of transient prefrontal-parietal 40 Hz binding at P300 onset documented in non-averaged cognitive brain potentials. Neurosci Lett 1998; 255: 163–6.
115. Kotchoubey B, Lang S, Baales R, et al. Brain potentials in human patients with extremely severe diffuse brain damage. Neurosci Lett 2001; 301: 27–40.
116. Giorgianni R, Lo Presti R, D'Aleo G, Mondo N, Di Bella P, Bramanti P. Event-related potentials in patients in persistent vegetative state. Electroencephalogr Clin Neurophysiol 1997; 103: 149.
117. Keren O, Ben Dror S, Stern MJ, Goldberg G, Grosswasser Z. Event related potentials as an index of cognitive function during recovery from severe closed head injury. J Head Trauma Rehabil 1998; 13: 15–30.

6 Therapy

Leon Sazbon and Giuliano Dolce

Medical Therapy

As treatment for the vegetative state (VS) has become more and more effective, the number of patients surviving in conditions that make them largely or totally dependent on others has steadily increased. Recently, concerns have been raised as to whether the traditional aims of preserving life, recovering consciousness, and management of complications in this patient group are indeed justified [1]. This process has been accompanied by a growing preoccupation with public expenditure and the optimal usage of limited health-care resources. As a result, there has been a shift from the conservation of life per se to an emphasis on quality of life. Attention is being redirected toward reducing the risks of secondary cerebral lesions in the early course of VS and creating conditions that allow maximum recuperation of nervous functions and social rehabilitation [1,2].

Recovery from the vegetative state depends on several factors: the severity of the brain damage; the degree of dysfunction; successful activation of the neural systems blocked by ischemia, edema, or diaschisis; reconstruction of systems through regeneration or substitution with related intact systems; and transfer of functions to distant neural systems. Giacino and Zasler [3] distinguished between two types of intervention. Standard interventions include the assessment and treatment of basic medical problems such as skin breakdown, autonomic system dysfunction, muscular contractures, gastrointestinal problems, cardiopulmonary and genitourinary complications and infections; prophylactic management of high-risk complications such as deep vein thrombosis, pulmonary embolism, and heterotopic ossification; and treatment of late neurological complications that inhibit neurological recovery, such as normotensive hydrocephalus and post-traumatic epilepsy and agitation, and of electrolyte disturbances and neuroendocrine disorders. Supplementary interventions include enriched environmental stimuli, such as playing audiotapes of voices of loved ones or videocassettes showing family members, hanging posters displaying the patient's favorite pastimes, introducing contact with domestic animals or objects the patient would appreciate (for example, a basketball), use of sensory regulation or stimulation, administration of centrally active agents, and implantation of electrodes in deep brain structures. High-quality nursing is essential to optimize the chances of recovery.

The Quality Standards Subcommittee of the American Academy of Neurology [4] recommends that patients in the vegetative state receive appropriate medical, nursing, or nursing home care to maintain their personal dignity and hygiene.

Physicians and the family must determine the appropriate levels of treatment with regard to the administration or withdrawal of medications and other commonly ordered treatments; supplemental oxygen and antibiotics, complex organ-sustaining treatments such as dialysis, and administration of blood products and artificial hydration and nutrition.

Before any therapy is instituted, the risks must be weighed against the benefits. Drugs are often used in patients in the vegetative state, but since neuronal destruction is inevitable and irreversible, no specific pharmacotherapy exists. So far, the benefits have proven modest. There have as yet been no double-blind or placebo-controlled trials, and the results that have been reported are inconsistent. Indeed, medication may even have an adverse effect on the recovery rate. Giacino and Zasler [3] recommended that drug administration be kept to a minimum (preferably not polytherapy) to avoid inhibiting neural recovery or blurring the neurobehavioral presentation.

Types of Drug Used in the Vegetative State

Although none of the drugs available today can restore lost neural cells or influence one specific cerebral function over another less impaired one, some have been found to be of limited benefit. Those most worthy of consideration are the neurometabolic regulators and neurotransmitters, which activate cerebral metabolism or favor the transmission of nervous impulses in the synapses. The most extensive attention has been directed to levodopa or L-dopa, a dopaminergic agonist that has an activating effect on subcortical mechanisms involved in consciousness, behaviors related to the sleep–wake cycle, and motor regulation. By promoting the restoration of aminergic activities in the brain, L-dopa induces the recovery of damaged systems. Its use is supported by findings of a marked decrease in dopaminergic metabolites in the cerebrospinal fluid of patients in the vegetative state [2,5–10].

In addition, Vecht et al. [7] described changes in the metabolism of dopaminergic and serotonergic neurotransmitters in the chronic phase of the disease, while others authors [11–15] have reported a direct correlation between the severity of brain damage in the vegetative state and the level of homovanillic acid in cerebrospinal fluid.

In two clinical studies, Lal et al. [16] and Haig and Ruess [17] demonstrated the efficacy of levodopa/carbidopa (Sinemet) in the treatment of patients with severe brain damage. Using systemic administration of L-dopa, Higashi et al. [18] reported that at least two patients in the vegetative state in their series showed good recovery. Both responders were young adults with good cortical function, according to the initial electroencephalography (EEG) findings. Haig and Ruess [17] presented a similar anecdotal case of recovery from vegetative state in a 24-year-old man after 6 months of L-dopa treatment.

A similar action to L-dopa was reported for amantadine sulfate, which works presynaptically and postsynaptically, inducing the release of dopamine from its peripheral or central depots and elevating dopamine sensitivity in effector cells [19–22]. It reportedly clears neuroreceptor sites that have been blocked by false neurotransmitter substances [21] and is often used to antagonize the hypnotic effect of barbiturates. Zafonte et al. [23] reported on one patient in minimally responsive state who was successfully treated with amantadine five months after brain injury. In an interesting case report, Ross and Stewart [6] described the unsuccessful outcome of 2 months of treatment with methylphenidate (Ritalin) and carbidopa/levodopa in a patient in the vegetative state. Replacement of these drugs with lergotrile mesylate (amantadine) and bromocriptine, a dopamine agonist, led to progressive improvement and recovery of consciousness. Kugler [20] presented 16 patients in coma who were treated with amantadine intravenously and/or per os, with a remarkable brightening of the consciousness in six cases, while in another four the improvement was slight and transient. A successful response to bromocriptine alone was reported by Passler and Riggs [24], Müller and von Cramon [25], Pulasky and Emmett [26], and others [27,28]. Other neurotransmitters or their precursors, such as atropine [29], physostigmine [9], and galanthamine, a cholinesterase inhibitor [30], could theoretically produce similar results.

Amphetamines, which release dopamine and norepinephrine from storage vessels in the central nervous system, have shown promise in the treatment of agitation. Agitation is manifested by thrashing of the extremities, truncal rocking, dislodging of catheters, yelling, combativeness, and attempts to get out of bed. Reyes et al. [31] reported that patients with agitation in the vegetative state have a good outcome. This has been our experience as well. Haloperidol may also be effective in reducing aggressiveness in these patients and increasing attention and alertness [32]. However, it blocks or disrupts dopamine receptors in the brain. So far, there is no concrete evidence that patients who are treated with haloperidol have a better outcome than those who are not. Jackson et al. [33] used tricyclic antidepressants to treat agitation. Antidepressants have also been used in other phases of coma [34], but there is little chance that they substantially influence either the level of consciousness or the contents of the vegetative state.

Hornstein et al. [35] advocated the use of dextroamphetamine to enhance recovery in severely brain-damaged patients. The mechanism of action of the sympathomimetic amines is still unclear. They appear to increase the release of norepinephrine from the presynaptic neurons and block the synaptic reuptake of both norepinephrine and dopamine, thereby increasing catecholaminergic activity. They excite not only higher nervous structures, but also lower centers and peripheral receptors [23,35]. This results in improved alertness, concentration, initiative, and motor activity [35], but it also warrants stringent control of patients. Kaelin et al. [36] and Plenger [37] used methylphenidate to improve attention in brain-injured patients. However, negative results with stimulants were reported by Speech et al. [38] and Gualtieri and Evans [39]. Uranova et al. [40] noted that in patients with vegetative state, stimulants may augment neuronal plasticity and regeneration.

Calliauw and Marchau [41] and Hakkarainen and Hakamies [42] suggested the use of piracetam, a cyclic derivative of γ-aminobutyric acid (GABA), in the treatment of the restlessness preceding recovery. Piracetam is known to increase the adenosine triphosphate (ATP) turnover of cortical nerve cells, thereby increasing their energy potential and normalizing the lowered polyribosome/ribosome ratio. This protects the cerebral cortex against hypoxia. These authors reported that patients given piracetam regained a state of consciousness significantly superior to that of patients given placebo. However, clinicians should beware of prescribing piracetam to patients with hepatic or severe renal dysfunction. Once treatment is initiated, the drug should not be withdrawn abruptly. Another agent, meclofenoxate hydrochloride (Lucidril), may improve cellular metabolism in the presence of diminished oxygen concentration [43].

The lazaroids (21-aminosteroids), which have no glucocorticoid activity, are thought to promote neurological recovery by inhibiting lipid peroxidation at the cell membrane level [44–46]. However, these assumptions were not supported by Huang et al. [47] in a clinical trial. Although several therapeutic attempts have been made with exogenous gangliosides (glycosphingolipids) on the assumption that they increase neuronal sprouting or plasticity [48–50], there is little evidence that their use in humans is effective [51].

Cytidine diphosphate choline (CDP-choline, citicoline) is a chemotherapy regimen used experimentally and clinically in Japan that can apparently be safely administered by intrathecal infusion in therapeutic doses [52]. Citicoline is believed to induce the synthesis of lecithin, passing through the cerebrospinal fluid (CSF) barrier and acting directly on nerve tissue. It targets sites around the cerebral hemisphere and brain stem [43], making it a feasible agent for study in the treatment of vegetative state.

With regard to anticonvulsants as treatment of the vegetative state, Chatham and Netsky [53] recently treated a series of 13 patients with severe brain injury with lamotrigine, which has been found in animal studies to block sodium channels and inhibit glutamate release for up to several weeks after injury. This is the only study so far with this drug.

McClain et al. [54] reported on exaggerated urinary zinc secretion with concomitant hypozincemia in severely brain damaged patients, and Sandstead et al. [55] observed reduced DNA and RNA in male rats exposed to intrauterine zinc deficiency. Zinc alters neuroexcitability, thereby modifying the affinity of neurotransmitter receptors. This could be clinically manifested by alterations of consciousness [56]. Young et al. [57] stated that zinc supplementation is associated with a decreased rate of mortality and improved rate of neurologic recovery in patients in the vegetative state.

Sedatives are often prescribed to treat epilepsy or spasticity. Great care must be taken to ensure that the drug being used has the lowest feasible sedative activity, combined with the highest potential effectiveness. Rigorous and unrelenting control is mandatory with regard to both drug choice and dosage. Giacino and Zasler [3] suggested that spasticity be managed by physiotherapy, positioning and tone-reducing casts, motor point or nerve blocks, followed by enteral drugs. Muscle stimulants should be avoided, particularly in the early stages of vegetative state, when sleep is qualitatively and quantitatively reduced, and hypotonia is present.

Among other methods tried, the results of hyperbaric oxygenation seem to be encouraging in cases of acute coma; however, not enough experience has yet been gathered in patients in the vegetative state [58,59].

Our experience suggests that drug therapy does not influence the recovery of consciousness or the final functional outcome. The current state of knowledge is poor, however, and further research is needed to determine the precise value of drugs.

Deep Brain Electrical Stimulation

The role of neurostimulation therapy is probably one of the most controversial issues in the management of VS and low-level consciousness. Its use is based on the rationale that stimulation of the ascending reticular system will activate the cerebral cortex and facilitate recovery of consciousness [3].

The first attempt at neurostimulation therapy in VS was reported by Hassler et al. [60] in 1969. In this study, stereotactic electrical stimulation was applied to the internal lamella pallidi and base of the contralateral ventroanterior nucleus in two patients. The protocol was repeated several times daily for 3 weeks. A slight transitory arousal was achieved. Several years later, Stern et al. [61] reported on one patient successfully treated with chronic stimulation of the reticularis polaris nucleus of the thalamus.

More recently, Katayama et al. [62] noted that stimulation of the mesencephalic reticular formation led to transient increases in pain-related P250 in four of eight patients in VS. A persistent increase in P250, with clinical improvement, was produced by chronic stimulation of the mesencephalic reticular formation or nonspecific thalamic nuclei for more than 6 months. Definite improvement with some degree of interpersonal communication was also reported by Cohadon and Richer [63] in 13 of 25 patients who underwent bipolar stimulation with stereotactically implanted electrodes in the centrum medianum parafascicularis complex. Treatment was applied for 2 months, 12 h daily. In another study of eight patients, thalamic stimulation was applied every 2 h in the daytime for 30 min each time, over a period of 6 months [64]. Four of the patients showed apparent activation of the ascending reticular system, with a consequent increase in cerebral blood flow and glucose metabolism in both the cortex and thalamus, in addition to some neural plasticity in the central nervous system. The authors suggested that the treatment needs to be applied for at least 3–4 months to achieve emergence from VS.

Dorsal column stimulation was applied by Kanno and colleagues [65] for 4 h a day in four patients, three of whom showed an improvement in clinical condition and EEG findings. This study suggested that the underlying mechanism of stimulation therapy is a change in cerebral blood flow.

Finally, one group assessed the effects of cervical spinal cord stimulation in a patient in VS using positron emission tomography (PET) and single-photon emission computed tomography (SPECT) [66]. They found that that this technique activates glucose metabolism and increases cerebral blood flow.

Information on deep brain electrical stimulation in VS is still lacking. Before definitive conclusions can be reached on the value of this intervention, further studies are needed to determine the optimal timing of treatment after injury and methods of patient selection, and to define appropriate outcome measures.

Surgical Therapy

Severe brain injury may be associated with complications or sequelae that require surgical treatment. One of the most well-known complications is ventricular enlargement, or ventriculomegaly. This term is sometimes confusing, as it is an anatomic or imaging description. The clinical condition is referred to as hydrocephalus, and it results from an imbalance between the production and absorption of cerebrospinal fluid. According to Jennett and Teasdale [67], post-traumatic ventricular dilatation can be divided into three types, according to cause:
- Ex vacuo hydrocephalus, due to wasting of the white matter
- Obstructive hydrocephalus, due to meningeal adhesions and circulatory CSF abnormalities
- Normal-pressure or communicating hydrocephalus, due to CSF malabsorption

The dilatation may be widespread, involving the whole ventricular system, or it may be concentrated in the lateral ventricular system (central atrophy) or cortical sulci (cortical atrophy). Radiologically, empty images of the porencephalic type may be observed on brain computed tomography (CT) scans, with the cavities communicating with CSF passages [2,68].

Post-traumatic hydrocephalus usually occurs between 1 and 3 months from the date of injury. Diagnosis is based on a combination of clinical imaging findings and physiologic data. The majority of patients (81%) in the series reported by Matshushita et al. [69] showed subarachnoid hemorrhage on the first CT scan. In obstructive hydrocephalus, the presence of blood breakdown products in the CSF interferes with the normal rate of CSF absorption by the arachnoid villi [70]. In 1965, Adams et al. discovered that certain patients developed hydrocephalus despite a relatively normal CSF pressure [71]. They hypothesized that the decreased rate of CSF formation reaches an equilibrium with the impaired rate of absorption. Katz et al. [72] concluded that in these cases, the hydrocephalus was apparently the result of impaired CSF flow and absorption round the cerebral convexities, or of arachnoiditis due to blood in the subarachnoid space.

Incidence of Hydrocephalus

The reported incidence of post-traumatic ventricular enlargement ranges widely, from 0.7% to 86% [72–78]. Using a CSF dynamics technique, Marmarou et al. [79] found a 44% incidence of ventriculomegaly in survivors of severe brain injury. However, only 20% of these patients had true post-traumatic hydrocephalus (PTH), and their outcome was significantly worse.

There are only a few reports on ventricular enlargement specifically in patients in patients in the vegetative state. The reported rates were 25% in the study of Tribi and Oder [80], 37% in the study by Kaliski et al. [81], and 51% in the study by Sazbon and Groswasser [82,83]. Kaliski et al. [81] explained the wide differences among studies by the use of different methodologies to determine ventricular size.

Diagnosis and Treatment

The detection and correction of true PTH pose a challenge to clinicians.

Communicating hydrocephalus may be managed by ventricular shunting. It is particularly important to distinguish it from ex vacuo hydrocephalus, which is less responsive to shunting and for which there is no real treatment [3,67,75]. At the same time, patient selection for shunting is complicated. Communicating hydrocephalus is impossible to recognize clinically, because the classic triad of dementia, incontinence, and gait disturbances is not applicable in unconscious patients [80] and is often absent [67]. In cases of PTH, the CT scan typically shows enlarged ventricles without cortical atrophy, with maximal expansion in the frontal horns, an increase in the content of interstitial fluid in the periventricular tissue, and fibrosis and flattening of the choroid plexuses [84]. However, the etiologic accuracy of CT is uncertain, and the diversity of results is not encouraging [85,86]. Gudeman et al. [74] used CT to diagnose PTH on the basis of enlargement of the frontal and temporal horns and the third ventricle in the presence of normal or absent sulci. They reported that the presence of a periventricular translucency with dilatation of the fourth ventricle is not conclusive, because these findings are observed in the majority of patients with brain atrophy and do not distinguish an atrophic process from true hydrocephalus with transventricular edema. In addition, the abnormalities in CSF flow provoked by subarachnoid hemorrhage develop slowly. According to Marmarou et al. [79], 45% of patients with PTH show the characteristic dynamic CSF changes on CT scan. These become evident in 93% of those with ventriculomegaly within 2 months and then reach a plateau. Therefore, using CT to check for progressive changes in ventricular size as the only indicator of communicating hydrocephalus is misleading. Serial measurements are also not trustworthy, because patients with cerebral atrophy will also show an augmentation in ventricular size [79].

Radionuclide cisternography, a popular diagnostic technique, shows reflux into the ventricles and delayed pericerebral diffusion, with no radioactivity in the region of the superior sagittal sinus. However, some researchers, such as Narrayan et al. [87], failed to find any value in cisternography. Another potential diagnostic tool is continuous drainage or aspiration of large amounts of CSF in the lumbar space.

Pneumoencephalography is not currently used, because it often worsens the clinical state.

Marmarou et al. [79] introduced a novel approach, using an intrathecal bolus injection of 2–5 mL saline solution at a rate of 1 mL per second to evaluate CSF dynamics, which is correlated with ventricular size and outcome. Prior to the study, baseline intracranial pressure (ICP) was measured, and the pressure volume index (PVI) and resistance to CSF absorption (RO) were calculated. CSF pressure was measured just before each injection, and maximal pressure immediately after and some time later. The authors found that patients with communicating hydrocephalus (9.3% of the total sample of brain-injured patients) were characterized by normal baseline ICP, high RO and progressively decreasing PVI.

Jennett and Teasdale [67] recommended that the decision to perform shunt procedures should be based on the clinical evolution – arrest or regression in clinical progress – combined with progressive ventricular enlargement with ballooning of the third ventricle, without a clear dominant brain atrophy or massive loss of brain tissue.

The rationale for shunting is based on the fact that the insertion of one-way valves set at the desired pressure allows the escape of CSF into the pleural or peritoneal cavity or into the cardiac atrium, leading to a decrease in intraventricular pressure to the predetermined level. Katz et al. [72] stated that shunting is generally successful if the lumbar CSF pressure is above 180 mmH$_2$O and there is a progressive increase in ventricular size on the CT scan. They claimed that ventriculoperitoneal shunting is the treatment of choice, because of the ability of the peritoneal cavity to accept a large loop of tubing, combined with the relatively benign complications of the procedure and the ease of shunt revision. Ventriculoatrial shunting is indicated in the presence of abdominal abnormalities (previous extensive surgery, extreme obesity, etc.).

Outcome of Surgery

There is little information about the outcome of severe traumatic brain injury after shunt implantation. Usually, the ventricles decrease in size within 3–4 days, and clinical improvement occurs in the next few weeks [84].

Cardoso and Galbraith [85] reported a marked improvement in consciousness in 50% of 17 patients and a slight improvement in 25%. In the series reported by Sazbon and Grosswasser, 41% of patients recovered consciousness [83]. Improvement rates of 50% were also reported by Noubourg et al. [88] and Narrayan et al. [87]. More recently, Tribl and Oder [80] noted a 52% rate of improvement of various degrees at 3 months after shunting. The highest rates were reported by Matshushita [69] (77%) and Meyer et al. [89], Stein and Langfitt [90], and Vasshiloutis [91] (100% recovery of consciousness).

Graff-Radford [92] reported a 30% rate of complications, and Tribl and Oder [80] reported 41%. Complications of shunting include subdural hygroma or hematoma due to rupture of the bridging dural veins. This tends to occur when drainage is done too rapidly. Ventricular hemorrhage is also possible due to technological problems. Infection of the catheter or the valve can lead to encephalitis, peritonitis, pleural empyema, or sepsis [71,84]. The majority of infections occur 2–3 months after surgery [72], and the most common culprit organisms are *Staphylococcus epidermidis* and *S. aureus*. Treatment consists of removing the infected shunts and administering appropriate antibiotics. According to Katz et al. [72], infections occur in 5–39% of cases.

Another frequent complication is occlusion of the catheter tip by brain tissue or choroid plexus, resulting in revision of the shunt. In the study of Tribl and Oder [80], 31% of patients required shunt revision. These authors also reported the occurrence of epileptic seizures in 10% of patients immediately after shunt implantation and in 35% at a mean of 23 weeks later.

Stimulation Techniques

The last 20 years have witnessed a growing interest in sensory stimulation for the treatment of patients in the vegetative state. Together with the current high-technology approach of monitoring, machine support, and aggressive medical care, stimulation programs have found a place in the rehabilitation of acute and long-term unconscious patients. Their use is based on the rationale that both the degree and quality of recuperation is increased when attention is directed to the whole patient, and not to bodily well-being alone [93–96].

The concept of sensory stimulation programs for brain-injured patients was prompted by early studies on cognitive growth showing that children who were exposed to stimuli-enriched environments had better neurophysiological development than children who were not [97]. Later support was provided by experimental data from animals with cerebral lesions or after sensory deprivation [98–100]. In 1977, Greenberg et al. [101] and Hume et al. [102] independently reported that comatose patients respond to certain sensory stimuli. To explain this finding, Kater [103] suggested that head injury causes a disorganization of neuronal accessory pathways essential for cognitive functions and that sensory stimulation could activate those parts of the nervous system on which consciousness depends. This assumption was supported by the study by Walsh [99] confirming that the brain increases in both dimension and weight in a stimulus-rich environment. In addition, in the work of Finger and Stein [104], brain-injured patients exposed to a wide variety of stimulating experiences were found to develop an extensive functional neuronal circuitry that was lacking in restricted subjects. LeWinn and Dimancescu [105] argued that if sensory deprivation could change cerebral electric activity and produce widespread impairment of intellectual and perceptual processes in non–brain-damaged patients, we could expect that in brain-injured patients, the greater and richer the stimulation, the better the prospects for recovery.

Sensory stimulation in comatose patients is directed at the reticular system, which has a much higher sensory-stimulation threshold than other systems in the body, lowering it and thereby reducing deprivation levels. Because unconscious patients have short potential reactivity periods, the stimuli are given for very short periods of time, and efforts are made to avoid overstimulation. Apparently, better cognitive functioning is achieved when stimulation is focused on previously learned or recognized patterns [103].

Recently, Wood [106] introduced a new technique of sensory regulation (not stimulation) to prevent patient overstimulation and consequent habituation to stimuli. The technique involves limiting all sources of continuous ambient noise, such as television and radio, so that the environment is kept quiet and restful. The staff are instructed to regulate their activities and movements and to speak slowly and quietly to the patient, using certain key words (telegraphic speech). The author claimed that for best results, patients need to be exposed to long periods of silence interspersed with therapy sessions.

There are certain preliminary conditions for the success of sensory stimulation. The presence of a brain-stem lesions might block the path of the sensory stimuli [107]. In addition, prior to initiating the program, clinicians must ensure that patient use of sedatives and antiepileptics is minimized, because these drugs tend to lower sensory stimulation thresholds and reduce the efficiency of the environmental input [107].

Types and Techniques of Sensory Stimulation

There are two types of sensory stimulation, and it is important to differentiate between them. Environmental stimulation is based on the assumption that sensory deprivation should be prevented. Patients are subjected to ongoing, variable, unstructured stimuli of all types, which are presented in an unsystematic fashion [3,108]. Some activities for higher-functioning patients encourage passive participation. Environmental treatment strategies continue to be widely used in clinical practice, despite the absence of any published reports on their effectiveness. By contrast, structured stimulation introduces stimuli in a labor-intensive, systematic fashion [108]. Both types apply stimuli directed at all five senses: auditory (familiar voices, radio, music), visual (familiar members and friends, posters, familiar objects), tactile (personal clothing, blankets, stuffed animals, and real pets), olfactory (favorite odors, perfumes, foods), and gustatory (favorite flavors, sharp spices such as lemon, cinnamon) [103,105–107,109–114].

In 1990, Aldridge et al. [109] developed a form of stimulation therapy using music for the rehabilitation of comatose patients. The concept was based on the belief that the self is more than a corporeal entity and that human beings are organized not mechanically, but musically, "in a harmonic complex of interacting rhythms and melodic contours." To maintain our coherence with the world, we must creatively improvise our identity, and "music therapy is the medium by which a coherent organization is regained, i.e., linking brain, body and mind." This method yielded a range of reactions, from a change in breathing and fine motor movements to grabbing movements of the hands and turning of the head, to opening the eyes and the regaining of consciousness.

On the basis of this study, Sazbon (personal communication) recently applied six different types of melody in a sensory stimulation program. He used classical pieces broken into 15-min segments of quiet and constant listening periods. Each piece had a different tempo and rhythm. In each patient, the rhythm used was lower than the individual heart rate. This method is still in the experimental stage.

Wood [106] postulated that in normal individuals, a neural system can be "dishabituated" by exposure to an alternative stimulus or a more intense stimulus, either in the same or a different modality.

The effect of unimodal versus multimodal stimulation was examined using stimuli of known personal salience to the patients. Arousal was measured by the total frequency of eye-opening and spontaneous eye movements. Significant changes were noted immediately after treatment in four patients subjected to multimodal stimulation; in some of them, the effect continued to be observed as late as 28 months after injury [112]. Older patients showed a greater frequency of eye-opening. There was no relationship between time since injury or magnitude of response and mode of stimulation, although some individuals seemed to be particularly responsive to the unimodal type [106].

The frequency and duration of sensory stimulation vary considerably among the published reports [115,116]. For example, LeWinn [95] advocated at least 36 repetitions of the stimulation procedure per day, and Wilson et al. [113] used two treatment sessions daily 3 weeks apart, repeated with certain variants. The program used by Kater [103] was conducted for 5 min, 6 days a week for 3 months, whereas that of Mitchell et al. [111] was applied for 1 h twice daily, with no limit on duration. The music therapy program described by Aldridge et al. [109] lasted 12 min. By contrast, Feldman [107] used music stimulation for 25 min or 45 min, depending on the intensity and frequency of the sound, once or twice daily. These authors reported that after 20 min, a decrease in patient agitation could be observed (not reaching the level of relaxation), with a decrease in cardiac rhythm and arterial pressure. The reaction lasted 2–3 h after termination of the stimulus.

Assessment and Outcome

The response to treatment is measured by the reflex responses to auditory stimulation, voluntary motor response, phonation, recognition capability, and reduction of spasticity [107]. Sensory stimulation may provoke the appearance of a K-complex in the EEG. Many researchers have reported a positive influence of sensory stimulation programs in comatose patients [105,111,117–119]. Sisson [120] obtained a behavioral or alerting response on EEG in five treated patients, and Kater [103] reported a significant effect in 15 patients. Wilson et al. [113] noted a significant increase in arousal in 24 subjects immediately after treatment. The group who emerged from VS showed higher rates of spontaneous movements. However, these kinds of response may show up only during stimulation, and they do not imply clinical improvement [107]. Indeed, the effectiveness of sensory stimulation remains a strongly controversial issue [108,121], and there is as yet no evidence that sensory stimulation leads to a better outcome than conventional treatment [115]. The major problem is the lack of comparability between studies, due to wide differences in the intervals since the onset of brain injury, poor descriptions of cognitive status and of complications, and lack of information on patient selection. In addition, a great number of the studies conducted to date have been methodologically poor, with small samples, lack of a control group, and absence of peer review [111,117–120]. These factors are compounded by the difficulty, specific to this patient group, in distinguishing the effect of sensory stimulation from spontaneous recovery, possible effects of environmental stimuli, and effects of other treatments over which the coma therapist has no control [112,122]. Two other major areas that require clarification are the standards for identifying progress secondary to treatment and for decision-making with regard to continuation or reduction of treatment [96]. Some of these problems could be resolved by stringent examination of patients before and immediately after sensory stimulation sessions. Moreover, examiners must be made aware that they need to assess changes in awareness, not in arousal.

Several scales have been designed specifically to evaluate the response to sensory stimulation in patients in the vegetative state and to standardize assessments. These include the Coma/Near-Coma Scale erase [124], the Coma Recovery Scale [125], the Disability Rating Scale [123], the Sensory Stimulation Assessment Measure [116], the Western Neuro-Sensory Profile [126], the Rancho Los Amigos Levels of Cognitive Functioning [127], the Sensory Modality Assessment Rehabilitation Technique [110], and the Coma Exit Chart [128,129].

It should also be stressed that the results of sensory stimulation may be affected by many injury-related, treatment-related, or patient-related factors, as well as environmental factors. These include the type and severity of brain damage, time since trauma, and neurological status; the rate and duration of sessions; the patient's age and educational level; and frequency of family visits. Studies by Rader et al. [96] indicated that some of these factors may be predictive of improvement over time. For example, earlier initiation of rehabilitation programs after injury can maximize the ultimate potential for recovery [111,130,131]. With regard to external factors, studies have shown that better results are achieved in patients who were exposed to an enriched environment prior to the head injury [132]. Kater [103] reported that patients with moderate scores on the Glasgow Coma Scale, of between 7 and 10, achieved the highest mean cognitive scores, similar to those in patients who came from an enriched environment. Accordingly, patients who have strong family support seem to do better than those who do not [132]; and today, clinicians tend to encourage visible active intervention by the family in the programs [96]. Finally, optimal responsiveness cannot be achieved without a high degree of interpersonal (verbal, emotional enthusiasm) relatedness on the part of the therapist.

Other Potential Advantages

Clinicians should not overlook the comfort that participation in a structured stimulation program provides to both staff and family members. It gives them the sense that everything possible is being done to help the patient. It also helps relieve the anxiety and feelings of impotence that are sometimes accompany continuous passive care [133]. Family members feel more control over the situation, and staff members enjoy greater job satisfaction. These in turn lead to a better level of care for the patient.

Conclusions

Despite the few positive findings reported in the literature, there is at present no concrete evidence that sensory simulation definitively alters or facilitates the course of recovery [108,125]. The *International Working Party Report on the Vegetative State* [134] recently concluded that sensory regulation by itself does not lead to mental recuperation, although it may enhance sensory conditions by regulating the environmental noise with alternate periods of treatment and nursing care. Wood [106] cautioned that the use of sensory stimulation is not endorsed by current knowledge on brain processes and sensory input in normal and damaged brains. This problem is exacerbated by the lack of standardization and poor methodology. Clinicians should therefore beware of raising unreasonable expectations among family and staff members.

Further, better-controlled studies are needed on this subject.

References

1. Bricolo A, Turazzi S, Feriotti G. Prolonged post-traumatic unconsciousness. J Neurosurg 1980; 52: 625–34.
2. Bricolo A. Prolonged post traumatic coma. In: Vinken P, Bruyn GW, editors. Handbook of clinical neurology, vol 23. Amsterdam: North-Holland, 1975: 699–755.
3. Giacino JT, Zasler ND. Outcome after severe traumatic brain injury: coma, the vegetative state, and the minimally responsive state. J Head Trauma Rehabil 1995; 10: 40–56.
4. Quality Standards Subcommittee of the American Academy of Neurology. Practice parameters: assessment and management of patients in the persistent vegetative state. Neurology 1995; 45: 1015–28.
5. Higashi H, Sakata Y, Hatano M, et al. Epidemiological studies on patients with a persistent vegetative state. J Neurol Neurosurg Psychiatry 1977; 40: 876–85.
6. Ross ED, Stewart RM. Akinetic mutism from hypothalamic damage: successful treatment with dopamine agonists. Neurology 1981; 31: 1435–9.
7. Vecht CJ, Van Woercom TC, Teelken AW, et al. On the nature of brain stem disorders in severe head injured patients, 1: changes in cerebral neurotransmitter metabolism. Acta Neurochir 1976; 34: 11–21.
8. Binder H, Getstenbrand F. Post-traumatic vegetative state. In: Vinken P, Bruyn GW, editors. Handbook of neurology, vol 24. Amsterdam: North-Holland, 1976: 575–98.
9. Van Woerkom TC, Minderhoud JM, Gottschal T, et al. Neurotransmitters in the treatment of patients with severe head injuries. Eur Neurol 1982; 21: 227–34.
10. Sazbon L. Prolonged coma. Prog Clin Neurosci 1985; 2: 65–81.
11. Korf J, van Praag HM. Amine metabolism in the human brain: further evaluation of the probenecid test. Brain Res 1971; 35: 221–30.
12. Lakken JP, Korf J, van Praag HM, et al. Clinical significance of probenecid test. Lancet 1971; 1: 614–5.
13. Olsson R, Roos BE. Concentrations of 5-hydroxyindoleacetic acid and homovanillic acid in the cerebrospinal fluid after treatment with probenecid in patients with Parkinson's disease. Nature 1968; 219: 502–3.
14. Sachs E. Acetylcholine and serotonin in the spinal fluid. J Neurosurg 1957; 14: 22–7.
15. Bowers MB. CSF homovanilic acid: effects of probenecid and alpha-methyl thyrosine. Life Sci 1970; 9: 691–4.
16. Lal S, Merbitz C, Grip J. Modification of function in head-injured patients with Sinemet. Brain Inj 1990; 2: 225–33.
17. Haig A, Ruess J. Recovery from vegetative state of six months' duration associated with Sinemet (levodopa/carbidopa). Arch Phys Med Rehabil 1990; 71: 1081–3.

18. Higashi H, Hatano M, Abiko S, et al. Five-year follow up study of patients with persistent vegetative state. J Neurol Neurosurg Psychiatry 1982; 44: 552–4.
19. Opel F, Klaes H. Die Amantidinsulfat-infusion in der Akut-Behandlung des Morbus Parkinson. Klinikarzt 1982; 10: 559–62.
20. Kugler J. Action of aminoadamantane sulphate on vigilance and consciousness. Aktuelle Neurol 1975; 2: 43–51.
21. Wallnofer H, Schiller L. Aminoadamantane treatment of comatose patients. Med Welt 1974; 25: 703–6.
22. Horiguchi J, Inami Y, Shoda T. Effects of long term amantadine treatment on clinical symptoms and EEG of a patient in a vegetative state. Clin Neuropharmacol 1990; 13: 84–8.
23. Zafonte RD, Watanabe T, Mann NR. Amantadine: a potential treatment for the minimally conscious state. Brain Inj 1998; 7: 617–21.
24. Passler MSA, Riggs RV. Positive outcomes in traumatic brain injury–vegetative state: patients treated with bromocriptine. Arch Phys Med Rehabil 2001; 82: 311–5.
25. Müller U, von Cramon DY. The therapeutic potential of bromocriptine in neuropsychological rehabilitation of patients with acquired brain damage. Prog Neuropsychopharmacol Biol Psychiatry 1994; 18: 1103–20.
26. Pulasky KH, Emmett L. The combined intervention of therapy and bromocriptine mesylate to improve functional performance after brain injury. Am J Occup Ther 1994; 48: 263–70.
27. Luciana M, Depue RA, Arbisi P, et al. Facilitation of working memory in humans by a D2 dopamine receptor agonist. J Cogn Neurosci 1992; 4: 58–68.
28. McDowell S, White J, D'Sposito M. Differential effect of dopaminergic agonists in traumatic brain injured patients. Brain 1998; 121: 1155–64.
29. Faden AI. Pharmacological treatment of central nervous system trauma. Pharmacol Toxicol 1996; 78: 12–7.
30. Luria AR, Naydin VL, Tsvetkova LS, et al. Restoration of higher cortical functions following local brain damage. In: Vinken PJ, Bruyn GW, editors. Handbook of clinical neurology, part 3: disorders of high nervous activity. Amsterdam: North-Holland, 1969: 368–433.
31. Reyes RL, Bhattacharyya AK, Heller D. Traumatic head injury: restlessness and agitation as prognosticators of physical and psychologic improvement in patients. Arch Phys Med Rehabil 1981; 62: 20–3.
32. Rao N, Jellinek HM. Agitation in closed head injury: haloperidol effects on rehabilitation outcome. Arch Phys Med Rehabil 1985; 66: 30–4.
33. Jackson RD, Corrigan JD, Arnett JA. Amitryptiline for agitation in head injury. Arch Phys Med Rehabil 1985; 66: 180–1.
34. Reinhard D, Whyte J, Sander M. Improved arousal and initiation following tricyclic antidepressant use in traumatic brain injury. Arch Phys Med Rehabil 1996; 77: 80–3.
35. Hornstein A, Lennihan L, Seliger G, et al. Amphetamine in recovery from brain injury. Brain injury 1996; 10: 145–8.
36. Kaelin D, Cifu D, Maithes B. Metylphenidate effect on attention deficit in the acutely brain injured adult study. Arch Phys Med Rehabil 1996; 77: 6–9.
37. Plenger P. Subacute metylphenidate treatment for moderate to moderately severe brain injury: a preliminary double blind study. Arch Phys Med Rehabil 1996; 77: 536–40.
38. Speech T, Rao SM, Osmon DC, et al. A double-blind controlled study of methylphenidate treatment in closed head injury. Brain Inj 1993; 7: 333–8.
39. Gualtieri CT, Evans RW. Stimulant treatment for neurobehavioral sequelae of traumatic brain injury. Brain Inj 1988; 2: 273–90.
40. Uranova NA, Klinzova AJ, Istomin VV, et al. The effects of amphetamine on synaptic plasticity in rat's medial prefrontal cortex. J Hirnforsch 1989; 30: 45–9.
41. Calliauw L, Marchau M. Clinical trial of piracetam in disorders of consciousness due to head injury. Acta Anaesth Belg 1975; 26: 51–60.
42. Hakkarainen H, Hakamies L. Piracetam in the treatment of post-concussional syndrome: a double-blind study. Eur Neurol 1978; 17: 50–5.
43. Parfitt K, editor. Martindale: The complete drug reference. 32nd ed. London: Pharmaceutical Press, 1999: 1599.
44. Braughler JM, Hall ED, Jacobsen EJ, et al. The 21-aminosteroids: potent inhibitors of lipid peroxidation for the treatment of central nervous system trauma and ischemia. Drugs Future 1989; 14: 143–52.
45. Hall ED, Yonkers PA, McCall, et al. Effects of the 21-aminosteroid U74006F on experimental head injury in mice. J Neurosurg 1988; 68: 456–61.
46. McCall JM, Braughler JM, Hall ED. A new class of compounds for stroke and trauma: effects of 21-aminosteropids on lipid peroxidation. Acta Anaesthesiol Belg 1987; 38: 417–20.
47. Huang H, Patel PB, Salahudeen AK. Lazaroid compounds prevent early but not late stages of oxidant-induced cell injury: potential explanation for the lack of efficacy of lazaroids

48. Karpiak SE, Li YS, Mahadik SP. Ganglioside treatment: reduction of CNS injury and facilitation of functional recovery. Brain Inj 1987; 1: 161–70.
49. Karpiak SE. Exogenous gangliosides enhance recovery from CNS injury. Adv Exp Med Biol 1984; 174: 489–97.
50. Sabel BA, Slavin MD, Stein DG. GM1 ganglioside treatment facilitates behavioral recovery from bilateral brain damage. Science 1984; 225: 340–2.
51. Nobile-Orazio E, Carpo M, Scarlato G. Gangliosides: their role in clinical neurology. Drugs 1994; 47: 576–85.
52. Ogashiwa M, Takeuchi K. Intrathecal pharmacotherapy in coma. Acta Neurochirurg 1976; 34: 37–44.
53. Chatham PE, Netsky D. Stimulating consciousness and cognition following severe brain injury: a new potential use for lamotrigine. Brain Inj 2000; 11: 997–1001.
54. McClain CJ, Twyman DL, Ott LG, et al. Serum and urine zinc response in head-injured patients. J Neurosurg 1986; 64: 224–30.
55. Sandstead HH, Fosmire GJ, McKenzie AR, et al. Zinc deficiency and brain development in the rat. Fed Proc 1975; 34: 86–8.
56. Kassarskis EJ. Regulation of zinc hemostasis in rat brain. In: Frederickson CJ, Howell GA, Kassarskis EJ, editors. The neurobiology of zinc, part A: physiochemistry, anatomy and techniques. New York: Liss, 1984: 27–37.
57. Young B, Ott L, Kassarskis E, et al. Zinc supplementation is associated with improved neurologic recovery rate and visceral protein levels of patients with severe closed head injury. J Neurotrauma 1996; 13: 25–34.
58. Artru F, Chacornac R, Deleuze R. Hyperbaric oxigenation for severe head injuries. Eur Neurology 1976; 14: 310–8.
59. Phillippon B, Munsch RC. Etude des variations de débit sanguine cerebral après oxigenation hyperbare dans le coma traumatique. Neurochirurgie 1975; 21: 483–92.
60. Hassler R, Dalle Ore G, Dieckman G, et al. Behavioural and EEG arousal induced by stimulation of unspecific projection systems in a patient with post-traumatic apallic syndrome. Neurophysiology 1969; 27: 306–10.
61. Stern V, Kuhner A, Schmitt HP, et al. Chronic electrical stimulation of the thalamic unspecific activating system in a patient with coma due to midbrain and upper brain stem infarction. Acta Neurochir 1979; 47: 235–44.
62. Katayama Y, Tsubokawa T, Yamamoto T, et al. Characterization and modification of brain activity with deep brain stimulation in patients in a persistent vegetative state: pain-related late positive component of cerebral evoked potential. Pacing Clin Electrophysiol 1991; 14: 116–21.
63. Cohadon F, Richer E. Deep cerebral stimulation in patients with post-traumatic vegetative state: 25 cases. Neurochirurgie 1993; 39: 281–92.
64. Tsubokawa T, Yamamoto T, Katayama Y, et al. Deep-brain stimulation in a persistent vegetative state: follow-up results and criteria for selection of candidates. Brain Inj 1990; 4: 315–27.
65. Kanno T, Kamei Y, Yokoyama T, et al. Neurostimulation for patients in vegetative state. Pacing Clin Electrophysiol 1987; 10: 207–8.
66. Momose T, Matsui T, Kosaka N, et al. Effects of cervical spinal cord stimulation on cerebral glucose metabolism and blood flow in vegetative patients assessed by positron emission tomography (PET) and single positron emission computed tomography (SPECT). Radiat Med 1989; 7: 243–6.
67. Jennett B, Teasdale G. Management of head injuries. Philadelphia: Davis, 1981.
68. Sazbon L. Prolonged coma. Prog Clin Neurosci 1985; 2: 65–81.
69. Matshushita H, Takahashi K, Maeda Y, et al. A clinical study of post-traumatic hydrocephalus [abstract]. No Shinkei Geka 2000; 28: 773–9.
70. Ellington E, Margolis G. Block of arachnoid villus by subarachnoid hemorrhage. J Neurosurg 1969; 30: 651–7.
71. Adams RD, Fisher CM, Hakim S, et al. Symptomatic occult hydrocephalus with "normal" cerebrospinal pressure. N Engl J Med 1965; 273: 117–26.
72. Katz RT, Brander V, Sahgal V. Updates on the diagnosis and management of post-traumatic hydrocephalus. Am J Phys Med Rehabil 1989; 68: 91–6.
73. Bontke CF, Zasler ND, Boake C. Rehabilitation of the head-injured patient. In: Narayan RK, Wilberger JE, Povlishock JT, editors. Neurotrauma. New York: McGraw-Hill, 1996: 841–58.
74. Gudeman KS, Kishore PR, Becker DP. Computed tomography in the evaluation of incidence and significance of post-traumatic hydrocephalus. Radiology 1981; 141: 397–402.
75. Guyot LL, Michael DB. Post-traumatic hydrocephalus. Neurol Res 2000; 22: 25–8.
76. Herrmann HD. Neurotrumatologie. Weinheim, Germany: VCH, 1991: 185–6.
77. Kampfl A, Franz G, Aichner F, et al. The persistent vegetative state after closed head injury: clinical and magnetic resonance imaging find-

ings in 42 patients. J Neurosurg 1998; 88: 809–16.
78. Kishore PR, Lipper MH, Miller JD. Post-traumatic hydrocephalus in patients with severe head injury. Neuroradiology 1978; 16: 261–5.
79. Marmarou A, Montasser A, Abd-Elfattah F, et al. Post-traumatic ventriculomegaly; hydrocephalus or atrophy? A new approach for diagnosis using CSF dynamics. J Neurosurg 1996; 85: 1026–35.
80. Tribl G, Oder W. Outcome after shunt implantation in severe head injury with post-traumatic hydrocephalus. Brain Inj 2000; 14: 345–54.
81. Kaliski Z, Morrison DP, Meyers CA, et al. Medical problems encountered during rehabilitation of patients with head injury. Arch Phys Med Rehabil 1985; 66: 25–9.
82. Sazbon L, Groswasser Z. Outcome in 134 patients with prolonged post-traumatic unawareness, 1: parameters determining late recovery of consciousness. J Neurosurg 1990; 72: 75–80.
83. Sazbon L, Groswasser Z. Medical complications and mortality of patients in the postcomatose unawareness (PC-U) state. Acta Neurochir 1991; 112: 110–2.
84. Adams RD, Victor M. Principles of neurology. 4th ed. New York: McGraw-Hill, 1989: 507–9.
85. Cardoso ER, Galbraith S. Post-traumatic hydrocephalus: a retrospective review. Surg Neurol 1985; 23: 261–4.
86. Zander E, Forogou G. Post-traumatic hydrocephalus. In: Vinken P, Bruyn G, editors. Handbook of clinical neurology, vol 24: injuries of the brain and skull, part II. Amsterdam: North-Holland, 1976: 231–53.
87. Narrayan RK, Gokaslan ZL, Bontke CF, et al. Neurological sequelae of head injury. In: Rosenthal M, Griffith ER, Bond MR, editors. Rehabilitation of the adult and child with traumatic head injury. Philadelphia: Davis, 1990: 94–106.
88. Noubourg Y, Garcia C, De Mol J, et al. Normotensive hydrocephalus: retrospective clinical study of 47 cases. Ann Med Psychol (Paris) 1982; 140: 1077–95.
89. Meyer JS, Kitagawa Y, Tanahashi N, et al. Evaluation of treatment of normal-pressure hydrocephalus. J Neurosurg 1985; 62: 513–21.
90. Stein SC, Langfitt TW. Normal pressure hydrocephalus: predicting the results of cerebrospinal fluid shunting. J Neurosurg 1974; 41: 463–70.
91. Vasshiloutis J. The syndrome of normal-pressure hydrocephalus. J Neurosurg 1984; 61: 501–9.
92. Graff-Radford NR. Symptomatic or normal pressure hydrocephalus in the elderly. In: Feinberg TE, Para MJ, editors. Behavioral neurology and neuropsychology. New York: McGraw-Hill, 1997: 627–37.
93. De Young S, Grass RB. Coma recovery program. Rehabil Nursing 1987; 12: 121–4.
94. Johnson DA, Roethig-Johnston K. Coma stimulation: a challenge to occupational therapy. Br J Occup Ther 1988; 51: 88–90.
95. LeWinn EB. The coma arousal team: procedures for the patient's professional attendants and for his family. R Soc Health J 1980; 100: 19–21.
96. Rader MA, Alston JB, Ellis DW. Sensory stimulation of severely brain-injured patients. Brain Inj 1989; 3: 141–7.
97. Bruner JS. The course of cognitive growth. Am Psychologist 1964; 19: 1–15.
98. Schwartz S. Effect of neocortical lesions and early environmental factors on adult rat behaviour. J Comp Physiol Psychol 1964; 57: 72–7.
99. Walsh R. Sensory environments, brain damage, and drugs: a review of interactions and mediating mechanisms. Int J Neurosci 1981; 14: 129–37.
100. Will BE, Rosenzweig MR. Effets de l'environnement sur la récupération functionelle après lésions cérébrales chez les rats adultes. Biol Behav 1976; 1: 5–16.
101. Greenberg RP, Mayer DJ, Becker DP, et al. Evaluation of brain function in severe human head trauma with multimodality evoked potentials. J Neurosurg 1977; 47: 150–62.
102. Hume AL, Cant BR, Shaw NA. Central sensory conduction time in comatose patients. Ann Neurol 1977; 5: 379–84.
103. Kater KM. Response of head-injured patients to sensory stimulation. West J Nurs Res 1989; 11: 20–3.
104. Finger SA, Stein DG. Brain damage and recovery. New York: Academic Press, 1982.
105. LeWinn EB, Dimancescu MD. Environmental deprivation and enrichment in coma. Lancet 1978; 2: 156–7.
106. Wood RL. Critical analysis of the concept of sensory stimulation for patients in vegetative states. Brain Inj 1991; 5: 401–9.
107. Feldman D. [Lecture presented at Ospedale Don Calabria, Verona, Italy, 1992.]
108. Zasler ND, Kreutzer JS, Taylor D. Coma stimulation and coma recovery: a critical review. Neurorehabilitation 1991; 1: 33–40.
109. Aldridge D, Gustorff D, Hannich HJ. Where am I? Music therapy applied to coma patients. J R Soc Med 1990; 83: 345–346.
110. Gill-Thwaites H. The sensory modality assessment technique: a tool for assessment and treatment of patients with severe brain injury

in a vegetative state. Brain Inj 1997; 11: 723–34.
111. Mitchell S, Bradley VA, Welch JL. Coma arousal procedure: a therapeutic intervention in the treatment of head injury. Brain Inj 1990; 4: 273–9.
112. Wilson SL, Powell GE, Elliots K, et al. Sensory stimulation in prolonged coma: four single case studies. Brain Inj 1991; 5: 393–400.
113. Wilson SL, Powell GE, Brock D, et al. Behavioural differences between patients who emerged from vegetative state and those who did not. Brain Inj 1996; 10: 509–16.
114. Wilson SL, Powell GE, Brock D, et al. Vegetative state and responses to sensory stimulation: an analysis of 24 cases. Brain Inj 1996; 10: 807–18.
115. Pierce JP, Lyle DM, Quine S, et al. The effectiveness of coma arousal intervention. Brain Inj 1990; 4: 191–7.
116. Rader MA, Ellis DW. The Sensory Stimulation Assessment Measure (SSAM): a tool for early evaluation of severely brain injured patients. Brain Inj 1994; 8: 309–21.
117. Boyle ME, Green RD. Operant procedure and the comatose patient. J Appl Behav Anal 1983; 16: 3–12.
118. Rosadini G, Sannita WG. Inter- and intra-hemispheric topographic analyses of quantitative EEG in patients in coma. Res Commun Psychol Psychiatry Behav 1982; 7: 97–107.
119. Weber PL. Sensorimotor therapy: its effects on electroencephalograms of acute comatose patients. Arch Phys Med Rehabil 1984; 65: 457–62.
120. Sisson R. Effects of auditory stimuli on comatose patients with head injury. Heart Lung 1990; 19: 373–8.
121. Wilson SL, MacMillan TM. Review of the evidence of the effectiveness of sensory stimulation treatment for coma and vegetative state. Neuropsychol Rehabil 1993; 3: 149–60.
122. White J, DiPasquale MC, Vaccaro M. Assessment of command-following in minimally conscious brain injured patients. Arch Phys Med Rehabil 1999; 80: 653–60.
123. Rappaport M, Hall KM, Hopkins HK, et al. Disability Rating Scale for severe head trauma patients: coma to community. Arch Phys Med Rehabil 1982; 63: 118–23.
124. Rappaport MD, Allison Dougherty BA, Devon L, et al. Evaluation of coma and vegetative states. Arch Phys Med Rehabil 1992; 73: 628–34.
125. Giacino JT, Kezmarsky MA, Deluca J, Cicerone KD. Monitoring rate of recovery to predict outcome in minimally responsive recovery. Arch Phys Med Rehabil 1991; 72: 897–901.
126. Ansell B, Keenan JE. The Western Neuro Sensory Stimulation Profile: a tool for assessing slow-to-recover head injury patients. Arch Phys Med Rehabil 1989; 70: 104–8.
127. Hagen C, Malkmus D, Durham P. Rehabilitation of the head injured adult: comprehensive physical management. Downey, CA: Professional Staff Association of Rancho Los Amigos Hospital, 1979.
128. Freeman EA. The Coma Exit Chart: assessing the patient in prolonged coma and vegetative state. Brain Inj 1996; 10: 615–24.
129. Freeman EA. The catastrophe of coma: a way back. Buderim, Queensland: Bateman, 1987.
130. Cope N, Hall K. Head injury rehabilitation: benefit of early intervention. Arch Phys Med Rehabil 1982; 63: 433–7.
131. Rush HA, Block JM, Lowman EW. Rehabilitation following traumatic brain damage: immediate and long-term follow-up results in 127 cases. Med Clin North Am 1969; 53: 677–84.
132. Clum NM, Ryan M. Brain injury and the family. J Neurosurg Nursing 1981; 13: 165–9.
133. Jacob HE, Muir CA, Klein JD. Family reactions to persistent vegetative states. J Head Trauma Rehabil 1986; 1: 55–62.
134. Andrews K, Beaumont JG, Danze F, et al. International Working Party report on the vegetative state. London: Royal Hospital for Neurodisability, 1996 (http://www.comarecovery.org/pvs.htm).

7 Practical Guide to the Management of Patients in the Vegetative State

Maria Quintieri and Sebastiano Serra

General Considerations

The recuperation of conscious activity is the main therapeutic goal and prevailing task in the treatment of patients in the vegetative state. A variety of approaches, ranging from intravenous amphetamine administration to the electrical stimulation of thalamic structures, have been followed in recent decades. Intense and prolonged sensory stimulation has been used as well, but this method is still a matter of debate (see p. 81). The recuperation of conscious mental activity requires individualized planning and relies on an empirical approach, based mostly on the inventiveness and goodwill of therapists and family members.

The physician needs to follow a scientific approach in order to devise a therapeutic plan that takes into account all the functional systems regulating vigilance and consciousness (p. 11). The theory of coherence suggests that a certain degree of simultaneous stimulation of the four functional systems regulating consciousness is required. It has been noted, for instance, that isolated auditory–tactile sensory stimulation can provoke a state of alarm, accompanied by a diffuse vegetative response. Similarly, a persistent supraliminal stimulation can provoke a state of hypervigilance, which can interfere with perception and the processing of each stimulus. With this in mind, we will put forth some general rules (derived from our practical experience, but also justified in theory) that are based on the knowledge of the neurological mechanisms described. These so-called "rules of thumb" [1] have been summarized as follows:

- First rule: before eliciting any type of performance, it is mandatory to obtain relaxation – so never work under alarm conditions.
- Second rule: assist in the recuperation of circadian rhythms.
- Third rule: passively induce ipsilateral and contralateral motor systems prior to any sensory stimulation, by passively turning the head toward the source of the stimulus.
- Fourth rule: stimulation must at first be simple – a caress on the face or hand. Never repeat a stimulus if a response is not obtained from the first stimulus.

Although based primarily on experience and common sense rather than on scientific evidence, these rules may suggest the choice of proper actions.

There is no particular technique or method for helping the patient to resume conscious activities during the vegetative state, but we would contend that the "method" by which therapeutic procedures are conducted can determine the efficacy of the treatment. In addition, it should be borne in mind that "the patient is locked in the only state of being that is possible to him or her at the moment, and is unable to use the forms of expression we would otherwise expect in different conditions; we must come forward to meet this new structure of existence and let it express itself, possibly also by helping its expression wherever we can" [2]. The observation of a sign, and above all its interpretation, should be shared by the whole team of attending nurses, therapists, technicians, and physicians, in a collective rather than individual effort to achieve objectivity and reliability. Beyond the individual techniques and methods, it is also necessary to establish unequivocal guidelines for use in analyzing each action.

Each single procedure and its modalities of application will be described as derived from the general strategy developed by Zylberman and Vichi [3].

Observation of the General State

Experience is a major source of know-how in the treatment of patients in the vegetative state. It should be noted once again that these patients have no way of interacting with the attending staff and are unaware of the therapeutic approach to be taken. This is a physician's responsibility, and a consensus from the family members should be obtained according to ethical requirements and local regulations.

The clinical picture is extremely complicated and includes pathologies due to cranial trauma, as well as acute complications [4,5] involving in varying combinations the osteoarticular, respiratory, gastrointestinal, genitourinary, and hemopoietic systems. Also, pathologies and symptoms otherwise not observed in other diseases sometimes have to be dealt with in the vegetative state, which is thus a distinct condition in its own right. Clinical observation and maintenance of the general state are the cardinal aspects of any action to be taken. To make this approach feasible and to some extent standardized, predefined procedures need to be established, and any progress should be detailed in the patient's records, which must be easy to consult and made available to all members of the staff. Predetermined procedures also make it possible to proceed with a global treatment schedule, which should be common to all patients in the first phase, and thereafter to follow a more detailed and personalized plan based on evaluation by the staff over several days of observation. In this initial phase, continuous monitoring of vital signs (also intended to avoid a wide range of life-threatening complications) and the drawing up of a complete clinical chart form the basis of treatment for patients whose conditions have a similar origin and tend to proceed in a predictable manner, although they may rapidly become different from patient to patient at a later time.

Survey of Vital Parameters

- The vital parameters to be monitored are blood pressure, heart rate, temperature, respiratory rate, and peripheral oxygen saturation.
- The vital functions to be monitored are diuresis, hydration, stool, and sweating.
- Monitoring procedures should be carried out by nursing staff and therapists during treatment in order to evaluate potential changes in vital parameters.
- Monitoring should be continuous throughout the duration of intensive care.
- Data should be recorded on the progress sheets and patient charts by both the nursing staff and therapists. Data that deserve further consideration are forwarded to the department physician.

Pharmacological Therapy and Drug Administration Modes

Particular attention must be paid to the use of pharmacological therapies, which should be reduced to a minimum to comply with essential needs only. Parenteral drug administration using central venous access should be switched to peripheral venous administration as soon as practicable, with a preference for the minimal possible number of administrations per day (possibly once daily). Intramuscular administration should be avoided whenever possible in order to minimize the risks of local infection, which often goes undetected, but may provoke abscesses or fever. The ultimate goal is enteral pharmacological administration via a nasogastric tube or percutaneous gastrostomy. Powders are preferable, while effervescent or oily formulations are not advisable. Subcutaneous administration is reserved for prolonged treatment (e.g. low molecular weight heparin) and should be on a single daily administration. It is only in this way that patients can be treated without the encumbrance of tubes.

Procedure: before Drug Administration

- The patient must be identified.
- An administration schedule for the drug or drugs must be established and detailed in the patient's charts as required, to ensure compliance by both nursing staff and physicians.
- The modalities for drug administration must be established: parenteral, enteral, aerosol, sublingual, etc.

- Communication with the patient should be established in any way possible in order to inform him or her about what is being undertaken and to avoid any feeling of being threatened.
- Administration.
- Recording of drug administration on the patient's chart or progress sheets.

The access routes must be monitored and maintained. Enteral nasogastric tubes and percutaneous gastrostomies must be rinsed with 20 mL water before and after drug administration. Parenteral infusions must be checked for drip speed and type of solution. A permanent cannula should be positioned whenever long-term administration or repeated administration are required (e. g., in the case of patients receiving heparin). Central venous catheters are to be replaced every 7 days. Once removed, catheters must be sent in for bacterial culture. Peripheral catheters must be replaced periodically and rotated. When possible, enteral access is preferred to other administration routes.

Treatment Program

Once a treatment plan has been established, the following must be carried out:
- Neurological examination
- Evaluation by an appropriate scale of the degree of communicative functions
- Evaluation by each member of the team
- Elaboration of a treatment plan
- Periodic staff meetings, with evaluations of each patient by each staff member

All staff members should be actively involved in the treatment. It is advisable that the treatment plan be carried out at scheduled times, as this allows reevaluation, monitoring, updating, and adaptation of the treatment plan to the patient's clinical progress. All colleagues should be provided with the patients' documentation.

Hygiene

The patients' hygiene is the responsibility of the nursing staff, and hygiene procedures need to be carried out accurately and according to schedule, after the patient has been informed about what is to be done using a suitable communication mode (if any). The patient is bathed on a fitted stretcher in the room if his or her vital signs are unstable, or otherwise in the bathroom and always at a warm ambient temperature. Soaps and shampoos that do not produce excessive foam should be used with hot water. In cases when communication is possible and there is partial autonomy, the nurse should ask the patient if he/she requires help. In fact, the nurse's gesture may possibly induce a response or voluntary movements in answer to a simple command. The presence of a gastrostomy or fever and the absence of consciousness are not impediments to this practice. Hot water, tactile stimulation, and repetition of a type of situation the patient might recognize from his or her own life all represent ways of resuming contact with the environment and favor communication. In addition, these procedures allow passive mobilization of all joints, changes in posture, and initial mobilization from the hospital bed. The patient is washed and dried; the use of hydrating and emollient substances allows olfactory and tactile stimulation, besides helping prevent decubitus ulcers and thromboembolic risks. Medications for decubitus ulcer are then reapplied to the skin around the tracheostomy and gastrostomy. In the morning, nurses shave patients, cut their hair, and clean their nails. Next, they dress the patients – again allowing passive mobilization and movements (such as putting on a T-shirt, socks, etc.) that are familiar to the patient and therefore of particular significance. Underwear with elastic or buttons should not be worn in the initial phase, as it produces localized skin pressure and can be an obstacle in emergency situations. Everyday hygiene (oral hygiene using a toothbrush, combing the hair, make-up) is performed at some centers by the therapist, with the patient seated in front of a mirror (Fig. 7.**1**). In the early phase, the patient passively follows the therapist's movements, until recuperation occurs at a level involving greater complete autonomy in everyday activities for self-care.

Procedure

The staff is responsible for skin hygiene and for performing procedures which also stimulates the patient's tactile perception and favors microcirculation through passive mobilization.

7 Practical Guide to the Management of Patients in the Vegetative State

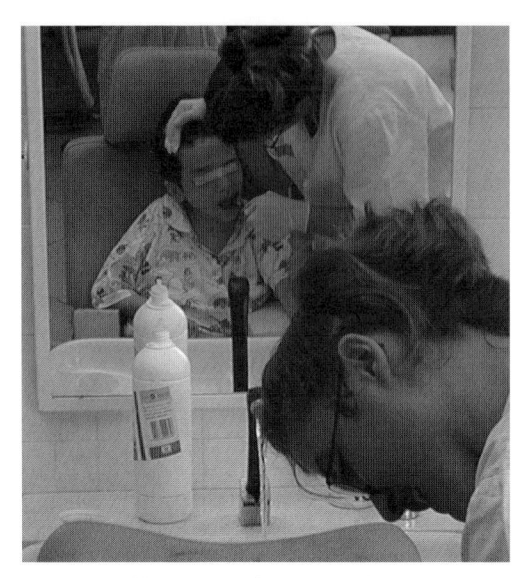

Fig. 7.1 Oral hygiene performed by the patient with the help of a mirror and assistance from the therapist

Preliminary procedures. Washing is part of the daily schedule and includes bathing or showering. The bathroom must be properly prepared, with optimal water and air temperature, and whatever may be needed for any individual patient (shampoos, sponges, sponge pieces, gauze to renew medications, diapers for incontinence, clothes, perfumes, emollient creams, etc.)

Shower. The patient is moved from his or her room to the bathroom by means of a lifting device. He or she is then undressed and medication tubes are removed. Care is taken to protect the tracheostomy cannula. The patient is washed by immersion or shower, with proper control of the position in space of each body segment. The nurse sprinkles the whole body surface with soap and asks the patient to follow the massage and washing movements of each body part. Particular care must be shown on surfaces with increased contact with organic liquids (urine, feces, vomit, bronchial secretions, sweat) or surrounding decubital sores. The nurse then rinses the whole body surface in the same manner as described above and dries it gently with a cotton towel. Emollients and hydrating creams are applied, and oral, ulcer, and decubital medications are renewed. Nails are cleaned and hair dried. The patient is dressed, and the entire procedure is documented, as are signs of relief during the shower. The presence of skin damage and anything of potential relevance needs to be noted in the patient's chart.

Prevention and treatment of decubitus sores. Patients in the vegetative state are by definition unable to care for their own personal needs, nor are they able to move or show appreciation or discomfort which makes them completely dependent on professional care. There are guidelines for the proper management of sphincters and cutaneous trophism in relation to hygiene procedures. In particular, decubitus sores are frequent, and their formation (and development directly proportional to the progression of the clinical picture and metabolic condition) should be prevented. Extreme attention must be given to the revival and maintenance of blood proteins through correct nutrition and integrated therapy. Patients often present with a tendency toward immunodeficiency (see p. 24). Treatment of decubitus lesions is of primary importance, as is the prevention of new sores. Antidecubitus mattresses are critical for this purpose (latex, hollow silicone fibers, air or water stuffing, computerized systems for differential regulation of pressure on skin and muscles, etc.), and remain the best strategy for prevention and therapy, even compared to topical medications. Before treatment, the patient's general state, skin hydration, and possible mobilization must be checked. The number of lesions, their positions, and their characteristics (depth, margins, secretion, color, odor) should be recorded. Continuous photographic documentation can be helpful in observing the progression of skin lesions.

General Procedures

- Showering and bed hygiene are to be performed daily by the nursing staff (see above).
- Application of hydrating creams, using gentle massage, will avoid maceration of skin areas where there is a risk of sores developing, for example due to continuous position-related pressure.
- Reduction to the minimum possible of any contact with urine and feces.
- Mobilization through frequent changes of position in bed, avoiding constant pressure on areas where there is a risk of sores developing (occipital bone, shoulder blades, trochanters, sacrum, ischial tuberosity, ankles, and any other areas potentially subjected to decubitus sores).

- Mobilization in a wheelchair, at least once a day.
- Progressive upright positioning in an electric bed, for relatively short periods but several times every day.
- Proper hydration and food intake compatible with the patient's caloric requirements. A hypercaloric diet is advised (estimated requirement for catabolic patients with decubitus sores up to 60 kcal/kg/day), using commercial products that ensure the daily intake of proteins, carbohydrates, fats, and minerals, following allowances detailed in the chapter on nutrition.

Local Treatments

The following methods cover the possible treatment options:
- Cleanse decubitus sores with saline for lesions in the granulation and reepithelialization phases, or with oxygenated water for necrotic or fibrinous lesions.
- Disinfect with 5% chlorine oxide electrolyte solution, rinsing infected lesions with saline.
- Apply occlusive medication with hydrocolloids for lesions in early or reepithelialization phases.
- Apply highly absorptive hydroactive medication for deep granulating, exudative, and infected lesions.
- Apply occlusive medication with hydrocolloid gels for necrotic and fibrotic lesions.

Management of Sphincter Activity

Again, the entire team should be involved in the effort to restore the patient's sphincteral continence. Use of a urinary catheter should be restricted to cases in which it is unavoidable and limited to the initial phase of recovery. The procedure involves removal of the catheter and use of an external collector once autonomous miction is reestablished. Defecation must also be controlled. A certain degree of sphincter control and appropriate aids have innumerable advantages, such as allowing the patient to leave the room during rehabilitation.

Constipation and diarrhea can be controlled by a proper diet and the regular application of enemas, whereas the long-term administration of laxatives has proved less effective. Controlling and regularizing stool avoids the danger of fecalomas, hemorrhoids, and autonomic reactions possibly due to the patient's discomfort. Loose stool is usually related to nutritional problems and can be prevented (after adequate chemical examination and a search for parasites) by means of a proper food plan focusing on food quality, amount, and speed of administration. In cases of diarrhea, the suspension of enteral feeding for a few hours, fecal cultures and parasite examinations, and the resumption of 250 mL enteral water administration (every 150 min up to a quantity of several liters, if allowed by the clinical heart and blood pressure conditions) are useful.

Procedure. First, the existence of sphincteral incontinence should be noted. Fecal and urine specimens should be collected for physicochemical examination and culture. The progress sheets should document the comprehensive water balance (intake, elimination, routes, infusions, hydration, nutritional volume). In case of permanent catheter the urine produced over 24 h should be assessed for diuresis control; contact between organic liquids (such as urine or feces) and skin should be avoided in order to prevent decubitus sores. The reasons for keeping the catheter in place are documented on progress sheets and patient charts.

The urinary catheter should be removed as soon as possible, and an external urine collector (in males) or diapers (in females) should be favored. The catheter needs to be repositioned in the few patients with urinary retention (globoid bladder) or neurological hypertonic bladder, with or without sphincteral incontinence, as well as in cases of urinary retention due to spastic bladder sphincter (as often seen in urinary infections). In the absence of spontaneous miction with urinary retention (globoid bladder) catheters are used extemporaneously or at fixed times. Catheter use should always be documented in the progress sheets.

If there is constipation, an enema is given within 3 days at the latest, with documentation in the progress sheets. In cases of loose stool or diarrhea, care must be taken to ensure immediate removal of feces and application of hydrating and protective substances in the perineal region.

Evaluation of Nutritional Aspects and Methods

Patients in the vegetative state often present with metabolic imbalances, such as increased metabolic processes, appearance of catabolic processes, alterations in the relationship among the different metabolic pathways, or water-electrolyte imbalances with resulting instability of vital signs [6]. Distinct strategies are required for stable patients, whose caloric requirements are estimated in the range of 40–50 kcal/kg/day, and cachectic patients, whose caloric requirement is 60 kcal/kg/day or more. Fat content is about 28% of total caloric requirements. It should be noted that oleic acid is the most readily oxygenated among dietary fats and that glutamine is the most important amino acid for enterocytes, which use it as their principal energy substrate. Enterocyte glutamine metabolism constitutes the most important role of the intestine in the metabolism of nitrates, which are excreted as urea. Vitamins and minerals should be administered in excess of the daily requirement under physiological conditions. In patients in post-traumatic vegetative state, the autonomic system is highly stimulated, therefore favoring the occurrence of nonspecific phenomena (such as hyperventilation, hemodynamic changes, fever, hypertonus, and convulsions) that all call for increased metabolic requirements. On the other hand, hypothalamic–hypophysial damage can alter the neuroendocrine response significantly.

Attaining a proper metabolic balance is usually possible within a short time. The patient's general state should be evaluated, however, also by monitoring the anthropometric (starting weight, periodic weight checks, tricipital plica, hydration conditions, and hydration loss) and laboratory (blood albumin, total proteins, transferrin, hemoglobin, creatinine, nitrate and glucose, creatinine clearance, etc.) indices.

Procedure for Body Weight Monitoring

Patients are weighed every 2 weeks in the morning (fasting), following a detailed procedure:
- Determine the scale net weight.
- Determine the weight of the wheelchair and safety belts.
- Remove the patient's clothes and incontinence aids (urinary sac and diapers).
- Position the belt.
- Position the patient on the wheelchair using a lifting device.
- Weigh the patient.
- Dress the patient and document the weight data in the progress sheets, possibly also noting the presence of any rigidity or temporarily unmovable orthoses.

Feeding: Routes of Administration

The main routes of administration are through a central venous catheter, a nasogastric tube, or gastric tubes (percutaneous endoscopic gastrostomy, PEG). The route of administration and amount may vary according to the protocols in use in the unit, using either continuous or scheduled feeding protocols consistent with the circadian cycles. Enteral feeding eliminates the risks connected with the protracted presence of central or peripheral venous catheters.

Meals are given on a schedule and if possible in a habitual environment, which can contribute to the resumption of biological rhythms and relationship. Oral feeding should be attempted in all patients showing some awareness of swallowing and should be resumed when bronchial aspiration becomes a minimal risk. Small amounts of pureed and jellied food, preserves, and purees, should be administered first, as swallowing liquids remains a persistent deficit. If there is insufficient swallowing, a nasal tube should be positioned.

Procedure for Enteral Feeding

This procedure can be applied in the absence of contraindications such as regurgitation, vomiting, diarrhea, and if there are organic gastrointestinal problems. If patients are fed parenterally at admission, it is necessary:
- To position a nasogastric feeding tube or a PEG, with the patient leaning 30° backward.
- To suspend parenteral feeding progressively and start enteral feeding gradually, in accordance with the assigned quantities and quality.

It is advisable to shift from parenteral to enteral feeding starting with a maximum amount of 500 mL/day, to be increased on the basis of the assigned diet plan. The advised speed of feeding is 160–250 mL/h; in cases of gastrointestinal intolerance, enteral feeding can be discontinued for a few hours and then restarted at the lowest speed tolerated. After feeding, the tube must be cleaned with 50 mL of water, to be subtracted from the amount of total water allowed.

Treatment in the Gym

Gym treatment plays an important role in the day schedule of any patient in the vegetative state, and should include most of the exercises done during

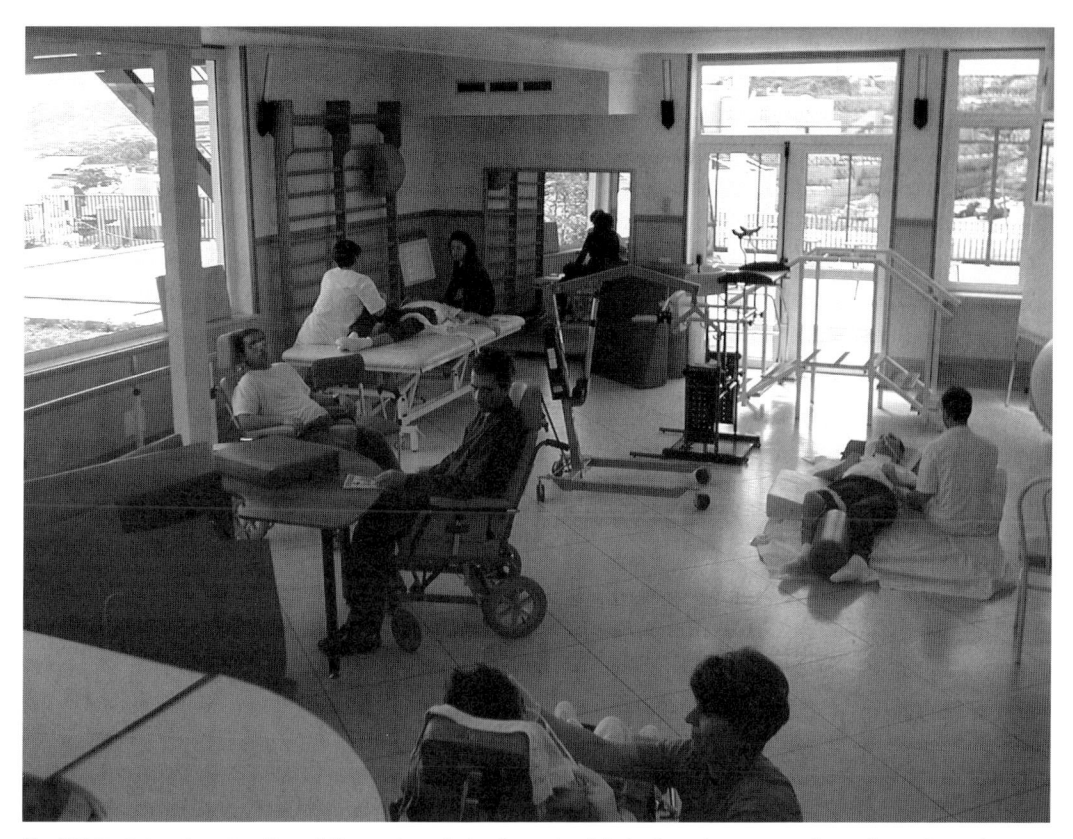

Fig. 7.2 Training the attention of the patient sitting in a wheelchair: first elementary signs of an oriented gaze

nursing care. However, the gym schedule should be tailored to each patient's needs, with one therapist attending each patient (Fig. 7.2).

Passive Mobilization

At the start of treatment, mobilization can only be passive. Treatment can begin very early, as it does not interfere with any medical procedures and represents an effective method of patient care and prevention of neuro-orthopedic complications, while also helping establish channels for communication between the patient, the therapist, and the outside world.

Objectives

- To maintain movements of the joints
- To prevent contractions
- To prevent trophic cutaneous disturbances
- To stimulate proprioception
- To promote awareness, relationships and exchanges between the patient and the therapist

Passive mobilization of the joints should be carried out bilaterally several times every day, each time for at least 20 min. This needs to be done slowly, with the therapist talking to the patient and explaining to him or her which part of body is going to be moved.

Positioning

It is mandatory for the patient to be in an appropriate position, as this is believed to prevent the appearance of muscle tonic disturbances and spasticity and to avoid secondary complications. Changes from supination to pronation and from side to side are warranted. Positions can be maintained with the help of different types of orthosis made of foam rubber with thermoplastic elements, the position of which should be chosen to allow the

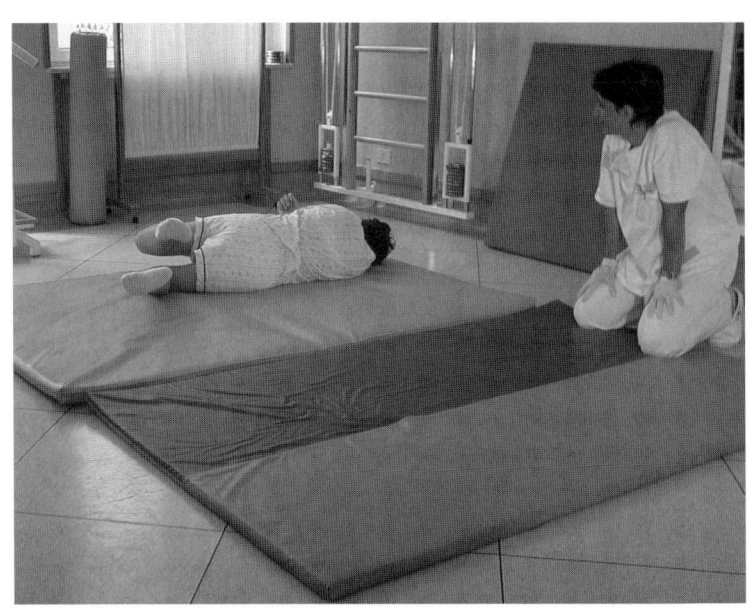

Fig. 7.3 Exercise: rolling

least number of restrictions possible. Dynamic positioning is very useful – for example, when the limb is positioned on spring supports that allow sub-continuous, intermittent small movements of the joints.

Rolling

Rolling constitutes the most important physiokinetic therapeutic approach in the treatment of patients in the vegetative state, and is mostly indicated when spontaneous motion is absent. Mechanisms regulating rolling along the longitudinal axis have been described and depend on the activity of the interstitial nuclei of Cajal in the mesencephalon, which are very active during wakefulness. This is the first motor system that reaches full myelination, as early as in the sixth month of pregnancy, and it is responsible for fetal intrauterine movements. The axial and belt musculature is innervated bilaterally. The kinetic chain responsible for the movement sequences for rolling is therefore the oldest and the one that first appears in motor development. Passively, both superior and inferior belt transverse axis rolling is seen.

The patient starts from a supine position with trunk and head in axis, with the therapist adducting an upper limb (with the elbow being semi-flexed) while holding the shoulder and gently starting the rolling movement. It is important that the patient complete the kinetic sequence with movements of the automatic motor sequence. The same results are elicited with forced adduction of the thigh while the knees are bent (Fig. 7.3). Rolling exercises are useful for eliciting postural reactions, such as tonic and labyrinth reflexes of the neck or straightening reflexes. The therapist must simultaneously stimulate auditory and visual afferents in order to promote communication, stimulate attention, and call out functions relative to the body scheme.

Respiratory Treatment

The patient in the vegetative state frequently suffers respiratory problems. A series of pathological conditions develop that can induce secondary respiratory disturbances: immobility in bed (often in a fixed position with hardly any mobility of the ribcage, occasionally also due to rib fractures), bronchial stagnation, and susceptibility to infection, should all be considered. The resultant incapacity of the respiratory function, with greater production of secretions and alterations in the rhythm and depth of breathing, often accompanies serious alterations in gaseous exchange, hypo-oxygenation, and sometimes pneumonia due to stasis. Treatment strategies to diminish secretion stasis include techniques based on clapping, vibrations, and shaking when the patient presents with an insufficient cough reflex but there are no rib fractures – as many times a day as deemed necessary for sufficient drainage. Postural drainage is another technique used when the patient is properly stabilized. Staff must periodically change the patient's position. Gradual verticalization of the patient should be attempted whenever the clinical conditions allow, with the aid of electric beds (see below) and then wheelchairs. The expansion of the rib cage should be improved as soon as possible by periodic mobilization of the upper limbs and by means of respiratory exercises that are able to lower the ribs and favor passive and (consciousness permitting) active expiration. A patented device that can be suitably attached to the tracheostomy cannula has been developed and is routinely used in some highly specialized centers. The device, based on a fitted diaphragm with changeable and progressively decreasing diameter, allows air inspiration only after a progressive increase in the inspiration strength and thoracic expansion. In this way, the patients who have gradually lost elasticity of the respiratory muscles over a period of months gradually recuperate by breathing against resistance and under controlled conditions, with monitoring of the number and depth of breaths, the P_{CO_2}, and gas analysis.

All patients who have undergone tracheostomy should be treated with humidification and aerosol therapy several times every day, and the condition of the large bronchi should be checked by bronchoscopy. In general, patients in the vegetative state are also monitored using a pulse dosimeter, and action is taken to maintain the peripheral oxygen saturation (measured from the finger or ear) at values of 95–100%, with periodic check-ups with gas analysis.

Verticalization

It is important in the treatment plan for patients in the vegetative state and, if properly carried out, combines simplicity of exercise with a valuable treatment, while at the same time allowing the application of the treatment approach suggested by the "rules of thumb" (Fig. 7.**4**). Early positioning of the patient in an erect position, while still in the vegetative state, involves a series of considerations and serves multiple objectives.

Considerations

The upright position is the best condition for space exploration. The patient is helped to recover and readapt to seeing, grasping, and recovering the

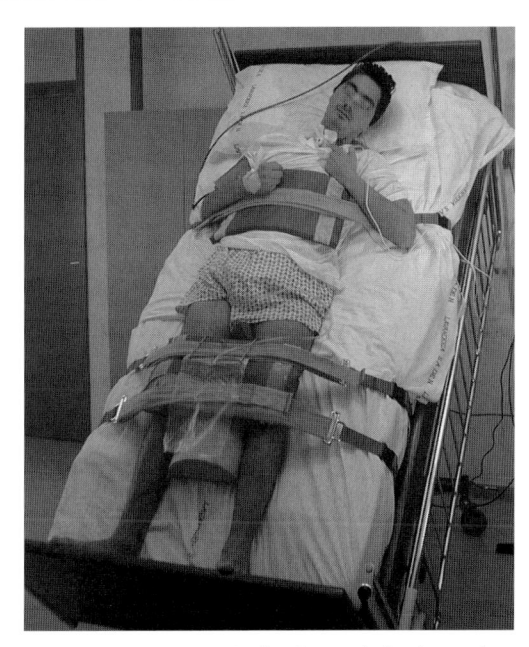

Fig. 7.**4** Exercise: verticalization to help the patient explore the surrounding space

body orientation in space by means of which humans relate to the external world. In a vertical position, the four anatomical systems sustaining the state of consciousness are simultaneously involved and, in particular, are "synchronized" with the ipsilateral and contralateral primitive motor systems. The position also helps reestablish or recover the reflexes for straightening the head and trunk.

Objectives

- Verticalization helps prevent complications due to prolonged immobilization, such as deep vein thrombosis, and favors frequent changes of the patient's position and body parts that suffer prolonged pressure from supports, stimulation from vessel receptors, reduction of smell stimuli, etc.
- It stimulates the mechanisms that regulate vegetative functions in a controlled way.
- Contraindications to verticalization include:
  - Serious orthopedic problems that impede correct positioning
  - Unstable vital signs
  - Signs of neurovegetative alarm
  - Endocranial hypertension
  - Deep venous thrombosis

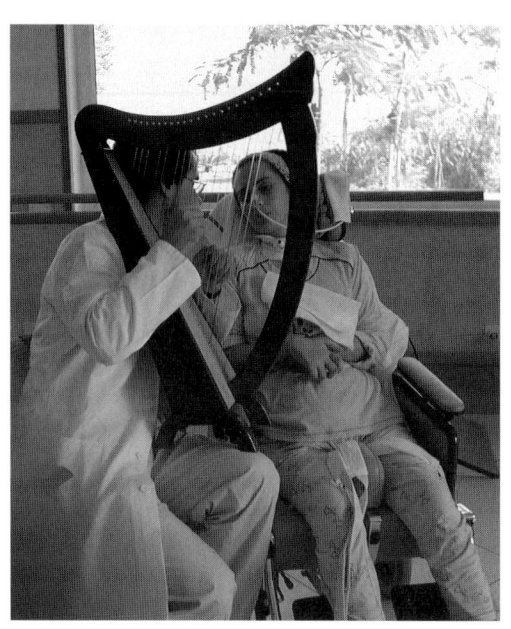

Fig. 7.5 In this position, the patient's head is rotated toward the therapist, and monomodal stimulation can be started

Procedure

The following equipment is necessary: electric beds (for passive verticalization in the hospital room), static plan, standing device, dynamic standing device (for active verticalization in the therapy room). Accessories (such as elastic socks, belts and straps to hold the patient, foam rubber aids and sand-filled bags for positioning) should be prepared. The vital signs need to be monitored continuously during verticalization.

Methods for Verticalization

- First position the patient in a supine position with the body properly in axis.
- Position wedges beneath the trochanters to avoid lateral rotation of the lower limbs and to improve supination of the feet.
- Place a foam or rubber pillow in the popliteal cavity to prevent hyperextension of the knees.
- Position the feet at 90° onto the lower board of the verticalization bed.
- Apply a strap around the thorax to prevent anteroflexion of the trunk and at the knee level to avoid flexion of the legs.
- Check that the positioning does not produce compression of vessels or nerves.

Following this type of arrangement, the patient can attain complete verticalization (up to 90°) progressively within 4–5 days. Verticalization treatments should be 30 min long at the beginning, progressively increasing up to 1 h (whenever possible), and should be performed several times every day at approximately the same time. The therapist (who must also prevent the patient's head from falling onto the chest) stands on one side of the patient, calming the patient by explaining the treatment or using tactile stimulation, and monitors the vital signs. Once the patient is relaxed, his or her head is turned over to one side, and a monomodal stimulation is performed (Fig. 7.5). The treatment can be performed simultaneously in several patients, providing a "mirror" effect that is therapeutic in itself. In the absence of other patients with indications for this treatment, a mirror placed in front of the patient during the treatment serves the same purpose and is as effective.

After a verticalization treatment, the horizontal position should be reached gradually (within about 10 min). If neurovegetative alarm reactions occur, horizontalization should be started over again after normalization from the last tolerated angle. The therapist must report in the progress sheets the duration of treatment, degree of verticalization reached, and all the observed changes in vital parameters or mimicry, as well as all responses obtained during the treatment.

Hydrotherapy

Hydrotherapy has been widely used for several years in the rehabilitation of deficits due to various neurological disorders. In patients in the vegetative state, hydrotherapy is the method of choice for obtaining muscular relaxation and a natural psychophysical condition of well-being. It is easily accepted by patients and therapists and represents a simple way of gradually increasing communication without excessive costs or requirements for complex equipment. In addition, hydrotherapy has trophic effects that go beyond reestablishing neurovegetative balance, and produces slight peripheral vasodilatation (with increased peripheral distribution of oxygen and nutrition) that is compensated for by the peripheral blood pressure with a resulting increase in venous return. It should also be noted that floating and hydrostatic effects promote stimulation

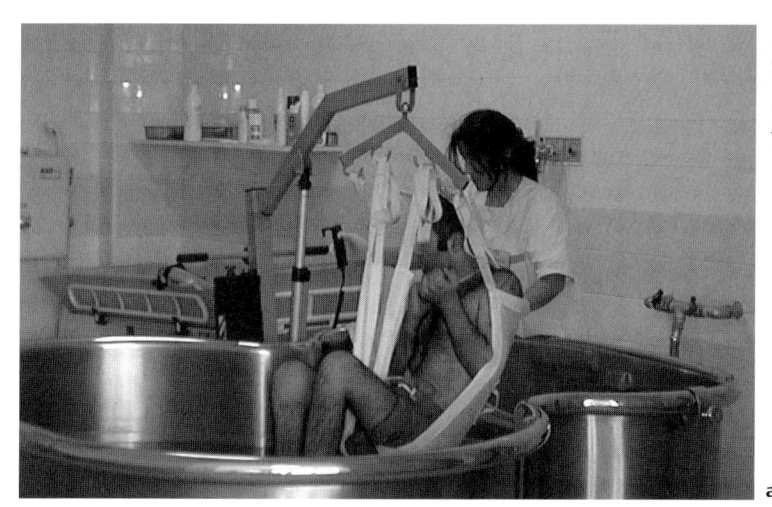

Fig. 7.**6a, b** Relaxation suitable for facilitating simple responses is best obtained by exercising the patient in the swimming pool at 32 °C

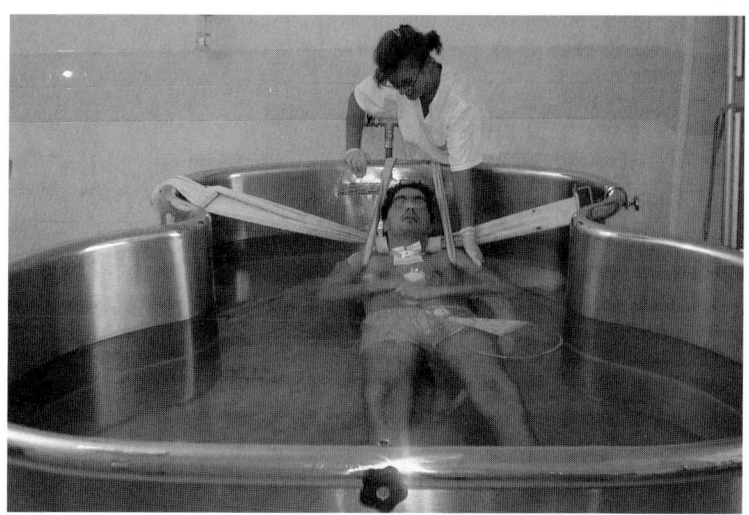

of motor responses otherwise unobtainable (Fig. 7.**6**).

Equipment Needed

- A pool or (in case of space limitation) a butterfly tub, with water at body temperature and with no variations in the external microclimate
- Electrical lifting device, complete with pouch
- Tub cleaning, with local disinfection with liquid products and ambient disinfection with UVA for 12 h
- Attending staff in charge and possibly assisted and helped by family members

Absolute contraindications to hydrotherapy are hyperthermia and serious hypertension or hypotension. Localized infective lesions and psychomotor agitation are relative contraindications, which should be evaluated in each case.

Treatment Methods

The total duration should be about 1 h, with an optimal frequency of three sessions or more every week. For the first 15 min of treatment, the therapist should encourage relaxation in the patient and improvement spastic hypertonia; then passive mobilization and inhibitory maneuvers are performed for about 20 min. Every movement performed is first explained to the patient while touching the part of his or her body that is to be mobilized. This has a calming effect and is favorable for the patient, who has to obey simple commands aimed at ob-

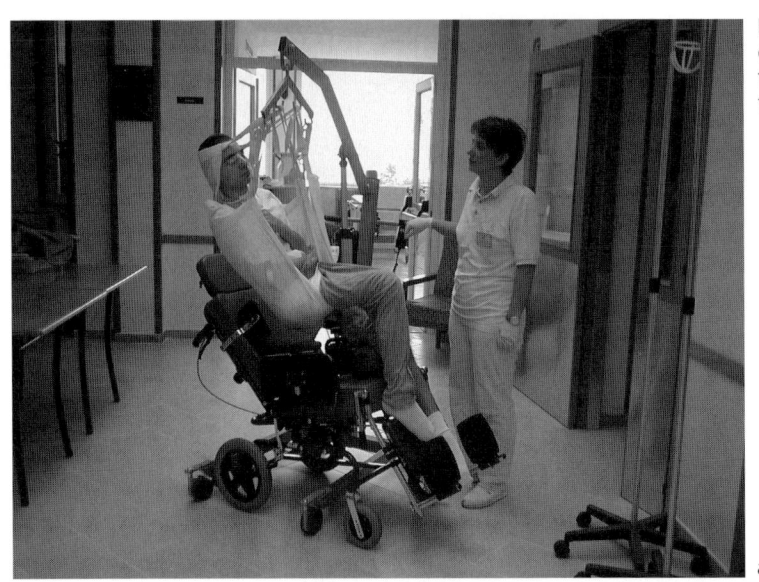

Fig. 7.**7a, b** The therapeutic effects of positioning the patient in a wheelchair are detailed in the text

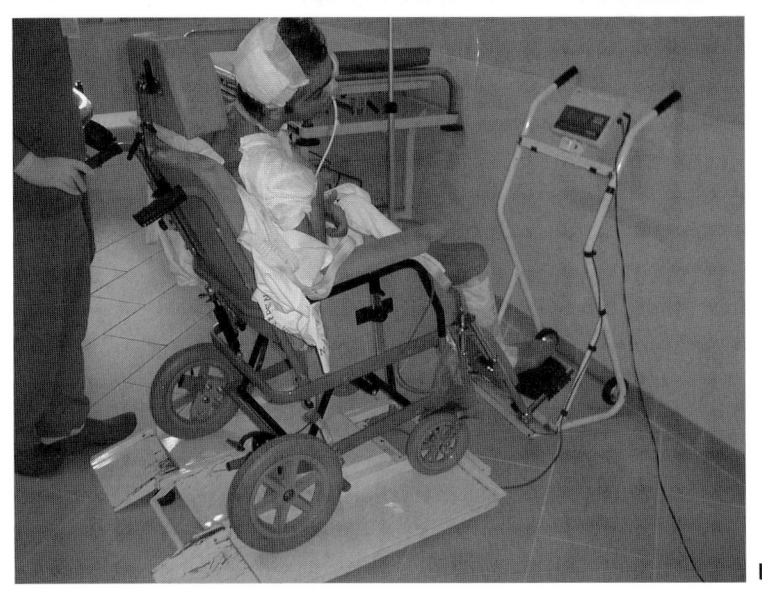

taining motor responses and maximal limb movements. Orders are given in expectation of a response. In general, the first effects obtained are a change in the patient's facial expression, together with a reduction in the pathological body posture.

Positioning the Patient on the Wheelchair

Positioning the patient on the wheelchair is basically a continuation of the rehabilitation treatment. There may be substantial differences between patients and they may require different types of assistance. Patients with cerebral lesions often require continuous monitoring of vital signs over long periods of time, which keeps the patients linked to monitor devices even in the wheelchair.

Why put a patient in the vegetative state in a wheelchair? The main purposes are to achieve improvement in or encourage the appearance of attentive functions, to stabilize and gradually achieve control over trunk posture and movements, to start the ipsilateral and contralateral primitive motor systems functioning, to reorganize the system regulating pressure and the vestibular system, to establish new proprioceptive inputs and conjugated gaze in the vertical position, to reduce the risk of decubital sores, to achieve better drainage of bronchial secretions and improve lung capacity, to allow a different body response to gravity, to improve sphincter functions (defecation, miction), and to reduce regurgitation due to esophageal sphincter insufficiency. The expectations (sometimes excessive) of the patient's family, who are able to see improvements as a pathway leading to a possible recovery (Fig. 7.**7**), are also satisfied. It should also be noted in this regard that adequate positioning of the patient on the wheelchair (with proper pressure on the seat, wedges and containing or corrective bands) is a fundamental step in achieving improved balance for posture and movement [7,8].

Clinical conditions, joint impairment, and the existence of cutaneous lesions should be taken into proper account so as to give the patient the correct position in the wheelchair. The use of buckles and belts should always be discouraged, unless warranted by a state of psychomotor agitation and the need to limit the patient's movements in or from the chair. The trunk is the main source of stability of the body and is therefore fundamental for correct movements of the head and limbs [5]. Inadequate alignment of the vertebral column affects the trunk and creates compensatory curves, which may erroneously be corrected at the cost of other sections of the column and with other resultant deviations. Optimal distribution of the weight over a wider base is also important, and extensive or excessive pressure against the ischial tuberosity and sacral bone should be avoided. Once the trunk is realigned with the pelvis, the base of support changes, with a resultant equal distribution of weight between the ischial tuberosities, thighs, and the feet. Combining all the elements and finding the best position for each patient's numerous requirements also needs imagination and creativity on the part of staff. It should be noted how tolerance and comfort in the wheelchair may become fundamental. Chairs with rigid backs and providing a solid base are preferable to "very comfortable" chairs, which according to reports by several physicians can even favor the development of decubitus sores. Pillows on solid bases can be provided at a later time.

The normal position of the trunk is the erect posture, with a slight anterior pelvic inclination and the weight equally distributed on both ischial tuberosities. Any incorrect positioning of the patient will cause flexion of the trunk and pelvic rotation (most likely backward), resulting either in scoliosis, an accentuated lateral inclination, or flexion of the thigh on the pelvis. Possible adverse effects of inadequate positions are decubitus sores, thoracic restraint with reduced ventilation and respiratory difficulties, decreased visual perception of the environment, proprioceptive and vestibular changes, antalgic posture and tension in the back muscles, and pain in the joints. A common method of preventing the patient from sliding off at the front is to hold the pelvis against the back of chair with a bilaterally adjustable belt on the pelvis or thighs. With regard to lateral trunk and pelvic inclinations, it is preferable to use wedges (three-point system) and supports placed on both parts of trunk to balance the angle. Also useful are support systems for the thighs (Fig. 7.**7**). On occasions, it may be necessary to produce a disparity using foam or rubber pillows (about 5 cm or thicker) positioned beneath the pelvis on one side, possibly with a softer pillow positioned contralaterally.

The alignment of the head with the trunk should also be taken into account, to avoid abnormal tonic reflexes in the neck. A collar supporting the head can be used, but may cause chin lesions, dysfunctions of the temporomandibular joints, and lesions on the sides of the neck. Wide straps placed between the forehead and a support on the chair are preferred. The latter arrangement is less traumatic but also less efficient, as the belts often tend to slide away, sometimes also covering the patient's eyes. Using slight angulation of the back of the chair also does not resolve the problem completely. Rigid lateral supports, similar to headrests, are sometimes used, but often cause microlesions or macrolesions on the temples and ears. A great deal of attention needs to been given to the contact between the occipital region and the support, which should be lined with a satin-type material, sheepskin fleece, or a similar material to avoid abrasions and alopecia due to friction. A support at the back of the head also minimizes muscular tension in the neck (Fig. 7.**8**).

With regard to the pelvis, the best position is flexion at about 90°, with abduction and spontaneous femoral rotation, which in turn influences trunk alignment. Excessive flexion of the upper hip

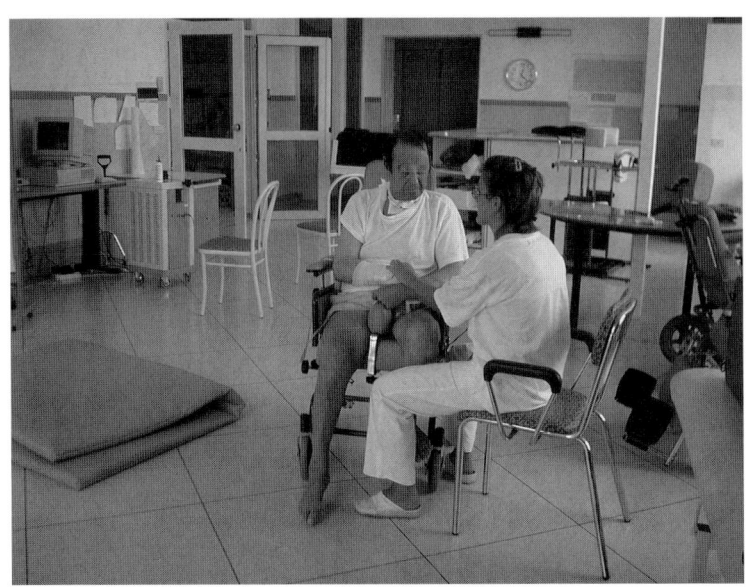

Fig. 7.8 A wheelchair and implements allow appropriate positioning of the head and trunk, while at the same time reducing muscle tension

at angles of more than 90° often depends on spasticity of the flexor muscles and warrants careful positioning with the knees higher than the pelvis, as obtained by reclining the back of the seat. A quite frequent problem is excessive femoral abduction and external rotation, with skin irritation and possible lesions due to tights continuously rubbing against the wheelchair metal. This is generally avoided by providing padding along the sides of the thighs. An abducted or externally rotated thigh, with the other one adducted and internally rotated, or a retracted limb and difficulties in the alignment of the limbs are also common observations. In particular instances, it may become necessary to construct appropriate structures to maintain an optimal joint position. Such structures are usually made out of rigid plastic, wood, foam rubber, plaster, etc. Correct positioning of the feet on the footrests should never be neglected, and abnormal positions should be corrected whenever possible.

The upper limbs pose different problems, depending on whether the paresis is flaccid or spastic. A flaccid limb requires adequate support, which also prevents subluxation of the shoulder, a frequent complication in the vegetative state. This disturbance must be cared for with functional electrical stimulation (FES) in addition to the use of figure of eight–shaped ortheses and dynamic ortheses. In general, patients with spastic upper limbs have little benefit from the use of restrictive devices, which instead are counterproductive and aggravate the already abnormal motor model in some cases. It is preferable to approach the problem on the basis of the limb's potential range of motion, its functional limitations, and the extent to which these may alter the entire alignment with the trunk [9]. Customized structures can be made using padded arms, which reduce the risk of skin lesions without interfering with correct positioning. It is also important to note in this regard how important it is to train physicians, physiotherapists, and any other health professionals involved with patients in the vegetative state to carry out accurate observation. One must ensure an ability to foresee potential future needs, progressive clinical and functional changes, and one must adapt any corrective treatment from time to time to suit each individual patient.

Treatment of Swallowing Disturbances

The total or partial loss of the physiological ability to swallow and the resulting inability to eat are common among patients in the vegetative state, especially in those presenting with serious medical conditions. Swallowing problems may be critical and may need to be dealt with by experienced professionals. Both the evaluation of swallowing disturbances and their treatment require a small, dedicated team, which should be organized by the attending physician with proper expertise and equipment (possibly also including fibrobronchoscopy and video fluoroscopy; see p. 108). Video fluoroscopy (which can only be carried out in cooperative patients) allows direct viewing and photographic documentation of possible malformations and pathologies in the oropharynx. It provides indications about the tracheostomy cannula and whether it is possible to remove it when the patient has an adequate laryngeal reflex according to the physiotherapist's and nurse's observations. The most frequently observed deficits are: lost or inadequate control of tongue movements, reduced esophageal peristalsis, and uncoordinated chewing movements. Primitive motor schemes, including mastication, sucking, lockjaw, and facial spasms are also observed in the first 3–4 months. Many patients already have a nasogastric tube or PEG in place. A reflex swallowing mechanism can often help in the vegetative state, as food placed in the proper position at the back of the pharynx triggers reflex swallowing movements and allows natural feeding. Some risks nevertheless exist, and anamnestic or direct knowledge of possible fractures of facial structures, respiratory disturbances, or food intolerance may be helpful. The position of the head and primary airways is important. The patient should be seated, with the trunk perpendicular to the seat plane, and the observer should continuously check for facial asymmetries (indicative of deficits of the involved musculature), changes in mimicry or respiration, or hypersalivation [10,11]. Forward flexion of the head is frequent in tracheostomized patients. In other cases, the head is forced to one side or hyperextended which makes evaluating the swallowing reflex a complex and sometimes difficult procedure, even when the therapist can manually move the head.

A proper examination must also include an accurate evaluation of head, neck, and trunk control in order to devise a treatment plan; information on whether the patient can be seated in a chair for feeding is important, for instance. The strength and mobility of perioral structures should be examined, and opening and closing of the patient's mandibles should be evaluated in order to establish whether food can be introduced into the oral cavity. The jaws open as wide as 35 mm in healthy subjects, with a lateral displacement of about 10 mm, but these figures are significantly reduced in patients with the bulldog reflex.

The physiotherapist is often confronted with patients who show signs of serious regression, such as a bulldog reflex, oculo-oral reflex, automatic sucking, mastication, teeth gritting, etc. The persistence of these signs (see p. 32) beyond 200 days after trauma is generally indicative of severe impairment. In patients in the vegetative state who show a bulldog reflex, for example, there is a considerable reduction in the capacity of the mouth to open. All these factors contribute to residual food remaining between the teeth and cheeks, or to an inability to keep food in the oral cavity. The strength of the muscles closing the mouth should also be evaluated (as it impedes hypersalivation). Possible imitations of visual or oral commands must be checked for. We also evaluate intraoral sensitivity to tastes by means of a pad moistened with flavored water and observation of changes in mimicry. Proper evaluation of the teeth and tongue is important too, as is the examination of the soft palate and posterior pharynx (often difficult in patients in the vegetative state). Presence of the cough reflex must also be noted.

The success of any program for the rehabilitation of swallowing depends on several variables and requires above all a proper, attentive observation of the responses to different types of stimulation. A specific position, an abnormal movement, any change in facial expression, and any other sign, can indicate that a stimulus can be perceived by the patient as abnormal, harmful, or bothersome in some way (the response to a stimulus can be delayed). Often, the rehabilitation of swallowing begins with delicate maneuvers, such as caresses on the cheeks with a cloth dipped in cold or tepid water, which are thought to help the patient relax (see the "rules of thumb," p. 89). Lips, and at times gums, are gently stroked with sterile pads or a tongue depressor. Firm pressure on the masseter muscles can be useful to obtain relaxation and opening of the lips in case a bulldog reflex appears. A tongue depressor or a gauze pad inserted between the teeth will encourage progressive opening of the mouth; this exercise in regulating muscular tone can be associated with pressure on the masseter muscle and needs to be repeated several times every day. Passive mobilization of the tongue in different directions is carried out using a velvet glove.

Several techniques have been used in to treat reduced tonus in the soft palate and posterior pharyngeal wall, but none has proved applicable in patients in the vegetative state due to the collaboration that is required. Oral electrical stimulation is applicable in patients with reduced sensitivity; in these patients, a standard wave stimulus is applied to the pharynx in 5-second pulses at intervals of about 10–15 s. The same method can be used to evaluate recuperation of the oropharyngeal motor functions. When sensitivity improves, the patient does not tolerate the electrical stimulus and refuses it or expresses refusal. Electrical stimulation does not preclude other methods, such as stimulation with ice sticks pressed against the soft palate, uvula, and back of the throat. Starting a feeding program therefore requires that certain fundamental criteria should be met. For instance, some ability to manipulate food inside the mouth, no matter how weak, and some control over the posterior pharyngeal wall are indispensable. In our experience, lifting the larynx approximately 2–3 cm helps swallowing and reduces the risk of food aspiration. The presence of the cough reflex is paramount, as is instructing the family and staff that liquids should never be administered unless it is certain that the patient can adequately swallow. The therapist begins by placing sugar or fruit jelly on the patient's lips, with the aim of getting the patient to stick out the tongue. Next, a very small amount is placed above the patient's tongue using a tongue depressor, and movements that may possibly be the start of swallowing are checked for. The sequence is repeated several times every day for many days, and is always explained to the patient even if consciousness is apparently lacking. All of these maneuvers are carried out with the patient seated in a wheelchair, with the head and trunk in axis and the back straight. If the patient meets these basic requirements and there are no medical emergencies, pureed food (fruit and, at a later time, meat) can be administered. The food flavor and taste should be enhanced, depending on the patient's preferences as described by the family in the case history. In the next phase, the patient should be fed on food with a denser consistency, such as shakes or soft vegetables. As soon as possible, the patient should be fed on solid food. The eating schedule should not be restricted, and the quantity should be gradually increased until caloric requirements are covered, with initial integration with industrial products.

Evaluation and Treatment of Spasticity

Spasticity is frequent in patients suffering from neurological pathologies, especially those in the vegetative state. It is regarded as a type of hypertonus, an alteration of movement in which hyperactivity of tendon responses results from increased excitability of the normal stretch reflex and muscular tone. The distribution most commonly observed in patients with serious cranial trauma includes plantar flexion of the foot, elbow, wrist, hand and fingers, and flexion of the hip (very frequent) and knees. Hypertonus of the adductors is common and interferes with correct posture in bed or wheelchair. Hyperadduction of the shoulder and internal rotation of the arm impede cleaning and dressing. According to several authors, spasticity is also a major factor contributing to the development of heterotopic ossification (periarticular new bone formation, PNBF).

Treatment of Spasticity

As a general rule, spasticity should be treated after proper and detailed evaluation and based on a treatment plan precisely matching the patient's requirements [12]. Treatment for spasticity is required in the following conditions:

- When it limits the range of passive mobility of a joint or limb.
- When prolonged forced postures produce or favor decubitus sores, deformities, and notable difficulties in everyday hygiene.
- When it is necessary to prevent complications (pes equinovarus, pes equinovalgus, etc.).
- When small movements (otherwise hidden) used by the patient for communication need to be promoted and enhanced.

Treatment is based on physiotherapeutic, pharmacological, and physical measures.

Physiotherapeutic Measures

Highly competent physicians, nurses, and physiotherapists need to work together. Every stimulus potentially increasing reflex hypertonus and all sources of friction potentially damaging the skin should be avoided by proper positioning. An initial measure to be taken is passive muscle stretching, based on a suggested mechanism increasing central inhibiting processes, at least transiently. In general, the spasticity of a limb depends more on the agonist than on the antagonist muscles. Reinforcement of antagonist muscles may help reduce the tone through reciprocal inhibition. Passive mobilization of a spastic limb is known to produce changes in the neurophysiological responses of the central nervous system [12,13]. A good residual function of the joints is also important for controlling hypertonus. Plaster casts, preventive splints, and the like are not always accepted and tolerated by patients in the vegetative state. These preventive measures should therefore be of limited use or may become harmful in case of neurovegetative reactions, with a return of the initial condition of deformity after they are removed.

A second step in the rehabilitation of spasticity is an attempt to restore a postural realignment opposing gravity. A reflex decrease in spastic muscles can be obtained by applying warm or chilled water or comparable means. Vibration or electrical stimulation are occasionally used to strengthen on inhibit tonus of the agonist or antagonist muscles [14]. The muscle tone also changes in relation to different head, trunk, and body positions in space. In patients in the vegetative state, primitive reflexes (such as straightening reflexes, symmetrical and asymmetrical tonus of the neck, parachute reflex, stumbling, etc.) are often exploited to help treat spasticity. The use of electromyography (EMG) biofeedback remains limited to awake patients with sufficient cognition and collaboration.

Magnetic pulse stimulation is used although with little effect. All physical treatments alone are absolutely useless for controlling spasticity, with the exception of the good results obtained with hydrotherapy (see above). This method allows maximal relaxation lasting several hours, a period during which the patient in the vegetative state is freed from the prison of spasticity and can often respond to treatment with an initial motor response.

Pharmacological Therapy

The cerebral or spinal origin of spasticity determines the choice of medication based on the sites and mechanism of action. Often, medications need to be administered in combinations and, unfortunately, may interfere with wakefulness and cognitive processes, or may induce side effects. The optimal dosage always depends on weight, metabolism, and the tolerance of individual patients and should be tailored, with titration in case of side effects. Improvement can be appreciated at dosages high enough to guarantee efficacy in the absence of side effects. The most commonly used medications are:

- *Baclofen.* This is an analog of γ-aminobutyric acid (GABA) that binds to GABAergic receptors, thereby inhibiting monosynaptic and polysynaptic reflexes and the activity of the neuromuscular junction. The therapeutic dose is in the range of 10–75 mg/day. Side effects include sedation and confusion.
- *Dantrolene sodium.* This compound acts peripherally at the muscular level, where it interferes with calcium release from the sarcoplasmic reticulum. The main side effects are sedation, nausea, and a rise in hepatic enzymes. The therapeutic dose varies from 25 to 400 mg/day.
- *Diazepam.* This facilitates the effects of GABA at the postsynaptic level. Side effects include sedation, etc. The therapeutic dose varies between 4 and 40 mg/day.
- *Clonidine.* This has a main central action as the adrenergic agonist of $α_2$-receptors and inhibits spinal reflexes, through mechanisms of action that are still poorly understood. Side effects include lethargy and orthostatic hypotension. It can be administered transdermally at doses between 0.05 and 0.1 mg.
- *Tizanidine.* This is a noradrenergic $α_2$-agonist, which shares the side effects of clonidine but is in general better tolerated, at doses of 4–36 mg/day.

Alternative Techniques, Routes of Administration, Neuromuscular Blocking

Several compounds have been used for some years now to obtain partial relief of spasticity.

Anesthetic block. Distinct approaches can result in a temporary, local blocking of conduction, such as 1–2% lidocaine in water solution, 0.25% or 0.50% bupivacaine and mepivacaine. Procaine has proved less reliable, is difficult to obtain as a commercial product, and acts on both afferent and efferent fibers. In general, the nerve trunk to be injected is located by transcutaneous electrical stimulation (for 30 min, four times a day) with square waves at a current intensity of 1 mA. This stimulation provokes a strong muscle contraction, signaling that the stimulating needle is close to the nerve; alternatively, the drug can be injected at the nerve ending of the muscle.

Neurolysis is a similar technique, much less popular today, using phenol and ethyl alcohol [14,15]. Phenol is used at a concentration of 2% or 7%, with effects lasting longer after administration at the 7% concentration. It can also be injected, at doses depending on the size of the muscle and with electromyography monitoring; the result is a transient loss of spastic contraction. It should be noted that phenol toxicity (convulsions, arrhythmias, and cardiocirculatory collapse, as with all anesthetics at high doses) is to be expected after administration of approximately 1 g. It can also be injected at the nerve ending to produce a localized effect. Inflammation often develops at the injection point.

Ethyl alcohol is injected, at a concentration of about 45% in water solution, into distinct muscle areas and acts by causing degeneration of the muscle tissue. This effect last for about 1 year in patients in the vegetative state, due to the lower tissue regeneration compared to phenol.

Botulinum toxin. There is a growing consensus for this method, which has limited risks of a deafferentation syndrome. Botulinum toxin binds at postsynaptic neuromuscular receptors and is uptaken for reuse [16]. Several types of toxin (A, B, C, etc.) have been isolated from *Clostridium botulinum*, and all cause neuromuscular blocking by interfering with acetylcholine release at the distal nerve ending. Injections are administered under electromyographic control in the muscle body and nerve ending, at doses varying according to the muscle and protocol used. In general, one to four inoculation sessions are carried out. The lethal dose is about 40 U/kg, and doses not exceeding 300–400 IU can therefore be safely used in single sessions. When administered correctly, side effects are absent and the first effects are observed after 24–72 h, with a maximum effect after about 1 month and a duration of 3–4 months [16–18].

Physiotherapy or orthotherapy and occlusive bandages (favoring muscle stretching and larger toxin diffusion) improve efficacy, with repetitive stimulation increasing the toxin action and reducing the time span between inoculation and clinical results. Occlusive bandaging must be repeated after administration of the botulinum toxin and changed at least once per day for at least five or six consecutive days, while repeated stimulation varies in different institutes in the range of two to three times every day for 4–5 days after toxin administration. Antibodies are produced over time; these reduce the effect and have encouraged the isolation of new types in recent years. This method is unfortunately quite expensive, and the purified toxin must be conserved at low temperatures. In addition, the physician also must be competent in electromyography and neurophysiology.

Careful selection of candidate patients for botulinum toxin administration is important. The time window for expected toxin efficacy is in the range of 3–12 months from the appearance of spasticity, and should be relied on especially in cases of spasticity with flexion of the upper limb, elbow, and fingers of the hand. The main muscles to be treated are the biceps, brachioradialis, radial flexors, ulnar of the wrist, superior flexor of the fingers, pronator teres, etc. The adductor pollicis is always treated when holding movements need to be improved.

Orthopedic Surgery

There are important surgical procedures that can help reduce excessive contraction. In general, tendon elongation is sufficient to reduce the muscular tone, as well as possibly balancing forces. It is also used to correct functional deficits resulting from spastic contraction and the resulting abnormal posture. The most common techniques are: tendinoplasty, split anterior tibial tendon (SPLATT), lateral transposition of part of the tendon of the anterior tibialis muscle, tenotomy, arthrodesis, and osteotomy.

Neurosurgical Measures

The neurosurgical approach is complex, unreliable, and requires expert and dedicated personnel. It is therefore unusual in treatment and restricted to cases that are absolutely refractory to other therapies. One relatively common approach that has been in use for several years now is anterior and posterior rhizotomy [5]); the DREZ-otomy (dorsal root entry zone) is no longer used [8]); myelotomy and electrical stimulation of the spinal cord are also used.

A method that has acquired popularity in recent years is intrathecal administration of baclofen using a controlled-release pump implanted under the skin. This method is generally used when others have failed or when spasticity is diffuse [19]. An administration test is first carried out with an intrathecal baclofen reservoir after evaluation using the Aswort Scale. Administration is usually with 0.25 µg baclofen diluted in 1–2 mL saline, to be increased to a maximum of 1.5 µg within 3 days. If an improvement of at least two points on the Aswort Scale is seen within 2 h after administration, the next implantation is done. Unfortunately, baclofen can cause notable and dose-related side effects, including sleepiness, epilepsy, and exceptionally sudden death. One positive side effect, in the form of a remarkable attenuation of neurovegetative reactions, especially sweating, is frequent [20]. Appropriate equipment allows reprogramming of the pump to administer smaller or larger doses as needed. The results are relatively good in patients with spinal spasticity, with a variability of efficacy among patients in the vegetative state that requires further evaluation.

Heterotopic Ossification

A frequent complication among patients in the vegetative state is the abnormal formation of osseous tissue around the joints, that begins around the second month after head injury and blocks joint and musculature in a spastic contraction. The most common sites are the shoulders, elbows, hips, and knees. Contractures in flexion are often associated with the condition, and aggravate osseous neoformation. The etiopathogenesis is unknown (see p. 71), and not all patients are affected. Alkaline phosphatase is often elevated in the affected patients, without any observed relationship with the extent of heterotopic ossification. Radiographic examination demonstrates friable tissue of lower density, which expands around and within the joint space.

At present there are no valid pharmacological or physical treatments for reducing heterotopic ossification once it has developed, and no results are obtained by physical therapies such as ultrasound, radar, etc. Diphosphonates can prevent its formation but not block its growth. Passive manipulation is again an option for delaying ankylosis. Once osseous neoformations have formed and developed excessively within a time span of 12–15 months, surgical resection is indicated (earlier surgery should be avoided due to the risk of additional heterotopic ossification).

Management of Tracheostomy Patients in the Vegetative State

Paolo Scola

Tracheostomy has been used with increasing frequency in recent years, due to its efficacy in providing better ventilation and easier control on the respiratory functions and the development of simpler and safer surgical procedures. It becomes necessary (after a variable period ranging from 3 to 15 days in different institutions) whenever patients cannot correctly perform the distinct phases of spontaneous breathing.

A wide range of tracheostomy cannulas are available. A cannula selected to suit the needs of patients in post-traumatic vegetative state should have the following characteristics:
- It should have no cap, in order to avoid decubitus sores from mucous membrane.
- It should have an interchangeable countercannula.
- It should be made of a flexible and thermosensitive material that can adapt to the patient's anatomy and reduce the risk of encrusted secretions.
- It should be movable both horizontally and vertically.
- It should have flanges of minimal thickness for patients whose neck is short.
- It should have a diameter allowing easy management of the upper airways and occlusion compatible with phonation later on.

Countercannula Disinfection

The flowchart for disinfection of the countercannula includes substitution three times a day in order to avoid infections and occlusions caused by bronchial secretions. Countercannulas should be soaked in H_2O_2 for at least 15 min and then washed under running water, cleaned with a special brush, and then soaked in a suitable disinfectant solution for at least 2 h before being dried up with sterilized gauze.

Inhalation

Tracheostomy tubes increase bronchial secretions, partly due to the altered activity of the ciliary and mucous membrane of the trachea and partly because of the absence of the nose's protective functions such as filtration and humidification. Aspiration of tracheobronchial secretions is a basic maneuver that reduces slackness in the tube and the risk of respiratory infections, while ensuring accessibility to the upper airways. It is also a maneuver that in itself can potentially promote infections, however, and should be performed with adequate aseptic technique. Tracheostomy should be performed rapidly, when the patient's physical examination reports cough and production of abundant expectoration, and it should be as nontraumatic as possible. These goals are achieved when the aspiration pressure does not exceed 250 mmHg and the duration does not exceed 30 s. After careful introduction, the probe must be rotated to avoid adherence to the mucous membrane and injury to it. Aspiration can start only after the probe has been completely introduced. Correct hydration of patients and adequate humidification of the environment are factors affecting the quantity and fluidity of bronchial secretion; a direct spout and humidifiers are useful for this purpose, and can help keep secretions fluid and facilitate expectoration. Use of aerosol therapy and mucolytic compounds is common; in our experience, mesna for endotracheal instillation has proved a good choice.

Swallowing

Tracheostomy interferes with the swallowing mechanism; rehabilitation is often disturbed by dysphagia induced by the tracheal cannula, which impedes elevation and shifting forward of the larynx. On the other hand, a cannula protects the airways against aspiration pneumonia and allows the removal of any material that has been aspirated accidentally.

Fibrotracheal Bronchoscopy

A periodic examination of the upper airways and trachea (every 6 months) is advisable in patients in the vegetative state, as it allows observation of the larynx plane and the bronchi underneath it and evaluation of the morphology and the patient's breathing and swallowing.

Complications

Most complications are associated with the cap pressure from the orotracheal tube and cannula. The mucous membrane in the trachea is damaged by pressure greater than 30 mmHg, which causes ischemia. Tracheomalacia or granulation tissue protruding into the tracheal lumen can develop when there is necrosis of the cartilage rings. Stenosis, the most feared complication, can develop after physiological repair mechanisms, and may become clinically evident only when the lumen is reduced to one-third. Tracheoesophageal fistulas require surgical treatment and the positioning of a stent.

Cannula Removal

In patients in the vegetative state, the cannula should be removed as one of the first steps in the rehabilitation treatment plan. For obvious reasons, the cannula should always be removed following a flow-chart based on a specific sequence. The basic criteria for starting the process of removing the cannula are:

- At least 250 mL expired air volume/min measured by spirometry (Wright manometer)
- Values in the physiological range on blood gas analysis
- Values of blood electrolytes (including Mg) within the physiologically normal range
- Fibrotracheal bronchoscopy estimate (tested through stoma and nose) in the physiological range
- Active and efficient swallowing is not necessary at this point

Occlusion modalities:
- Two blood gas analysis recordings need to be performed, at the baseline and at the end of each occlusion process, respectively.
- Occlusion is performed for progressively longer periods of time (e.g., 4, 8, 12, 16, and 24 hours on five consecutive days). Blood gas analysis is carried out at the end of each occlusion procedure and recorded in a special chart (an example is shown in Table 7.1).

Table 7.1 Record of cannula removal

Days	Hours	pH	Po_2	Pco_2
1	0			
1	4			
2	8			
3	12			
4	16			
5	24			

- O$_2$ saturation needs to be continuously monitored; if any breathing problem appears during occlusion, blood gas analysis must be performed immediately and occlusion suspended if necessary.

References

1. Dolce G, Serra S, Quintieri M, Sarà M, Carlino F. L'unità di risveglio dal coma: l'esperienza di Crotone. In: Atti del XVI Corso Nazionale di Aggiornamento SIMFER (Gubbio, 8-11 September 1999).
2. Zylberman MR. Approccio neuroriabilitativo al paziente in stato vegetativo. In: Dolce G, Rosadini G, editors. Polo didattico permanente/Istituto Anna 2000: p 168-185.
3. Zylberman MR, Vichi R. Terapia intensiva post acuzie per traumatizzati cranio-encefalici gravi. In: Dolce G, Rosadini G, editors. Unità di risveglio dal coma. Crotone, Italy: Polo Didattico Permanente/Istituto S. Anna, 1997: 42-76.
4. Longman JA. Evaluation and treatment planning for the head-injured patient with oral intake disorder. J Head Trauma Rehabil 1989; 4: 24, 1989.
5. Fisher B. Effect of trunk control and alignment on limb function. J Head Trauma Rehabil 1987; 2: 72.
6. Cherney LR, Halper AS. Recovery of oral nutrition after injury in adults. J Head Trauma Rehabil 1989; 4: 42, 1989.
7. Letts RM. Principles of seating the disabled. Boca Raton, FL: CRC Press, 1991.
8. Peterson MJ, Adkins HV. Measurement and redistribution of excessive pressures during wheelchair sitting. Phys Ther 1982; 62: 990-4.
9. Fisher B, Akura J. Movement analysis: a different perspective. Orthop Phys Ther Clin North Am 1993; 2: 1, 1993.
10. Lazarus CL. Swallowing disorder after traumatic brain injury. J Head Rehabil 1989; 4: 34, 1989.
11. Winstein CJ. Neurogenic dysphagia; frequency, progression, and outcome in adult following head injury. Phys Ther 1983; 63: 1992-7.
12. Glenn MB. Nerve blocks. In: Glenn MM, White J, editors. The practical management of spasticity in children and adults. Philadelphia: Lea and Febiger, 1990: 227-67.
13. Hummelsheim H, Maurtiz KH. Neurophysiological mechanism of spasticity modification by physiotherapy. Heidelberg: Springer, 1993: 425-37.
14. Bodine-Fowler SC, Allsing S, Botte MJ. Time course of muscle atrophy and recovery following a phenol-induced nerve block. Muscle Nerve 1996; 19: 497-504.
15. Moore TJ, Andreson RB. The use of phenol blocks to the motor branches of the tibial nerve in adult acquired spasticity. Foot Ankle 1991; 11: 219-21.
16. Berardelli A, Abbruzzese G, Bertolasi L, et al. Guidelines for the therapeutic use of botulinum toxin in moviment disorders. Italian Study Group for Movement Disorders, Italian Society of Neurology. Ital J Neurol Sci 1997; 18: 261-9.
17. Montecucco C, Schiavo G, Tugnoli V, de Grandis D. Botulinum neurotoxins: mechanism of action and therapeutic applications. Mol Med Today 1996; 2: 418-24.
18. Simpson DM, Alexander DN, O'Brien CF, et al. Botulinum toxin type A in the treatment of upper extremity spasticity: a randomized, double-blind, placebo-controlled trial. Neurology 1996; 48: 1306-10.
19. Yablon SA, Agana BT, Ivanhoe CB, Boake C. Botulinum toxin in severe upper extremity spasticity among patients with traumatic brain injury: an open-labeled trial. Neurology 1996; 47: 939-44.
20. Coffey RJ, Cahill D, Steers W, et al. Intrathecal baclofen for intractable spasticity of spinal origin: results of a long-term multicenter study. J Neurosurg 1996; 78: 226-32.

8 Minimal Response Syndrome

Ofer Keren, Jacqueline Resnik

What is Minimal Response Syndrome?

An increasing number of severely brain-damaged patients survive as a result of improved technology, and face severe incapacitating disabilities [1]. Over the past 30 years, epidemiological studies have shown an increase in the survival of patients with both traumatic and nontraumatic brain injuries [2]. The numbers of patients who remain in an altered state of consciousness (ASC) – i. e., those in coma, in a vegetative or near-vegetative state, with postcomatose unawareness, with postcomatose cortical unresponsiveness, slow recovery, or those who are minimally responsive or with minimal activity – are therefore substantial [3]. The existence of so many "similar" names for these conditions suggests two possibilities – firstly, that there is disagreement regarding the nomenclature, or secondly, that ASC is a "basket" term including a spectrum of diagnoses, rather than being a single definite condition [4].

This chapter is deals with aspects of the treatment of one specific subtype of ASC patients – those who are termed "minimally responsive" (in "postvegetative state" or in a "low-awareness state"). No one clear unique definition for this "vague" entity is found in the literature. The definition of "minimal response" includes objective issues such as "measurable" parameters, as well as subjective issues, such as the decision as to which response may be called "minimal". Minimally conscious patients are those who can follow simple commands reliably, but are unable to follow complex commands [5].

Significance of the Syndrome

Few studies have been published concerning the clinical aspects of patients in the minimally responsive state. There have been many more reports on comatose patients and/or patients who succeed in recovering from coma to "active" life. Therapists get satisfaction and the recognition accompanying success when patients recover. The drama of treatment in the intensive-care unit, where the major emphasis is on saving the life of the patient, often ceases to interest the medical staff once the patient has gained "stability." The quality of the life that has been saved may be largely ignored; in other words, minimally responsive patients draw a "minimal response" from the medical and scientific personal in turn.

There are, however, two main reasons why it is important to focus on this group of patients:
- Developments in medicine have enabled more people to survive severe brain damage and to remain in this state.
- Focusing investigations on the life of a person who is in the minimally responsive state can enrich our understanding about what the term "consciousness" actually means.

Implications for Health Policy

A policy on the care of this group of patients needs to be developed, and it should be based on the following considerations: what is the optimum way of assessing the response and what level of consciousness does it actually reflect [5]? The answers to these questions should form the basis of the rationale and guidelines used in practical clinical management.

To better understand the meaning of the syndrome of "minimal response" it may be useful to interpret firstly the meaning of its components [6]. The response component is a measurable parameter, which means it has a quantitative value. To determine the meaning of "response" is not a purely medical and/or laboratory decision, but depends upon the "value" of the response (i. e., a qualitative statement). Thus, the decision that a response is minimal should not be taken only by the medical team. The response should be measurable and repeatable. Further questions then arise, for example: what kind of responses can be called meaningful ones? Who should decide this? How (using what tools) [5]? When and for how long? Since the answers to these questions are both qualitative and quantitative, they should be given by the medical team working together with other nonmedical personal such as "the family," religious personnel, and/or a legal representative.

Practically, since we are dealing with patients who suffer from very severe neural damage, their "minimal response" is not a constant one, but instead may change depending on various self and nonself influences [7]. The syndrome of minimal response therefore represents a wide range of conditions in patients and cannot be defined for some time after the initial neural insult (at least several months).

Diagnosis and Assessment Tools

Diagnosis is very much linked to definition. Coma is the extreme manifestation of severe brain insult. Loss of consciousness and coma are synonymous terms for the diagnosis of a patient who has no "connection" with his surroundings. "Coma is a profound or deep state of unconsciousness. The affected individual is alive, but is not able to react or respond to life around him/her. Coma may occur as an expected progression or complication of an underlying illness, or as a result of an event such as head trauma" [9]. The use of a practical method of assessing coma, such as the Glasgow Coma Scale (GCS) [10], enables the medical team to deal with these patients using more concrete (regular) medical terminology. It does, however, emphasize the complexity of this diagnosis, since "coma" is no longer a vague concept, but a measurable entity – i. e., it has a quantitative value. Farber and Churchland [11] stated that it is more fruitful not to define consciousness, but to describe the various subcategories that are included in the concept. These subcategories are:
- *Sensory awareness:* this includes stimuli from the sensory organs, but also "modality-specific imagery."
- *Generalized awareness:* this includes inner states with no clear link to any modality, such as "comfort."
- *Metacognitive awareness:* "there are all sorts of things one can be aware of in the realm of one's own cognition."

These subcategories give some insight into the concept of consciousness, since it is not only synonymous with awareness, but also carries with it an implication of agency and control. Included in it is the more vague term of "soul." Neural synchrony with a precision in the millisecond range may be crucial for conscious processing, and may be involved in arousal, perceptual integration, attention selection, and working memory [12]. Consciousness is a complex concept that incorporates several issues, such as wakefulness, the experience of oneself and one's surroundings, and the possession of intentions. Consciousness, in all its aspects, is a matter of degree.

Coma is a term for the acute phase after the insult. Jennett and Bond [13] developed an assessment for the postacute state in these patients. The Coma Outcome Scale consists of five global categories in an ordinal scale going from recovery, moderate disability, severe disability, and persistent vegetative state, to death. Jennett and Plum were among the first to introduce the concept of persistent vegetative state in describing the syndrome of wakeful unresponsiveness [14]. In 1991, Sazbon and Groswasser suggested an alternative term, "postcomatose unawareness" [15]. Glenn suggested a more direct term, "postcomatose cortical unresponsiveness" [16]. These semantic nuances emphasizes the complexity of this issue. The state of "minimal responsiveness" includes patients who are unable to respond to commands and communicate reliably [17]. "Minimal responsiveness" can be diagnosed under a general term, but it must be emphasized that this broad category may actually include different levels of brain functioning, both in terms of quality and quantity. The body of knowledge, precision of assessment, specificity of treatment, and effectiveness of communication might be improved if we had better tools for differentiating these particular patients [18,19]. Horn et al. [20], after presenting a review of the existing assessments for minimally responsive patients, concluded that their efficacy was based on short-term projects and that the tools required further validation in order to establish their usefulness in the long-term setting. The distinction between patients who are diagnosed as being in the vegetative state, as opposed to the minimally responsive state, depends not only on their functional status, but also on the tool by which they are evaluated

[4]. It is not surprising, therefore, that the diagnostic classification and assessment of patients who remain unconscious for prolonged periods and recover from coma only to demonstrate a very low level of response, has not yet been well developed [14–16].

Better tools for assessing, differentiating, monitoring treatment, and communicating about these particular patients should be developed [18, 19,21,22]. On the basis of multicenter data on patients with low-level brain injury (vegetative or near-vegetative), Berrol stated that there are substantial changes occurring that may not reflect the potential for functional improvement [23]. He also added that it might well be that evolutionary changes continue to occur over long periods of time. Ansell and Keenan introduced the term "slow to recover," which was used for patients who improve more slowly than most others with severe brain injury [24]. These patients do not follow the "normal recovery pattern," seen as the achievement of major functional improvement during the first 6 months after injury. Ansell and Keenan stated that these patients are considered ready for rehabilitation when they reach Ranchos level V [25], i.e. when "responses are prompt and consistent although not necessarily accurate or appropriate." The few reports about long-term follow-up in this population indicate gradual improvement [15, 24,26].

Rosenberg and Ashwal [28] suggested the following distinctions between patients who are in coma, vegetative, or minimally responsive:

- *Coma:* patients have no self-awareness, are not aware of pain, do not have sleep–wake cycles or purposeful movements, and may have depressed respiratory functions. The coma diagnosis does not last longer than 4 weeks; the possible outcomes are death, vegetative state, minimal response, and recovery.
- *Vegetative state:* patients have no self-awareness, do not feel pain or have sleep–wake cycles, have no purposeful movements, but do have normal respiratory function.
- *Minimal response:* patients have limited self-awareness, do feel pain, and have sleep–wake cycles. They may also have severely limited movement, and respiratory function may be depressed [28].

Clinical evaluation of awareness may be divided to subgroups such as: visual, auditory, somatosensory, and motor activity. To avoid misdiagnosis, it is recommended that information be gathered from a variety of sources, including interviewing family members [29].

The differential diagnosis becomes more questionable when sophisticated tools for evaluation are used [30]. Menon et al. used evoked a response of oddball (P300) study and a ^{15}O positron emission tomography (PET) subtraction paradigm to assess the response to familiar faces that were presented. These tests were used to demonstrate responsiveness in a patient who was otherwise diagnosed as being in the vegetative state [30].

Incidence and Prevalence

There have so far been no epidemiological studies dedicated to these patients. As mentioned above, there is no absolute agreement on which patients should be labeled under this diagnosis. It is therefore impossible to give any reliable numbers for the incidence and prevalence of minimally responsive patients. This task is especially complicated, since there are two possible ways in which patients may enter the minimally responsive state – firstly, those who "recover" from the vegetative state, and secondly, those whose mental function has deteriorated to a minimal response (e. g., patients suffering from severe degenerative brain disease). Although these two groups of patients are similar from the point of function, it can be expected that their "brain status" will react differently, since one group is on a "recovery path," while the other is on a "deteriorating path." The focus in this section is mainly on the first group. The incidence of this subgroup can be estimated from data for patients who were comatose following insult and did not die. When information from a local district in Japan was generalized, there was an estimated figure of approximately one per 100 000 population for traumatic brain injury patients with a very severe outcome [31].

The next question concerns the prevalence – an even harder issue, since it incorporates data on the incidence as well as data about the expected length of life. As mentioned before, these patients are fully dependent, so the expected length of life has a direct relationship to the quality of care and therapy provided. It is reasonable to assume that the reduction in motor activity has a negative influence on the cardiorespiratory system. In recent years, there have been many studies on the didactic relationship between the immune system and central nervous system (CNS) activity, but it is impossible to predict from these data what quantitative effect it may have on changes in lifespan. It is reasonable to estimate that life in "semi-isolated surroundings" would have influence on physiological and psychological elements, but since there are so many factors involved, no one can predict the "end-point" of their effects. These patients are unable to travel, for example, so that they are safe from many dangers that others are exposed to in life. It is impossible to use data concerning small groups of patients who are treated in a specific community to deduce "hard" data concerning the expected length of life of these patients. In practical terms, this is a very important medicolegal issue, since data of this type are needed to estimate the amount of compensation for these patients. Certainly, individual parameters such as age, sex, and premorbid medical condition will have an effect on lifespan.

More specific epidemiological studies have been performed concerning the follow-up in severely brain-injured patients admitted to neurosurgical departments. On the basis of such data, a prediction "tree" has been developed [32]. It is impossible to determine from these data any clear information concerning minimally responsive patients, since this group is usually included in the subgroup defined as "bad outcome."

Practical Management Recommendations

Clinical Management

By definition, these patients in the minimal responsive state are fully dependent for all their activities of daily living. Their cooperation is severely limited, as is their ability to ask for any specific needs or be involved in any decision-making concerning their life. The quality and quantity of their treatment will depend totally on their care-givers. Their lifespan is thus directly related to the quality of care.

Objectives of Treatment

There are three main aims of treatment for these patients:
- Care and management for basic maintenance (e.g., feeding, infection prevention, and preservation of general good health).
- Specialized therapeutic techniques aimed at improving quality of life. These may include a variety of stimulating techniques – motor, sensory, and communicative.
- Spiritual maintenance – e. g., the use of physical contact, such as massage, hydrotherapy, enhancement of the surroundings with art and music, human contact, and animal contact.

The separation between these aims of treatment (care and therapy) is not always so clear. The meaning of the word "recovery" can be interpreted two ways – either raising the level of responsiveness without changing the diagnosis, or achieving recovery to a point at which the patient can no longer be considered to be in the minimally responsive state.

Treatment Aimed at "Care"

Maintenance (Keeping the Patient Alive)

Nutritional intervention. Support all elements of nutrition under the guidance of a specialist in the field. The metabolic balance must be controlled so as to ensure that neither malnutrition nor obesity develops. All of these patients require feeding; this can be achieved either orally or via a feeding tube.

Hygienic care, including the bladder and bowel. Since none of these patients are expected to be able control their secretions, routine check-up and cleansing should be done. Care must be taken that there is no residual urine in the bladder and no difficulties in passing stool. Whenever there is any difficulty in controlling secretions, medical intervention should be involved, such as intermittent catheterization or administration stool softeners. These procedures should only be prescribed by a specialist and should be followed up with intensive monitoring.

Respiratory and skin care. These patients are very limited in self-movement, so their position should be changed every few hours, including during the night, to prevent skin lesions. The skin all over the body must be routinely checked and lubricated. Some of the patients breathe via tracheotomy tubes, and all are expected to have difficulty in expectoration. It is extremely important to position these patients in the sitting and/or standing position at least once daily. Some of these patients will require routine respiratory physiotherapy.

Pain control. The argument as to whether ASC patients have some conscious awareness at subcortical levels is as yet unresolved. There is therefore no reliable way of determining how much they can perceive pain and suffering [33]. In many cases, it is only possible to suspect that the patient is indeed suffering only by observing mimic reactions, hearing wailing, and/or observing changes in autonomic activity on monitors. It is critically important first to look for a possible cause for the observed changes, which may be reversible – e. g., smoothing out the bedsheet or removing any internal blockage.

Sleep control. Every few months, the patient's sleep–wake cycle should be monitored to test the quality of the sleep cycles. Treatment for sleep disturbances should be implemented whenever significantly abnormal sleep patterns are detected.

Prevention of Secondary Complications

Routine daily motor activity. Patients should spend part of the day sitting out of bed. Standing should be carried out whenever possible. Passive movements and stretching (under the direction of a physiotherapist) should also be performed daily, with the aim of preventing contractures developing due to muscle shortening or the development of new bone formation.

Continuous medical monitoring to prevent development of metabolic imbalance. Observation should ensure that any developing infection is noted as quickly as possible. Deep vein thrombosis or decubitus ulcers or osteoporosis should be prevented.

Pharmacological treatment should be provided, with anti-epileptic drugs to prevent seizures without the possible development of unwanted side effects.

Maintenance (Spiritual)

Family support. The families of these patients can expect to have to live for many years with a relative who is "minimally responsive." There is little or no communication with the patient as there was before the trauma. The patient's absence from the family's regular daily routines and the uncertainty of the future can all contribute to family distress.

Touch. The importance of touch in this group of patients cannot be measured objectively. Treatment should provide the patient with more than just the technical procedures required to maintain life. The families should be encouraged to touch and massage their loved one as much as possible.

Sexuality. Since this group of patients is frequently in the age group in which sexual relationships are an important aspect of life, this subject should be open to discussion with the families. If the patient's partner demonstrates a desire to have an intimate relationship with him or her, this should be encouraged. However, possible medical side effects such as overstimulation of the autonomic system should be monitored. No one can say how much positive stimulation such a relationship may provide.

Treatment Aimed at "Therapy"

Alertness

Cognitive malfunctions in these patients mainly involve arousal disturbances, attention, recognition, and memory disorders. There have been some attempts to improve these activities by therapy and/or pharmacological intervention. Various methods of stimulation are employed [34], and various medications have been used, such as stimulant antidepressants [35].

To stimulate recovery, many rehabilitation professionals recommend placing minimally responsive individuals in stimulation-rich environments [35]. They believe that exposure to frequent and varied sensory stimulation facilitates dendrite growth and improves synaptic conductivity in patients with traumatic brain injury (TBI). It is believed that these patients will gain improvement in their cognitive functions, environmental awareness, and interactions. There are two controversial ideas about the activation of the reticulolimbic system: the more widely accepted idea that external stimulation may stimulate recovery; or alternatively, that too much uncontrolled activation may actually interfere with the natural recovery processes.

In most rehabilitation facilities, it is now accepted that a certain degree of stimulation should be given. However, controversy persists as to the best method and the amount that is necessary [36].

Motor and Tonus Control

These patients may suffer from different types of motor control dysfunction. A specialist should follow any motor response, for use in communication. Basic reflexes should be stimulated to improve balance and body positioning. Abnormal muscle tonus is most likely to be in the form of spastic hypertonus. A multidisciplinary team, including medical, physiotherapy, and nursing personnel, should conduct the "battle" against these impairments. The therapy should include positioning the patient throughout the day. Specialized physical therapy includes techniques for reducing tonus manually, and the use of various modalities such as hydrotherapy, cryotherapy, and the introduction of neurolytic agents for muscle/nerve block.

Complementary Therapy

As mentioned above, these patients suffer from very severe brain damage, and the prognosis is poor. Since conventional medicine is unable to offer miracle cures for these patients, the families often are drawn to seek alternative solutions in the form of complementary medicine – such as acupuncture, homeopathy, reflexology, etc. However, controlled studies are still needed before such therapies can be legitimized.

Spirituality, Feelings of Satisfaction

The patients are individuals who may live for many years, but are unable to initiate any enjoyable activities. An effort should be made to look for a way to make them feel positive – emotionally and spiritually. It may be using music, visual stimulation, taste and smell, or an opportunity to be at home for short periods. The link between desire, motivation, and awareness is an interesting issue that has not yet been fully investigated.

Clinical Treatment Providers

Who should provide the treatments and for how long? Since the treatment is expected to be given for many years, the cost-effectiveness of interventions needs to be taken into consideration. Since the goals are dynamic, it is recommended that an expert in the field should monitor the patient over a long period of time and take the decision as to which is the treatment of choice. The chance of recovery from this state decreases as time progresses, so therapy for stimulation should be more intensive in the earlier stages – i.e., in the first 2 years post insult.

As was mentioned earlier, the line between what is care and what is therapy is not always clear. Every form of contact with the patient has a combined influence of therapy and care. Care-givers and family members carry out the majority of contact care. It is extremely important that this contact (with nonmedical professionals and family members) should be controlled and monitored by a specialist in the field, such as the physiotherapist, occupational therapist, speech pathologist, etc. The guidance provided by the specialist is intended to prevent complications and enable modifications to be made whenever needed (and it is recommended that he or she be a member of the team).

In many of these patients, the quality and quantity of the response can demonstrate functional progress over many years of treatment, but they nevertheless remain at tragically low levels of function. Other patients may make minimal progress, although that, however, becomes very significant in subjective terms for them and their families in terms of quality of life. Most of these patients do not make any conventional functional independent progress (i.e., reducing the assistance needed) after many years of treatment in their communication, social, or emotional functions. The single case design model appears to be the intervention of choice, with its great flexibility and tailored approach to each individual case [37]. "Recovery" from ASC does not appear to be a smooth, continuous process; those who remain in the vegetative state can show improvements and those who do recover from vegetative state may show little or no improvement, or even deterioration at times [38]. The degree and rate of recovery within different modalities varies between individuals; it will usually occur first in the auditory, communication, motor, or olfactory modality, or in a combination of these responses; visual responses are only rarely the first sign [38].

Debate is continuing regarding whether ASC patients have some conscious awareness at subcortical levels or not. There is no reliable way of determining the extent to which they can perceive pain and suffering [33].

Since there is only limited research evidence as to the long-term benefits of sensory stimulation programs, the recommendations rely on "agreed opinions" rather than "hard data." In order to prevent overstimulation, staff and relatives should use a consistent program of specific stimulation. A period of rest should be allowed before starting the specific controlled sensory input session.

Rehabilitation has been defined as "the development of a person to the fullest physical, psychological, social, vocational, avocation, and educational potential, consistent with his or her physiological or anatomical impairment and environmental limitations" [40]. The application of this definition to severely injured patients, with a guarded prognosis for functional independence, raises interrelated ethical, social, practical, and financial questions. There are no clear criteria for appropriate use versus abuse of rehabilitation resources in such patients.

In order to improve communicative behaviors in minimally responsive patients, Shiel and Wilson [41] adapted a structured interview that was developed for children with mental delay. A single case report demonstrated that this system was useful in enabling a patient to obey commands consistently when they were within the patient's ability and to interact with staff, primarily using facial expression. She was able to understand and retain simple information for a period of 10 min, but had no recall of this 2 h later [41].

Even at the "lowest" level of minimal response, if motor responses are evaluated and interpreted, then at least minimal degrees of movement can be observed [42]. The role of repeatable meaningful responses to commands has been proposed as a distinguishing neurobehavioral characteristic of the minimally responsive state [43]. Even these minimal movements can have huge importance, since they may serve as a communication tool. Extended observation can prevent misdiagnosis [5]; in their study of 49 vegetative patients, Childs et al. [44] found that 37 had been incorrectly diagnosed.

Policy and Ethics Related to the Minimally Responsive Patient

In a multicultural, pluralistic society, individuals may be members of several different cultures tied to ethnicity, religion, or business that share some values and differ in others. The rules of behavior for the providers of the rehabilitation services are based on three major cultural fields: the scientific, the humanistic, and the entrepreneurial [45].

Practical and ethical questions arise on a daily basis concerning the treatment of these patients, such as how long, how much, and in what way these patients should be treated [1,46,47]. Many articles have been written concerning the questions of legal and ethical aspects of patients in the vegetative state, usually concerning life and death and euthanasia [48]. Very few articles have been concerned with the question of what is the "meaning" of treatment for the minimal responsive patient. In the end, however, the question of treatment efficacy remains a moral, rather than a scientific one. Resolving the question of "what is treatment effectiveness?" hinges on the definition of effectiveness. Many of these patients will successfully gain functional improvement over time with the application of conventional methods of rehabilitation and the novel use of pharmacological agents. Usually, it is only several months after the insult that they began to respond in a consistent way. This recovery process is slow and does not change the patients' basic severe disabilities, as they are still fully dependent in all their activities of daily life. However, they may be able to communicate emotions and desires, and to become more involved in their family life.

The question of how long the treatment should be carried out is easier when the diagnosis is more definitive, as in the vegetative state, than in a group of patients whose abilities are much more diverse, as in the minimally responsive state. Based on reviews of clinical experience and scientific findings, the Multiple Task Force indicated that the odds of emergence from vegetative state are small after 1 year [49]. It is impossible to make such a statement about minimally responsive patients, since the question is not one of quantity (such as a return to consciousness, or emergence from the vegetative state), but of quality (what are the changes in the level of consciousness?).

Questions that involve combined parameters of ethical and practical issues include what the outcome of rehabilitation will be, and what the expected prognosis is. The answers to such questions can be based on statistical and pathophysiological data - for example, a statement such as: "the least recovery of function was seen in anoxic patients who remained comatose for 4 weeks and more" [46]. Comatose patients with traumatic brain injury recover over a period of months and even years after injury, whereas the period of recovery from anoxic brain damage was measured in weeks, with practically no functional gains after 4 months [50]. These widely accepted statements about the time course of recovery, and by inference the appropriate time for treatment, are based on "macroscopic" assessment of functional activity using extremely simple ordinal rating scales with extremely broad and vague categories, such as the Disability Rating Scale [18]. For a "minimally responsive patient," this "conventional" and simplistic approach of evaluation may not always be valid, since in the view of the patient and family some "microscopic" functional improvement has a "huge" significance.

There are no clear criteria for appropriate use versus abuse of rehabilitation resources in such patients. Who has the responsibility for deciding how much and for how long the treatments should be provided [51]? Often a patient does not gain any conventional functional independence (i. e., reducing the assistance needed) after several years of treatment, yet on the other hand gains significant improvement in communication abilities and social and emotional functioning. Is the goal of the rehabilitation process to achieve functional ability, or to improve the quality of life within the confines of the disability? Any attempt at defining the quality of life and "worth" of questionable functional gains will imply moral and ethical judgments. Some patients may achieve some rehabilitation, but nevertheless remain at tragically low levels of function. Others may obtain minimal progress, although it is very significant in subjective terms to their quality of life. There is no way at present to predict accurately how much recovery will occur, or when the recovery will plateau. Ansell reported that about half of these patients (classed as "slow to recover") reach a status of "rehabilitation-ready", as defined, between 2 and 48 months after injury; two-thirds of these patients had reached this status of "rehabilitation-ready" 6 months after injury [47].

Conclusions

According to conventional prognostic criteria, a "minimally responsive" patient is doomed to a very poor rehabilitation outcome, as measured in terms of functional independence and simple, ordinary category scales. A "microanalytic" approach to change may reveal that the long-term rehabilitation process has a more positive impact. Although in the eyes of family members this rehabilitation process is absolutely worthwhile, the gains may only decrease the global costs to society if the families care for patients outside of expensive institutions. With "the era of unlimited medical care over" [8], the view that society as a whole will take of the costs arising from full professional care for these patients is not clear. No definite answers are available to difficult questions such as for how long, and how much, patients with "minimal activity" should be treated. Each group has to make its own decisions on these issues, depending on resources and ethics. These dilemmas need to be discussed in future medical planning and training programs.

References

1. Gouvier WD, Blanton PD, LaPorte KK, Nepomuceno C. Reliability and validity of the Disability Rating Scale and the level of cognitive functioning scale in monitoring recovery from severe head injury. Arch Phys Med Rehabil 1987; 68: 94–7.

2. Jennett B, Teasdale G, Galbraith S, et al. Severe head injuries in three countries. J Neurol Neurosurg Psychiatry 1977; 40: 291–8.
3. Andrews K, Beaumont JG, Danze F, et al. International Working Party report on the vegetative state. London: Royal Hospital for Neuro-disability, 1996 (http://www.comarecovery.org/pvs.htm).
4. Gill-Thwaites H. The sensory modality assessment rehabilitation technique: a tool for assessment and treatment of patients with severe brain injury in vegetative state. Brain Inj 1997; 10: 723–34.
5. Whyte J, DiPasquale MC, Vaccaro M. Assessment of command-following in minimally conscious brain injured patients. Arch Phys Med Rehabil 1999; 80: 653–60.
6. Giacino JT, Zasler ND, Whyte J, Hate DI, Glenn M, Andaly M. Recommendations for the use of uniform nomenclature pertinent to patients with severe alterations in consciousness. Arch Phys Med Rehabil 1995; 76: 203–7.
7. Andrews K, Murphy L, Munday R, Littlewood C. Misdiagnosis of the vegetative state: retrospective study in a rehabilitation unit. Br Med J 1996; 313: 13–6.
8. Beck M. Rational health care. Newsweek, June 27, 1994: 30–35.
9. National Institutes of Health. What is coma, including persistent vegetative state? Bethesda, MD: National Institutes of Health, April 2000 (http://accessible.ninds.nih.gov/health_and_medical/disorders/coma_doc.htm#What_is_Coma,_including_Persistent_Vegetative_State).
10. Teasdale G, Jennett B. Assessment of coma and impaired consciousness: a practical scale. Lancet 1974; ii: 81–4.
11. Farber IB, Churchland PC. Consciousness and neuroscience: philosophical and theoretical issues. In: Gazzaniga MS, editor. Cognitive neuroscience. Cambridge, MA: MIT, 1995: 1295–1306.
12. Engel AK, Singer W. Temporal binding and the neural corselets of sensory awareness. Trends Cogn Sci 2000; 5: 16–25.
13. Jennett B, Bond LMR. Assessment of outcome in severe brain damage: a practical scale. Lancet 1975; i: 480–4.
14. Jennett B, Plum F. Persistent vegetative state after brain damage. Lancet 1972; i: 734–7.
15. Sazbon L, Groswasser S. Prolonged coma, vegetative state, post-comatose unawareness: semantics or better understanding? Brain Inj 1991; 5: 1–2.
16. Glenn MB. Post-comatose unawareness? Brain Inj 1992; 6: 101–2.
17. Giacino LOT, Kezmarsky MA, Deluca J, Cicerone KD. Monitoring rate of recovery to predict outcome in minimally responsive recovery. Arch Phys Med Rehabil 1991; 72: 897–901.
18. Rappaport M, Dougherty AM, Kelting DL. Evaluation of coma and vegetative states. Arch Phys Med Rehabil 1992; 73: 628–34.
19. Keren O, Groswasser Z, Sazbon L, Ring C. Somatosensory evoked potentials in prolonged unawareness state following traumatic brain injury. Brain Inj 1991; 5: 233–40.
20. Horn S, Watson M, Wilson BA, McLellan DL. The development of new techniques in the assessment and monitoring of recovery from severe head injury: a preliminary report and case history. Brain Inj 1992; 6: 321–5.
21. Rader MA, Alston JB, Ellis DW. Sensory stimulation of severely brain-injured patients. Brain Inj 1989; 3: 141–7.
22. Cossa A, Fabiani M, Farinato A, Laiacona M, Capitani E. The "preliminary neuropsychological battery": an instrument to grade the level of minimally responsive patients. Brain Inj 1999; 13: 583–92.
23. Berrol S. Evaluation and the persistent vegetative state. J Head Trauma Rehabil 1986; 1: 7–13.
24. Ansell B, Keenan J. The Western Neuro Sensory Stimulation Profile: A tool for assessing slow-to-recover head injury patients. Arch Phys Med Rehabil 1989; 70: 104–8.
25. Hagan C, Malkmus D, Durham P. Rehabilitation of the head injured adult: comprehensive physical management. Downey, CA: Professional Staff Association of Rancho Los Amigos Hospital, 1979.
26. Timmons M, Gasquoine L. Functional changes with rehabilitation of very severe traumatic brain injury survivors. J Head Trauma Rehabil 1987; 2: 64–73.
27. Ansell BJ. Slow-to-recover brain injury patients: rational for treatment. J Speech Hear Res 1991; 24: 1017–22.
28. Rosenberg J, Ashwal S. Recent advances in the development of practice parameters: the vegetative state. Neurorehabilitation 1996; 6: 79–87.
29. Wade TD, Johnston C. The permanent vegetative state: practical guidance on diagnosis and management. Br Med J 1999; 319: 841–4.
30. Menon DK, Owen AM, Williams EJ, et al. Cortical processing in persistent vegetative state. Wolfson Brain Imaging Centre Team. Lancet 1998; 352: 1148–9.
31. Sato S, Imamura H, Ueki K, et al. Epidemiological survey of vegetative state patients in the Tokohu district, Japan: special reference to the follow up study after one year. Neurol Med Chir (Tokyo) 1979; 8: 327–33.
32. Choi SC, Muizeilaar P, Barnes TY, Marmarou A, Brooks DM, Young HF. Prediction tree for se-

verely head-injured patients. J Neurosurg 1991; 75: 251–5.
33. Day L. Persistent vegetative state: important considerations for neuroscience nurse. J Neurosci Nursing 1996; 28: 199–203.
34. Jones R, Hux K, Morton-Anderson A, Knepper L. Auditory stimulation effect on a comatose survivor of traumatic brain injury. Arch Phys Med Rehabil 1994; 75: 164–71.
35. Zafonte RD, Lexell J, Cullen N. Possible applications for dopaminergic agents following traumatic brain injury, 2. J Head Trauma Rehabil 2001; 16: 112–6.
36. O'Dell MW, Jasin P, Lyons N, Stivers M, Meszaros F. Standardized assessment instruments for minimally responsive brain injury patients. NeuroRehabilitation 1996; 6: 45–55.
37. Piguet O, King AC, Harrison DP. Assessment of minimally responsive patients: clinical difficulties of single-case design. Brain Inj 1999; 13: 829–37.
38. Wilson SL, Gill-Thwaites H. Early indication of emergence from vegetative state derived from assessment with the SMART: a preliminary report. Brain Inj 2000; 14: 319–31.
39. Andrews K. International Working Party on the management of the vegetative state: summary report. Brain Inj 1996; 10: 797–806.
40. DeLisa JA, Martin GM, Currie DM. Rehabilitation medicine: past, present, and future. In: DeLisa JA, editor. Rehabilitation medicine: principles and practice. Philadelphia: Lippincott, 1993: 3–27.
41. Shiel A, Wilson BA. Assessment after extremely severe head injury a case of life or death: further support for McMillan. Brain Inj 1998; 12: 809–16.
42. Pilon M, Sullivan SJ. Motor profile of patients in minimally responsive and persistent vegetative states. Brain Inj 1996; 10: 421–37.
43. American Congress of Rehabilitation Medicine. Recommendations for use of uniform nomenclature pertinent to patients with severe alterations in consciousness. Arch Phys Med Rehabil 1995; 76: 205–9.
44. Childs NL, Mercer WN, Childs HW. Accuracy of diagnosis of persistent vegetative state. Neurology 1993; 43: 1465–7.
45. Malec JF. Ethical conflict resolution based on an ethics of relationships for brain injury rehabilitation. Brain Inj 1996; 10: 781–95.
46. Groswasser Z, Cohen M, Costeff H. Rehabilitation outcomes after anoxic brain damage. Arch Phys Med Rehabil 1989; 70: 186–8.
47. Ansell BJ. Slow-to-recover brain injury patients: improvement to rehabilitation readiness. J Head Trauma Rehabil 1993; 8: 88–98.
48. McLean SAM. Legal and ethical aspects of the vegetative state. J Clin Pathol 1999; 52: 490–3.
49. Multi-Society Task Force on PVS. Medical aspects of persistent vegetative state, 2. N Engl J Med 1994; 330: 1572–9.
50. Stern JM, Groswasser Z, Alis R, Geva N. Day center experience in rehabilitation of craniocerebral injured patients. Scand J Rehabil Med Suppl 1985; 12: 53–8.
51. Danja JD. Ethics, fraud, and the misallocation of rehabilitation resources. J Head Trauma Rehabil 1992; 7: 114–6.

9 Ethical Aspects

Giuliano Dolce and Leon Sazbon

Care for patients in the vegetative state involves particular aspects that also affect those professionals dealing with patients who have an "uninhabited body," lack consciousness for long periods of time, sometimes permanently, and have needs but no way of expressing them. These patients live an extremely critical clinical condition, and have no support from their previous experience and personality.

The most important aspect to consider among those that characterize human individuals (moral, legal, socio-economic, and, above all, medical and ethical) is the person himself or herself [1]. If we identify a person as a unit that combines rationality and responsibility, continuity and identity, and is a center of relationships and bonds (in agreement with Max Scheler) [2], then the person *is* his or her own consciousness, and especially his or her own moral consciousness. This person appears canceled, and therefore lost, when consciousness is abolished, as in the vegetative state. However, since the body is present, the person also exists in a "potential" form.

Following this argument, Cohadon [3] reminds us of the way in which the embryo is considered to represent a potential person and is somehow in a vegetative state, which in this case evolves toward developing consciousness, rather than recovering it. The strong bonds with family members that become evident in patients in the vegetative state as a kind of "emotional stubbornness" also indicate that a "person" exists.

The particular bond between the patient and the attending and caring staff – who also take important measures without the patient's consent, for a period of time often as long as several months – signifies a special relationship in which the patient's consciousness is not manifest, but is reflected in and participating in that of the professionals caring for him or her [4]. In a sense, this involves the transfer of a specific human quality, as a form of temporary custody of the consciousness of someone who is being cared for on a professional basis, which – as a result of the form of "emotional stubbornness" and dependence that comes into play – cannot be dismissed and is applied by the family to the patient and reflected onto the medical team. This approach to the moral aspects of the medical profession is not supported by scientific evidence, but is instead the result of a moral choice. Basically, it is therefore subjective.

However, there is agreement in all industrialized nations about the time window that needs to be considered. In general, patients in the vegetative state can be treated according to the (ordinary) rules of general medicine during the first 12 months after head injury (or 6 months in case of other etiologies). The attitude to assume becomes a problem after this initial period. It is for this reason that the issue of the person, as described above, is fundamental. It should be clearly stated that a great deal of hypocrisy is seen, especially on the part of opinion leaders, who often use, or abuse, the media to spread ethical – moral concepts among the population that are not only questionable, but are also based on erroneous interpretations of the pathophysiological evidence to begin with. We would therefore like to clear up all the issues we consider indisputable, especially since the concept of death has changed to the point that brain death is today recognized as "real" and defined by precise universally and legally accepted rules. It was this change of attitude that made transplant procedures possible.

The brain of the patient in the vegetative state is not only living, but also working [5]. In fact, complex neurophysiological functions can be documented by recording the electrophysiological correlates of higher brain functions. Not only can brain activity at rest be recorded during wakefulness or sleep (using electroencephalography) in patients in the vegetative state, but in addition brain potentials with "cognitive" significance (such as the P300, contingent negative variation, and mismatch negativity) are also recordable (see p. 65).

To resolve the issue of whether a patient in the vegetative state is a potential organ "donor" (for instance, after the first year in this condition), it would be necessary to first declare the patient deceased and then provoke rapid death [6]. Such a decision would therefore share all the characteristics of a homicide and would be a crime in any country. In addition, a decision to stop supplying nourishment would be an act of active abandonment. When such practices are used in patients in the vegetative state who in their earlier life have expressed a desire not to be kept alive under certain circumstances (the so-called "living will"), penal responsibility varies from country to country, depending on national legislation and legal precedents.

In a well-known law case, a court in Frankfurt am Main, Germany, gave a ruling on these matters in 1995. The treating physician and the son of an 85-year-old woman in the vegetative state following an illness lasting many months decided to suspend the patient's feeding, except for tea. The prosecution accused both of attempted homicide, but in the appeal trial, the validity of the lady's request not to be kept alive in case of coma (her "living will") was acknowledged. It may appear surprising that the court accepted the vague testimony presented. However, the principle of respecting the patient's will was established.

A sentence handed down by the Massachusetts Supreme Court was more precise and detailed, imposing on physicians the obligation to respect the will clearly expressed by a nurse, Paul Brophy, before surgery. He went into a coma due to problems arising from anesthesia, which later led to a vegetative state. The patient died 3 years later when his wife obtained from the court the right to stop feeding out of respect for her husband's living will.

However, discontinuing hydration and nutrition is an act that necessarily incurs the patient's death and involves great responsibility. It is important to clarify at this point that discontinuing nutrition cannot by any means be regarded as a passive (rather than intentional) act comparable to euthanasia, as the press and media have often suggested. The patient in the vegetative state cannot become the object of euthanasia (recently legalized in the Netherlands, in November 2000), as this would ignore the conditions that make euthanasia acceptable from a rational point of view. In fact, patients in the vegetative state cannot be considered to be in a terminal condition, and should be able, we believe, to live their life even though they may have been in a vegetative condition for more than 1 year. These patients neither appear to be suffering physically, nor are their moral rights restricted in any way. Above all, they have never requested to die, and no one is authorized to take such a decision for them. Also, it is not relevant to involve euthanasia in the argument in order to justify the demands of those who support the need for "active abandonment." The rational basis of today's ethics should be acknowledged.

A balanced distribution of the resources available for health care requires precise action when choices are to be made. From the ethical point of view, one can justify the use of public funds to support people forced by events to live a vegetative life, if the quality of their life can be expected to improve. Determining the quality of life is a task that cannot be considered merely from a medical point of view, but involves much broader categories, in which religious, philosophical, moral, ethical, legal, and social values need to be considered – values that express the level and type of civilization in the country concerned.

It is of primary interest to know what the actual costs are for patients who remain in the vegetative state for more than 6 months or a year, and whose expectation of vegetative life may be longer than this to an unpredictable extent. In France, these costs have been estimated to total more than € 100 000 [7]. In the absence of precise estimates from different countries, five new patients in the vegetative state resulting from head injury can be expected per million population per year [8], of whom about 15–20% remain in the vegetative state after a year, with an average life expectancy of 5 years. At a cost of approximately $ 200 per day in specialized units offering proper nursing care, the annual costs would amount to about $ 365 000 for five patients.

Costs can be calculated with sufficient reliability and are likely to be equivalent in most developed countries. By contrast, calculating the "advantages" is difficult and depends to a large extent on each nation's values and culture. The continuing process of cultural evolution itself depends on the importance assumed by the different values characterizing it and endorsed by citizens. Culture is strongly influenced by the media regarding issues that deal with the enforcement of new laws or changes in moral values; however, people are seldom provided with objective information, and news often break through because of their emotional appeal. For example, an American girl who died after spending 17 years in the vegetative state following a fall from a horse appeared in newspaper headlines as the "six million dollar woman."

There are two lines of thought concerning "calculating the value of the life" of a patient in (permanent) vegetative state, and both are respectable, although they lead to diametrically opposed conclusions. Based on the considerations outlined above about the human person, it appears that the respect given to a person's life is considered to be as inalienable in a vegetative condition as it is in conscious life by the French, Germans, Italians, and Spanish. By contrast, in relation to vegetative life quite different kinds of respect are attributed to conscious and unconscious subjects by the British, North Americans, Dutch, and perhaps also those living in northern Europe [3].

Jennett and Plum pinpointed this problem as early as 1972, stigmatizing the issue [9]. A high moral authority in the judgment of the value of life, Lord Walton of Detchant – a neurologist who chaired the Medical Ethics Committee of the House of Lords in the United Kingdom – stated in 1995 that "in such cases, not only is the quality of life weak, but it does not exist." Following legal deliberations over the case of Tony Blond, a new parameter was established: the patient's best interests. Following a head injury, Tony Blond lived in a vegetative state for many years. The treating physician, together with the family and other physicians, asked for legal permission to discontinue treatment and feeding, and this was denied by the court. Following litigation, the question was presented before the Law Lords (Britain's supreme court), who unanimously decided in favor of the right to remove the food cannula. Tony Blond died a few days later. The decision was justified on the basis of the "the patient's best interests," with reference to statements issued by the Medical Ethics Committee under the chairmanship of Lord Walton of Detchant, which established the legitimacy of interrupting all care (in this case meaning all food and water) if the act should serve to protect the patient's best interests [10,11].

Another famous case that helped set a precedent in the United States was that of Karen Ann Quinlan, who in 1975 (at the age of 20) suffered cardiac arrest due to alcohol and hallucinogenic drug abuse, and then progressed to a vegetative state with ventilator treatment. Her parents and a Catholic priest asked that she be allowed to die and requested authorization to discontinue artificial ventilation. The attending physicians refused, and following a lengthy legal controversy, the New Jersey Supreme Court authorized stopping artificial respiration. However, the patient did not die and survived another 9 years. The case of Nancy Cruson was similar. She died 12 days after artificial feeding was discontinued, following a United States Supreme Court decision to endorse her living will after 6 years in the vegetative state [12]. These and other similar cases started a widespread reaction in the United States that was echoed in the media, therefore leading to often inconclusive debates. Finally, as Cohadon [3] noted, discussion focused on the procedures used to put an end to vegetative life, rather than on the ethical principles that would justify active abandonment. In 1990, the American Medical Association (AMA) took a position that we consider incomprehensible, proposing the application of the same procedure to patients in the vegetative state as to terminal patients facing imminent death: to suspend life-prolonging pharmacological therapy, including nutrition and hydration [13]. Although never applied on a large scale, the attitude in the United States is generally in favor of discontinuing care, either because physicians are unable to meet the patients' needs or because the patients' families are overwrought by the sacrifice made in assisting them. In the United Kingdom, too, permission from the courts is required in order to proceed with active abandonment by interruption of feeding. Families face high legal fees, and this may be one reason why active abandonment is infrequent. The opposite attitude prevails in southern European countries, as indicated by the French National Consultative Committee of Ethics statement in 1986: "Patients in chronic vegetative state are human beings with even a greater right to human respect, as theirs is an extremely fragile state" [14].

Following a debate among bioethical and legal experts, a group of 50 Italian physicians (anesthesiologists, neurologists, and physiatricians) issued the Crotone Document in 1998 [15], in which the authorities are urged to establish ad hoc guidelines or otherwise forbid the suspension of artificial feeding and discard measures that might be imported from the United States, the United Kingdom, and other countries – i. e., measures intended to limit therapy, reduce it to a form of compassion, or accelerate death.

The way the issue is handled, at least in the public media, is not lacking in hypocrisy. In reality, there has been insufficient effort to define principles, and it appears easier (or the issue is deliberately distorted in this way) to speak of euthanasia, active abandonment, or implementation of a "living will." However, it is the maintenance of the patient that is regarded as worthless, and the costs of this maintenance are crucial. In our judgment, this is a very dangerous and even monstrous way of approaching the problem. In 1935, some 300 000 German citizens who had serious mental and neurological diseases (e. g., many children with hydrocephalus) and were therefore regarding as "having a life without value" (*lebensunwert*) were actively eliminated in Germany. This policy was endorsed by a democratically elected parliament and was proposed as an act of love for patients who would otherwise suffer uselessly. In reality, it was a rationalistic attempt to limit the costs of medical measures that were thought to be useless – perhaps in an anticipation of more recent ethical views.

No matter what values make a life worth living, the identification of them cannot be the responsibility of the attending physician. However, even when established by a democratic government, moral principles regarding life and health may have unforeseeable developments, which may also affect citizens who are not in the vegetative state.

The assessment of human and ethical values is not the concern of the physicians whose duties include caring for patients in the vegetative state. Physicians nevertheless have the duty to state clearly the extent of their professional expertise, so that those in a position to establish new rules can be fully informed.

- The patient in the vegetative state has a living brain. After a year, the patient is more often a minimal responder, although capable of expressing discomfort, pain, or a degree of relaxation, and therefore remaining an inexhaustible source of emotions for those who care for him or her.
- He or she is not terminally ill, and can continue to live in the vegetative state for many years.
- After a year, patients are generally no longer in need of special medical care, but only of nursing and feeding. In this sense, they are "cured" of the post-traumatic brain pathology that provoked an extreme degree of disability and forced them to live a vegetative life, but they are capable of experiencing strong emotions, and with a certain degree of probability, also able to provoke them. Even after one or more years, one can observe a partial resumption of conscious activity, corresponding to the clinical picture of the minimal responder (see p. 110).

References

1. Borthwick CJ. The permanent vegetative state: ethical crux, medical fiction? Issues Law Med 1996; 12: 167–85.
2. Scheler M, quoted in Cohadon F. Sortir du coma. Paris: Editions Odile Jacob, 2000: 337–8.
3. Cohadon F. Sortir du coma. Paris: Editions Odile Jacob, 2000: 219–20.
4. Dolce G. L'anima della coscienza. In: Dolce G, Rosadini G, editors. Lo stato vegetativo. Crotone, Italy: Polo Didattico Permanente/Istituto S. Anna, 1998: 53–61.
5. Dolce G. Critica allo stato dell'arte della riabilitazione nella fase di risveglio dal coma. In: Dolce G, Rosadini G, editors. Unità di risveglio dal coma. Crotone, Italy: Polo Didattico Permanente/Istituto S. Anna, 1997: 27–41.
6. Hoffenberg R, Lock M, Tilney N, et al. Should organs from patients in permanent vegetative state be used for transplantation? International Forum for Transplant Ethics. Lancet 1997; 350: 1320–1.
7. Sailly JC. Economic aspects of the care of patients in the vegetative state. Acta Neurol Belg 1994; 94: 155–65.
8. Richer E. Récuperation après traumatisme cranien grave: les différentes phases cliniques et leurs problématiques specifiques. J Readapt Med 1995; 15: 170–8.
9. Jennett B, Plum F. Persistent vegetative state after brain damage: a syndrome in search of a name. Lancet 1972; i : 734–7.
10. Walton, Lord. Dilemmas of life and death, 1. J R Soc Med 1995; 88: 311–5.
11. Walton, Lord. Dilemmas of life and death, 2. J R Soc Med 1995; 88: 372–6.
12. Snyder L. Life, death and the American College of Physicians: the Cruzan case. Ann Intern Med 1990; 112: 802–4.
13. American Medical Association. Persistent vegetative state and the decision to withdraw or with hold life support. JAMA 1990; 263: 426–30.
14. Comité consultatif national d'éthique pour les sciences de la vie et de la santé. Avis sur les expérimentations sur les malades en état végétatif cronique. In: Cohadon F. Sortir du Coma. Paris: Editions Odile Jacob, 2000: 206–215.
15. [Anon.] La carta di Crotone. In: Dolce G, Rosadini G, editors. Lo stato vegetativo. Crotone, Italy: Polo Didattico Permanente/Istituto S. Anna, 1998: 115–6.

10 Treating Families of Patients in Vegetative State: Adjustment and Interaction with Hospital Staff

Anat Shilansky and Rosemarie Weitz

Your soul, halfway between this world and the next,
Hovering above it, looking into the abyss,
Undecided whether to remain here, or to leave it all behind.
You find no peace of mind, moving between darkness
And light, between life and death, despair and hope.

And the days pass, one after another, and yet there is no conclusion
Whether death is final or hope will get a fresh infusion.
And while you hover between these two worlds,
Awaiting permission to enter the next
But still being refused to reenter this one,
I sit here and await your decision with pain and love …

Published with permission of the author
Rachi Brotman [1]

These lines are from a poem written by a father to his son lying in a vegetative state. With these words, the father is trying to describe the impossible reality experienced by him and other families coping with a member suffering from prolonged unconsciousness.

In order to cope with this complex reality, it is advisable to review the theoretical dynamics that are in motion in this unique world – a world with rules and logic of its own. This is the "twilight zone," unknown to the outside world, where patients and families live in "limbo", where death is disguised as life. In treating the vegetative patient and his family, there are no clear-cut answers or conventional rules with regard to accepted human behavior and reactions. Here there are different rules, when life and death become intertwined.

Staff members entering the realm of unconsciousness may experience a sense of confusion, or even alarm. Questions such as how to approach a family in such desperation, or to form a professional relationship and be supportive at the same time, are not easily answered. In this chapter, we attempt to present a broader perspective on the complex and intertwined undercurrents that make up the world of unconscious patients and their families, in their daily interactions and encounters with staff members. The chapter offers suggestions for more effective coping techniques that can ease the tension aroused by this extreme and almost impossible situation.

Focusing on the Families

Let us begin this section with a seemingly simple question. Who is your patient in the intensive-care unit (ICU)? Most medical professionals focus their treatment on the obvious subject – the patient. The family is important, but of secondary status. However, in the ICU, this natural assumption is not valid. While the patient's needs are of the utmost importance, dealing with the family's psychological difficulties is just as critical.

There are three main reasons for this assertion. In the first place, families in the ICU experience an extreme state of uncertainty. The need to control an uncontrollable situation will spur them to maintain an ongoing and intense connection with the staff – a need that cannot be ignored, despite the burden it creates for the staff members.

In addition, since scientific knowledge about vegetative patients and their recovery is still limited, it is not advisable to disregard the contribution the family can make to the patient's recovery process. Families spend endless hours trying to stimulate their loved ones back to recovery and must therefore be recognized as part of the treatment plan.

The above conclusion may create fundamental conflicts over issues of boundaries, responsibilities, and authority. This presents a unique challenge: how do you include and achieve family assistance without disrupting the staff's daily medical routine? How do the staff enable the family to fulfill its required role while keeping the professional boundaries clear?

The last factor, but by no means the least important, is the devastating situation itself and the ongoing nightmare experienced by the families, day in and day out. This acute situation must be addressed by the staff and may require immediate crisis intervention as urgent as the treatment of the patients themselves. In order to meet the challenges and complexities of this unique situation successfully, there is a need for proper professional assessment and treatment of the patient's family.

Family Assessment

A family is a complex and sensitive system of significant interrelations [2]. When one of the members undergoes a major change, it immediately affects every other member as well. Accordingly, when one of its members suffers from prolonged unconsciousness, the entire family becomes enveloped in this breakdown of the life cycle. Life, as the family knew it before, will never be the same again. Vital areas in their lives have been disrupted. Intimate relationships, emotional interdependencies, economic status, housing accommodation, and occupational hazards all cause major changes in their daily routines. Each family will react differently, depending on its own patterns of behavior, based on many factors. Among these are: the premorbid and current characteristics of the patient and family, the nature and severity of the injury, and the availability of community resources to assist with coping [3]. It is essential to assess each family as a unique system. A combination of individual evaluation of each member of the family, along with a comprehensive approach to the family as a whole, will produce a better rehabilitation process.

The life cycle is one scale by which we can identify a family's needs. The stage in a person's life, age, and marital or parental status, are all variables that are influenced and disrupted by the crisis. The reassignment of former roles requires many adjustments on the part of family members and can cause a major change in the family's balance of power and authority [4].

Another scale that can be helpful for assessing families is the subdivision of the following needs:
- Physical needs
- Emotional needs
- Spiritual needs

Physical needs include satisfying the family's most basic needs, such as nutrition, lodging, mobility between the hospital and home, and a reasonable source of income. These needs must be taken care of as quickly as possible, because they are the foundation on which higher-level and more demanding challenges can be achieved.

Emotional needs relate to the necessity to relieve or lessen the feelings of emptiness and loss that are part of the emotional upheaval experienced by the patient's family. These needs include a desire for affection, support, involvement, and belonging. These needs may be expressed in many different forms of behavior. Some family members tend to externalize their feelings through crying, anger, or intensive verbalizing. Others may turn inwards, building an inner wall of protection around themselves.

Spiritual needs are fulfilled when a family can give some meaning to the awesome situation that has befallen them. Religious faith, belief in the power of the injured member to heal himself, or even mystical hopes can all be of spiritual comfort.

Typical Psychological Reactions of the Family Members

Despite the fact that each family member will react uniquely in this crisis situation, there are certain common reactions that characterize most of them at some stage in the mourning process. All of these reactions are legitimate and natural, stemming from the difficulty to comprehend, digest, and cope with an unbearable situation. Some of these reactions include [5–8]:

- Anger and hostility
- Denial
- Guilt
- Overprotection
- Anxiety and depression
- Psychosomatic symptoms
- Social isolation

Let us elaborate on a few of these.

Anger and hostility are often expressed when a family member feels desperate and helpless. At the beginning, most of the anger is directed toward those who caused the injury, or even toward the patient himself, for not trying hard enough to recover. With the passing of time and the absence of proper channels into which legitimate anger can be unloaded, hostility may heighten. Unfortunately, staff members often become convenient and vulnerable targets for this hostility, since they have not been able to achieve the desired remedy.

Denial is a defense mechanism that assists family members in postponing the need to face up to a painful and undesirable reality. It lets them cope with the trauma gradually, enabling them to comprehend the changes in their lives, without depriving them of the right to hope. Often, it looks as if a family member is "ignoring" the facts, fantasizing about a quick recovery. Some of the expressions heard on the ICU may sound like this: "I know him, he'll wake up when it suits him. He was always stubborn like that." Or, "She's so weak after the trauma that she can't respond. Give her time and she'll be back on her feet." Phrases such as these are characteristic of a normal coping process and are considered to be adequate in the short term, but could become pathological if continued over a longer period.

With regard to anxiety and depression, studies have shown that over one-third of the care-givers of patients suffering from a severe head injury or from unconsciousness will develop significant levels of anxiety or depression [9,10]. Some of them, feeling burdened by the frustrating situation, may resort to outbursts of anger, considered to be a form of disguised depression [9,11,12].

In conclusion, the reactions of the family members may often be extreme, difficult to excuse, and maybe even frightening. They react this way because they are caught up in an unbearable situation. Under normal conditions, we would classify their behavior as pathological, but on the ICU this behavior is considered to be a normal and necessary stage in the beginning of the mourning process. A few examples are given below to illustrate some of the reactions and dynamics described.

Mrs. S., the mother of a 19-year-old boy, told her therapist, "I think that with the passing of time the staff members tend to forget just how painful it is to see one's child so helpless. I realize that the daily routine is necessary, but it is so hard for me to leave my child alone, all night long, unable to speak for himself. What if he needs something? Who will be there to watch over his every sign? Is the daily routine really more important than my being there with him? Who can really answer this question, honestly?"

This mother is expressing feelings of anxiety and helplessness, and a need for emotional support. Since the staff members set boundaries between her son and herself, she turns her frustration and pain towards them.

Mrs. I., the wife of A. (43 years old): "It took time to fully comprehend the ramifications of my husband's injury. At first I would come to the ICU for long days of futile anticipation that perhaps he would awaken, or at least show me some sign of awareness that I was there. At that time, anyone who tried to candidly prepare me for a bleak future was unable to penetrate the inner shield within me. Only time and the unchanging reality cracked that shield. I was overwhelmed with pain and fear. Although I knew it was essential for me to receive relevant information, to help me comprehend the confusing reality I was living in, only those who could understand and accept my pain and confusion helped me to survive a very traumatic period in my life."

This woman is describing the importance of the denial mechanism as a protective shield, essential for her emotional survival in the early stages of the mourning process.

Mr. and Mrs. G., the parents of Y., (27 years old, and 5 years after their son's accident): "When we first arrived at the ICU, we felt completely lost. We felt so helpless. And then when our son made signs to us with his eyes, we were discouraged and told that these were only reflexes. If we hadn't been insistent about our son's progress, who knows where he would be today. Our feeling was that instead of working together with us, the staff were 'fighting' us almost all the way. There must be a better way to cooperate and trust each other. We wanted more information to help us understand the source of the injury. Sometimes we even felt that some information was being hidden from us. We wanted to be more involved in his treatment, but seldom received direct instructions. Although we understand that the staff need to maintain a routine on the ward, they must never forget that 'no family, no rehabilitation!' "

Anger is the most frequent reaction among families on the ICU. It is undoubtedly the most difficult behavior for the staff workers to cope with and often leads to painful conflicts.

In conclusion, the family undergoes an excruciatingly difficult period of loss. This situation induces extreme reactions, stemming from their basic needs. It must be kept in mind that while family members will react differently from each other, identifying their needs and giving them support will improve the quality of the rehabilitation process.

Focusing on the Staff: Emotional Stress and Sources of Tension

Staff members treating the vegetative patient are exposed to never-ending traumatic situations and suffer from what is known as "secondary trauma effects" [13]. As a result, the everyday working conditions are saturated with ongoing stress and high levels of tension. Let us examine some of the components of this stressful situation.

To start with, none of us are immune to life crises, such as road accidents and illnesses. Repeated exposure to the patients' traumatic stories leaves its impact on the staff members' sense of well-being. Although the staff absorb these stories daily, they do not have permission to express their fears openly. On the contrary, they are expected to be "strong" and to contain the sorrow of the families. Accumulation of locked-in feelings can be a source of great frustration.

In addition, the very fact that the patient is unconscious adds complexity to an already tense and complicated situation. The staff attendants find themselves in a position in which they have to decipher every sign that the patient makes. This demands an ongoing state of alertness and an extreme sense of responsibility and sensitivity on their parts.

Team members are expected to cure patients – but in the case of the vegetative patient, a cure is not always possible, leaving staff members feeling impotent and useless.

The staff's own feelings of helplessness are exacerbated by the families' endless complaints about the treatment of their loved ones. Their unrealistic anticipation of the patient's quick recovery is often expressed by putting blame on the staff [5]. In summary, the immense responsibility and exposure to disaster situations faced by staff members, and the disappointment and accusations they meet with from the families, cause tremendous pressure on the team, creating continuous frustration, vulnerability, and burn-out.

Among the typical psychological reactions of the staff, the most common and natural reactions to the stress situation mentioned above are usually various forms of avoidance, or a variety of expressions of anger. A few examples are given below.

- The helplessness felt by a patient's family is often a common feeling for staff employees as well. When it hurts too much to bear the pain of a family member, the hospital members may develop a pattern of ignoring or avoiding real relationships with that person – for example, a patient's mother who repeatedly approaches the doctor for some sign of encouragement. Unable to bear these ongoing encounters, the doctor may often find excuses for postponing their meetings.
- Common reactions among the team members and families are to express anger toward each other. For example, families often object to certain demands from the staff, such as to leave the patient's room at certain hours. The nurse, instead of understanding the source of the emotions leading to the family's objections, feels frustrated herself and expresses hostility towards them, inducing a vicious circle of reciprocal anger.
- When caught up in the vicious circle of anger, it is not hard to become judgmental as well. Making moral judgments about people in stressful states is unproductive and should be avoided.
- The issue of boundaries between staff and families is a very complex one. If the staff are too firm with regard to ward regulations, the family may view it as being rigid and insensitive to their needs. If a staff member is too lenient and becomes overinvolved, this too can be confus-

ing and may be interpreted wrongly. These two prominent patterns of behavior – underdoing things or overdoing them – are two extremes of the same defense mechanism, and both are counterproductive. It is recommended that one should try to identify one's own dominant pattern in order to bring about the professional change needed on this complex ward.

Shaw and McMahon [14] state that the main contribution made by the staff to the conflict with families is failure to recognize that in most cases, the family is in a state of stress and need, rather than being "pathological" or troublesome.

In conclusion, on the ICU there are two parties with a common interest, but often with different or even opposed needs. This gives rise to conflicts about "control" and "moral" issues. The control issue is the more obvious one. The family wants to set the rules on the ward, or at least be included in them, while the staff feel a need to restrain them.

The moral question is: who determines the patient's quality of life? Who decides what is best for him or her? Most families believe that this is not only their right, but their obligation as well. Most professionals would claim that it is their prerogative, due to their medical knowledge and experience. A few examples of common reactions expressed by staff members are given below.

Mrs. S., a nurse: "The families do not fully comprehend the complexities and heavy demands that are involved in the ongoing management of the ICU. They expect us to fulfill their requests immediately, no matter what else we are doing. There is neither understanding of our duties nor consideration of the needs of other patients. I know that the family is in the middle of a crisis, but there are other professionals to assist them with their sorrow. They shouldn't disrupt our daily routine. Also, they should be encouraged to go back to their daily lives and leave their patient to us."

The ICU staff members' feelings of helplessness are in parallel with those of the families. In many instances, setting firm boundaries helps the staff avoid these feelings, which can be exacerbated by the daily, ongoing relations with the families.

Mr. N., paramedical staff member: "We are working in the most difficult ward. The responsibility is huge and our patients are considered 'high-risk.' I feel that the families expect miracles and place unrealistic demands upon us. They don't understand that a major part of the awakening process is just waiting to see if something develops spontaneously. They want active intervention, but that isn't always feasible." This staff member's frustration, caused by the patient's lack of progress, is being expressed through the use of a defense mechanism, such as accusing the family of having unrealistic expectations.

Dr. A.: "There is always the heavy burden of responsibility and constant anxiety about deterioration of the patient. The ICU is unlike any other ward. The 'heroic' parts of medicine are achieved before and after entering the ICU. In the acute hospital, the patient is fighting for his life. In the head-trauma rehabilitation ward, the patient is fighting to regain independent functions. But here, we are only striving to restore consciousness – a long and often pessimistic process. The families don't usually comprehend the consequences of the brain damage. Sometimes they ask for information that has no meaning for the patient's progress, and yet they are emotionally unprepared to listen to the facts as we see them."

Most medical staff members feel appreciated; not so on the ICU, according to this doctor. In spite of the enormous amount of effort put in, the devastating situation prevents families from expressing feelings of satisfaction and gratitude. This may be a contributing factor to the burn-out situation experienced by many.

Recommendations and Suggested Strategies

Broadening family involvement in the rehabilitation process. It appears that the most significant source of frustration for the family members is their need to cope with the unknown. The uncertainty and uncontrollability of the vegetative state makes them strive to receive as much information as possible. Although there is no real cure for uncertainty, we suggest that direct clarifications about the patient's progress should be conveyed and that the families should be consistently acquainted with the staff's plans.

Active inclusion of family members in the rehabilitation program should lessen their anger and minimize some of the potential conflicts. Regular, prearranged family/staff meetings should be maintained in order to exchange information and to clarify future goals in the treatment program, with an emphasis on the family's special roles.

Development of casual channels of communication. Having team members initiate invitations to the families for special events is another technique for enhancing their knowledge and improving the atmosphere. Lectures on relevant and crucial matters, such as the risks involved in feeding the vegetative patient, or extended physical training of the patient by the families, are a form of coaching and instructing that will be of mutual benefit to both families and staff. Also, this is an opportunity to change misconceptions that families may have about traumatic brain injury [15]. In addition, it is not only an educational plan [16], but also develops a closer and more interactive relationship between the mentor and the "protégé."

Psychosocial intervention for families. Needless to say, the families on the ICU need professional support, guidance, and help in reorganizing their lives. As already mentioned, each individual and family have specific needs. A psychosocial evaluation should help determine what some of these needs are. Once the predominant problems have been determined, they should be addressed by permanent, therapeutic interventions. The social worker will try to identify each family's difficulties and dilemmas and search for solutions that are relevant to the breakdown in their life cycle. The main goal is to help the family members rebalance their emotional and instrumental resources in such a way that they can function both in the hospital and in the outside world, enabling each individual to begin the healing process and adjustment to the crisis that has befallen him or her. Working through dilemmas, such as loyalty to the patient or to other family members, or enabling family members to be helpers and clients at the same time, are all significant components in the mourning process.

Supportive intervention with staff members. It is commonly perceived that the hospital personnel are healthy and strong, always devoted and yet detached from the daily traumatic environment. Although this may be expected of them, the reality is otherwise. It is therefore recommended that a support group should be set up that every team member may attend. The aim of this group would be to create a supportive atmosphere in which it is legitimate to raise and express hostile feelings, frustrations, distress, pain, etc. The discovery that others share in these feelings often helps reduce pressures that may have been bottled up inside. By expressing them in a legitimate setting, the staff can avoid releasing them during work in undesirable directions.

In conclusion, a combination of maintaining healthier interactions between the families and the staff members, while at the same time giving support to both, should produce a better sense of satisfaction among the family members and improved professionalism among the staff.

References

1. Brotman R. To my beloved son [previously unpublished].
2. Broom L, Selznick P. Sociology, 4th ed. New York: Harper and Row, 1968.
3. Florian V, Katz S. The other victims of traumatic brain injury: consequences for family members. Neuropsychology 1991; 5: 267–79.
4. Maitz E, Sacks P. Treating families of individuals with traumatic brain injury from a family systems perspective. J Head Trauma Rehabil 1995; 10: 1–11.
5. Stern M, Sazbon L, Becker E, Costeff H. Severe behavioral disturbance in families of patients with prolonged coma. Brain Inj 1988; 2: 259–62.
6. Florian V, Katz S, Lahav V. Impact of traumatic brain damage on family dynamics and functioning: a review. Brain Inj 1989; 3: 219–33.
7. Lezak M. Brain damage is a family affair. J Clin Exp Neuropsychol 1988; 10: 111–23.
8. Brooks N. The head injured family. J Clin Exp Neuropsychol 1991; 13: 155–88.
9. Nigel M, Kersel D, Havill J, Sleigh J. Caregiver burden at 1 year following severe traumatic brain injury. Brain Inj 1998; 12: 1045–59.
10. Gillen R, Tennen H, Affleck G, Steinpreis R. Distress, depressive symptoms, and depressive disorder among caregivers of patients with brain injury. J Head Trauma Rehabil 1998; 13: 31–43.
11. Douglas J, Spellacy F. Indicators of long-term family functioning following severe traumatic brain injury in adults. Brain Inj 1996; 10: 819–39.
12. Burgess E, Drotar D, Taylor G, Wade S, Stancin T, Yeates K. The family burden of injury interview: reliability and validity studies. J Head Trauma Rehabil 1999; 14: 394–405.

13. McCann I, Pearlman L. Vicarious traumatization: a framework for understanding psychological effects on working with victims. J Trauma Stress 1990; 3: 131–51.
14. Shaw L, Mcmahon B. Family–staff conflict in the rehabilitation setting: causes, consequences and implications. Brain Inj 1990; 4: 87–93.
15. Springer J, Farmer J, Bouman D. Common misconceptions about traumatic brain injury among family members of rehabilitation patients. J Head Trauma Rehabil 1997; 12: 41–50.
16. Blosser J, De Pompei R. Fostering effective family involvement through mentoring. J Head Trauma Rehabil 1995; 10: 46–56.

11 Covert Cognitive Abilities of a Person with Altered Consciousness

Levy Rahmani

This chapter outlines a prospective, rehabilitation-oriented investigation at the bedside of possible covert cognitive abilities of a patient in a vegetative state. This type of investigation is based on:
- Accumulating knowledge about partially conscious and controlled visual-perceptual responses induced experimentally in normal subjects.
- Extensive observations of restricted and implicit manifestations of memory registration and retrieval in patients with specific cognitive-behavioral deficiencies following restricted brain lesions who maintain a general state of consciousness.
- Recent advances in the functional study of brain structures that do not belong to the neocortex: the basal ganglia, cerebellum, and medial frontal structures.

We shall conduct the argument in the form of an imaginary dialog.

Question: Is it not strange to use an abstract term such as "loss of consciousness" for a medical diagnosis? Indeed, is it satisfactory to conclude the examination of a person who has suddenly, and in the most dramatic way, lost any manifest functional ability, with the statement that he or she has lost consciousness? Can this serve as a basis for the initiation of treatment? Consciousness is a psychological term. What is the meaning of its "loss" for therapy?

Answer: The concepts of consciousness, on the one hand, and coma and vegetative state (alterations of consciousness) on the other, are indeed very complex. Giacino wrote:

> Disorders of consciousness remain enigmatic and continue to present some of the most intriguing challenges faced by neurologists and rehabilitation specialists in clinical practice. Of particular interest are those states characterized by severe alterations in consciousness such as coma and the vegetative state. Remarkably little is known about the relationship between clinical features associated with these disorders and the corresponding pathophysiologic substrates underlying them. In addition, little attention has been paid to investigating the natural evolution of disorders of consciousness, although this seems a logical and necessary first step toward establishing greater diagnostic accuracy, better prognostic specificity and more effective treatment interventions [1].

No wonder that neuroscientists have avoided involvement in the field of consciousness. Searle [2] was puzzled by the resistance of neuroscientists to tackling the problem of consciousness. To him, "one of the chief functions of the brain is to cause and sustain conscious states. Studying the brain without studying consciousness would be like studying the stomach without studying digestion, or studying genetics without studying the inheritance of traits."

Q: Has it been possible to briefly yet meaningfully characterize a state of altered consciousness such as a vegetative state?

A: Persons with an altered consciousness resulting from extensive brain damage would pass through a sequence of phases from full loss of consciousness to a state of a mild disorder. These phases are still barely definable, and the characterization and labeling of them differ from one expert to another. Beyond the divergences that exist, the picture emerging is one of degraded or reduced input or reception of sensory to communicative stimulation; abnormal meaningfulness, lying between loss and distortion; and abnormal responsiveness, lying between disconnection from the input and minimal, undifferentiated responses to intensive stimulation and ranging from unawakefulness to arousal deprived of awareness of environmental events. The neocortical structures known to be prevalently involved in higher cognitive performances, such as predominantly conscious perceptual experiences, explicit and voluntary recall of information, controlled executive functions, are the most compromised by this damage. Recent years have documented previously obscure cognitive abilities of supplementary cortical and subcortical structures – notably the basal ganglia and the cerebellum. It is increasingly appearing that emotions play a modulating role in memory and learning. The amygdala has quite extensive connections with cortical structures.

Almost as a matter of principle, the effect of a behaviorally relevant environmental stimulus can be enhanced by associating it with emotions believed to be deeply rooted. It is worth mentioning here a point made recently in favor of "overlearning": "The shift between being nonconscious and being conscious during information processing depends upon the number of cells (and, consequently the volume of brain tissue) that participate in the underlying processes and constitute the same macronetworks, or the same networks with additional recruited neuronal populations" [3].

Q: Is it right to claim metaphorically that the traumatic brain injury which results so frequently in states of altered consciousness offers the opportunity to brain structures that do not belong to the elite neocortex to shop up and take the rostrum?

A: It is true that propensities of such brain structure are more readily demonstrable under particular circumstances. Investigators of normal behavioral capacities endeavor to design particular experimental conditions to elicit properties that are otherwise obscure. This may occur in the case of brain injury. Covert participation of such structures in normal functioning, masked by the predominant manifestation of high-level structures, becomes known at the patient's bedside. The stimulation and promotion of these structures might be considered in a prospective tentative intervention program for patients with an altered consciousness. Limitations resulting from extensive damage could be regarded as an extreme instance of cognitive reduction, along a continuum of performances from particular induced moments of reduced awareness during a general normal performance, through modular deficits resulting from localized lesions. The management of a patient in a vegetative state requires a measurable assessment of as yet undisclosed mental life, notably the characteristics of cognitive residuals.

Q: Are there currently any specific, documented pieces of information about the connection between neural structures known to be involved in some cognitive or motor function and structures that have a role in emotion?

A: One of the most recent findings about this type of integration regards the functioning of the medial frontal lobe, notably the anterior cingulate cortex (ACC): "Conceptually, the ACC is a prime example of a brain structure in which a regulatory network, composed of cells from the modulatory brain-stem nuclei, interacts with an executive network ..." [4]. It is believed that the ACC has a triple role in behavioral control. It is involved in motor control due to its connections with both the motor cortex and the spinal cord. Patients with medial frontal lobe lesions involving the ACC are described as showing deficits in spontaneous initiation of movement and speech. Akinetic mutism, which is caused by bilateral lesions, is an extreme example. In addition, it is thought to have a role in cognition through the reciprocal corticocortical connections with the lateral prefrontal cortex. Last but not least, there is strong evidence for a role of the ACC in arousal. The extensive afferents from the thalamus and the brain stem contribute to the ACC's involvement in an arousal drive state. In this context, the intriguing idea has come up that "different cognitive-affective events may lead to a transient synchronization of neural activity in the ACC."

Q: Are we already in a position to point clearly to phases of transition from one degree of altered consciousness to a milder degree?

A: We have to distinguish between an appreciation of the patient's emergence from unconsciousness from the neurological and neurorehabilitation perspective and the subsequent neurobehavioral or neuropsychological perspective. Wide agreement on the gradation at the first level has been achieved with the Glasgow Coma Scale. A patient's gradation on the 15-point scale is mentioned in his chart. Essentially, this is a scale of the patient's responsiveness to stimulation. At a higher level of assessment, many different terms have been used to describe the constituent brain activities that support consciousness; however, the application of terminology has not been consistent. The terms "arousal," "orienting," "alertness," and "wakefulness" have been used interchangeably to refer to the continuum between sleep and the awake state. At the diagnostic level, any effort to group individual signs of coma into syndromes associated with severe alterations of consciousness faces difficulties due to the lack of clinical methods for assessing consciousness, particularly self-awareness.

Q: Do the prospects for further investigating the mind of the person in a vegetative state appear gloomier now, in view of the difficulty of analyzing and grading the manifestations of the alteration in consciousness in the "hard" terms of neuropathology and clinical neurology? Returning to the concept of consciousness as a mental state or process, why shouldn't we be able to extrapolate from the way in which definite cognitive processes are defined? After all, perception, memory, thinking, and attention, are components of consciousness, as is language, and these have quite clear and accepted definitions. For instance, visual perception seems to be widely defined as a process of recognizing the features of things in the environment – their color, shape, size, position in space, and so on – by vision, as a sensory system. We recognize sounds using another sensory system. We are perfectly well aware that as normal individuals we use a definite and limited number of sensory systems. We even take it for granted that the brain operates in such a way that there are different regions separately involved for each type of sensory information. We can somehow easily define memory as our ability to register information, store it for short or long periods of time, and retrieve it when needed. These may not be simple processes at all, particularly when it involves recognizing objects, pictures, scenes, or remembering life episodes distinctly from fragments of knowledge. However, even laymen use understandable definitions of perception and memory. We even have a reasonably comprehensible definition for "thinking." Can this knowledge and the way in which it has been reached not be extended to the domain of consciousness? Is consciousness so clearly distinct, due to being an integrated entity, that an extrapolation of this type is not possible?

A: Now we are getting to the core of the matter! Firstly, we should be aware of the complexity of the processes of perception, memory, and thinking themselves. For instance, the visual recognition of objects, as well as naming them, involves not only the brain region that specifically receives the visual information – the so-called "visual cortex." It is believed that about 60% of the cerebral cortex is involved, although obviously not solely, in visual perception. The definition of perception given in the question above is a simplified one. For instance, a fuller definition was offered in the *MIT Encyclopedia of Cognitive Science* (1999): "Perception reflects the ability to derive meaning from sensory experience, in the form of information about structure and causality in the perceiver's environment, of the sort necessary to guide behavior" [5]. In addition, most contemporary theories of vision describe object recognition in terms of a comparison between the input image and stored models that represent known objects [6]. Finally, there is a well-documented influence of the environment on an observer's memory for things. Memory is the name given to the ability of living organisms to acquire, retain, and use information or knowledge. The term is closely related to "learning." The brain substrate for memory is a topic of vivid debate. A central issue is that of the "consolidation" of memory in the brain [7]. The point is thus that it is not only consciousness that is difficult to define; one should be aware that the extensive knowledge available about perception and memory – to mention only two of the more specific entities for which there are widely used "handy" or convenient definitions – has been obtained only thanks to extensive studies in both normal and pathological conditions.

Q: Now there is a bit of confusion. It turns out that everything in the human mind is complex and that when something happens to the brain, the distortion of any one single aspect is hard to grasp. Why is consciousness in particular said to be "enigmatic," "mysterious," eluding any attempt to capture the cerebral substrate for it? Is this because it is a monolithic entity that cannot be broken down into smaller units? Generally speaking, any entity that cannot be broken down for analysis is more difficult to comprehend. If there is no way of parceling consciousness, are there any ways of grading it, particularly with regard to the way it is transformed into more familiar entities, even though these are complex in themselves as well? Perception, thinking, memory, and attention are largely conscious activities. Their complexity is closely linked to their being part of human consciousness. Yet it seems that we are pretty advanced in investigating and understanding these. The argument boils down to the following question: since specific cognitive processes are components of consciousness – and indeed form the core of consciousness, its contents – while at the same time their structure is more accessible for analysis and grading, might this avenue of systematic clinical observation and investigation lead to better insights into coma and its gradations, before we obtain better neurological and neuropathological information?

A: This could indeed be a prospective path of investigation – the specific cognitive elements of the vegetative state. These should be looked at from the perspective of their manifestations in a normal person. We can take the example of visual perception. There is recent experimental evidence that visual perception takes a variety of forms, some of which may not be under voluntary conscious control. This depends on the conditions of presentation of the visual displays being recognized. Neuroimaging studies of visual awareness in normal subjects have shown that there at least two distinct aspects of perceptual experience: "First, the neural correlates of those mechanisms responsible for maintaining a particular level of awareness, and second, the neural correlates of the specific contents of consciousness" [8]. These functional magnetic resonance imaging studies have been able to demonstrate the different role of two mechanisms in the cerebral cortex, beyond the traditional view about the role of visual cortex, with the occipital lobe situated in the posterior part of the cortex. The studies distinguished between the neural bases of conscious experience and unconscious perception and behavior. As Rees puts it, "We all have first-hand knowledge of what it is like to be conscious, as opposed to not being conscious (e. g. dreamless sleep). Similarly, when we are conscious we experience something. Our conscious state may change, but at any moment our experience is distinguished by its phenomenal content. When phenomenal content is absent, then consciousness is (usually) absent" [8].

Q: At each and every moment that we are awake, we see, recognize, and are aware of things that are present in our environment. This seems a very natural and elementary fact. Is this an inseparable element of consciousness that is bound to disappear in a person in vegetative state? Much has been written about a lowering of this capacity in a variety of modes in patients with circumscribed brain lesions. These persons did not lose consciousness, or their consciousness was not altogether altered. What does the content of their visual-perceptual experiences consist of?

A: We now have a great deal of information about perception in general, and in particular about visual perception in normal individuals and in those who have damage in part of the brain, in one of the two halves (hemispheres) of the cerebral cortex, or in part of a hemisphere. This knowledge is expected to provide the starting-point for studies leading to better insights into possible residual perceptual capacities in a comatose patient. A few relevant points are detailed below.

It is generally believed that the processing of visual patterning information follows a hierarchical structure, proceeding along multiple parallel pathways in the brain. Recoding usually begins in the retina and proceeds through the lateral geniculate nucleus to primary visual cortex. Cortical processing is thought to begin with an elementary representation of local spatial frequency, orientation, and contrast, presumably represented by responses of simple ells in primary visual cortex (V1). Much less is known about how the early neural representations are transformed at higher levels to signal information needed to perform tasks on complex, real-world objects [9].

Two groups of studies have reached the conclusion that visual conscious experience is not spontaneous and unitary. It is the product of the activity of several systems, obtained in a certain sequence. Zeki and Bartels studied the brain's mechanisms of vision, and in particular the perception of color, and pointed out that:

The primate visual brain has been shown to consist of many separate visual areas, and the number of areas continues to grow. Central to the visual brain is area V1 of the primary visual cortex ... The different visual areas of the cortex surrounding area V1 are specialized to process different attributes of the visual scene. Prominent among them are motion and colour ... It follows from the above that one characteristic of the visual brain is the presence of spatially distributed, functionally specialized functional systems that deal with different attributes of the visual scene ... Moreover, psychophysical experiments show that different processing systems do not complete their tasks at the same time. Different attributes of the visual scene are not perceived at the same time. Instead, colour is seen before orientation and orientation is seen before motion, the difference between perceptual times for colour and for motion being 60–80 ms. Human studies confirm that the different processing and perceptual systems are fairly autonomous. Thus, specific damage to one system alone, such as colour, does not lead to a global deficit in vision ..." [10].

Treisman opened up a new avenue of research into clinical applications in neuropsychology with her ingenious experiments designed to reveal subtle aspects of the process of bringing together separate features of visual displays, and the ways in which this process can fail. Visual attention and awareness are at the center of her work. To start with, Treisman draws attention to evidence showing that the visual system analyzes the scene along a number of different dimensions in various specialized modules. During the perception of an object, we form multiple representations and encode different properties of objects at different levels. There may be as many as six different types of object representation. This means that varying types of discrimination are required to distinguish one view from another. Unattended objects may be only implicitly – i. e., unintentionally – registered. According to Treisman, "object perception may involve seeing, recognition, preparation of actions, and emotional responses – functions that human brain imaging and neuropsychology suggest are localized separately. Perhaps because of this specialization, object perception is remarkably rapid and efficient" [11]. Karni and Bertini studied the learning process for perceptual skills, using behavioral probes into adult cortical plasticity [12]. The authors studied issues such as where in the brain and under what conditions practice-related changes occur. There is considerable evidence for a hierarchical organization of information processing in sensory systems, such that the physical parameters for a sensory input are selectively represented only at low-level processing stages, whereas neurons in higher-order areas respond invariably to those parameters.

The evidence for separate channels of sensory information gave rise to the issue of the way in which they are connected. "The binding problem in perception deals with the question of how we achieve the experience of a coherent world of integrated objects and avoid seeing a world of dismembered or wrongly combined shapes, colours, motions, sizes, and distance" [11]. In brief, how do we specify what goes with what and where? The problem is not an intuitively obvious one – which is probably testimony to how well, in general, our brains solve it. We are simply not aware that there is a problem to be solved. Yet the findings from neuroscience and psychology all imply that there is one [13].

Q: On the basis of the studies by Zeki and Treisman, is it to be understood that the impression we have of an immediate and spontaneous representation of the world of familiar objects is an illusion? Can we infer that in a state of altered consciousness, there may not be a total loss of the ability to register some partial, isolated properties of objects, but that there is an implicit, covert representation of objects that we cannot observe? Moreover, does it actually turn out that under certain conditions of stimulation, even normal perceivers may not be in full control of what they perceive?

A:
Once upon a time it was widely believed that human observers built up a complete representation of everything in their visual field. More precisely, it was believed that the stable and richly-detailed world viewed by a normal observer gave rise to a stable and richly-detailed representation within a "picture" that could be used for all subsequent visual and motor operations. This representation was thought to be long-lasting ... its contents built up by the superposition of eye fixations, and the results held in a high-capacity buffer [13].

The review of recent literature and independent research presented by Rensink at the Third Annual Vision Research conference held in Florida in 1999 [13] led to the conclusion that the subjective visual-perceptual experience is not quite in accord with objective fact. For example, visual processing is split into two largely independent streams, one concerned with the perception and recognition of objects and the other with visuomotor action [14].

The study of the visual awareness of normal adults asked to recognize complex scenes has shown that the presentation of a stimulus does not lead automatically to awareness of its presence. Even though subjects reported being aware of the whole scene, it was only when their attention was drawn to a change in the scene that they become aware of that change. Focal attention is a necessary condition for awareness of detail within a scene, as well as a mechanism of voluntary control [15].

The development of visual perception in the child has in recent years turned out to be a relevant source of knowledge about the formation of our awareness of the sensory world. Posner and Rothbart [15] noted that in infants, visual orientation may precede the capacity for volitional self-regulation by at least a year. Following this line of thinking, it has been proposed that visual awareness is a simpler function of consciousness and the one most amenable to scientific analysis, placing awareness at the center of discussion of brain mechanisms of consciousness [16].

The implicit meaning of "seeing" is the requirement that knowing by looking should be accompanied by a sensory experience – or, more precisely, by a conscious visual experience. But it is not necessary for all aspects of visual processing to lead to visual experience. Indeed, a large body of experimental evidence points towards the existence of sensing, the processing of visual information, without accompaniment by visual experience or by any conscious awareness at all. Milner and Goodale [14] distinguished between an on-line stream in vision, concerned with immediate visuomotor action (e. g., movement of the eyes, maintenance of balance) and an off-line stream concerned with more time-demanding processes, such as the conscious perception and recognition of objects. Visuomotor responses and conscious experience may be separated not only as a result of damage to the off-line stream, but also in certain normal conditions. This topic has been addressed in experiments investigating change blindness – the failure of observers to detect large, sudden changes in a display.

Perception itself is susceptible to various forms of momentarily induced "blindness." Rensink [13] referred to the finding that large changes in a scene often become difficult to notice if made during an eye movement, image flicker, movie cut, or other such disturbance. This change blindness can serve as a useful tool for exploring various aspects of vision, to map out the attentional mechanisms involved. Rensink pointed out that these results show that the failure to experience highly visible stimuli is not a rare pathological condition. Rather, it is a much more widespread effect – so widespread that it strongly suggests that observers never form a complete representation of the world around them. Beck et al. [17] used functional magnetic resonance imaging to study the neural correlates of visual change detection in normal subjects. They concluded that, despite the fact that "detecting change in the visual environment is of considerable evolutionary importance … people are remarkably poor at detecting a change if it occurs during a brief visual disruption." In addition, the study documented the involvement of parietal and dorsolateral frontal activation for conscious detection of changes coded in visual pathways. This means that dorsal-ventral interactions have a key involvement in visual awareness.

Q: Are there in fact definite testing conditions for normal visual perception that elicit varying kinds or degrees of visual responses below the level of full awareness?

A: A few instructive examples can briefly be given here. Several students of the neural correlates of visual perception have been impressed by the effects of perceptual, or binocular "rivalry." This is believed to be a useful experimental paradigm for the study of the substrate of conscious perception [18]. When dissimilar images are presented to the two eyes, they compete for perceptual dominance, so that each of the two images is visible in turn for a few seconds while the other is suppressed. Because the perceptual transition between each monocular view occurs spontaneously without any change in the physical stimulus, the neural responses associated with perceptual processes can be distinguished from those that are due to stimulus characteristics. Functional brain imaging studies have demonstrated the activated cerebral cortical regions that reflect both rivalrous and non-rivalrous perceptual transitions. The frontoparietal cortex is specifically associated with perceptual alternation only during rivalry. This cortical region therefore appears to play a central role in conscious perception [18].

Further evidence was provided by Treisman's study of "illusory conjunctions" [11]. An experiment was designed to test the performance of normal subjects in conditions similar to those that prevent patients from integrating separate parameters of sensory information. The subjects were prevented from focusing their attention on a visual display by giving them a brief presentation and requiring them to spread their attention globally over the whole display. One such display contained four shapes varying in color, size, shape, and format (filled or outline). The patients were instructed to report the features of the display at definite locations cued 200 ms. afterwards, and the results showed that the subjects failed to bind the features. Instead, they seemed to form "illusory conjunctions," recombining features that in fact characterized separate objects.

Normal activities were studied in experiments in which consciousness was temporarily suspended [19]. A typical experiment analyzes the suppression of conscious visual experience during eye movements, or "saccadic suppression." In the latter case, visual perception is suspended, but information presented during this period of time influences behavior. By identifying the changes in the neural circuitry that occur when a conscious visual perception is momentarily suspended, it may be possible to identify the regions that contribute to conscious experience. Patients with blindsight are very important in relation to this topic. Such patients, who are fully awake and otherwise alert, are described as having lost the conscious perception of visual information presented to a blind hemifield. However, information entering his field still influences behavior. The inference drawn is that the area of the brain damaged by the lesion contributes to the content of conscious experience.

Q: It appears that attention holds a central role in the recognition of objects. What is known about specific "visual" attention, the loss of which may prevent a patient in the vegetative state from identifying things in the environment?

A: Attention is a very important process, and recent studies have even attributed a higher role to it. These studies distinguished between "pre-attentive and attentive mechanisms in vision" [20]. Pre-attentive mechanisms transform the visual input rapidly and in parallel, and pair the image into coherent parts. One of these pairs may pop out and trigger a behavioral response. In many cases, pre-attentive mechanisms are not sufficient, and proper visual attention is needed. This involves focal attention, which can be targeted only on one part or a few parts of the scene. In addition, there is neuropsychological and psychophysiological evidence that there is a distinction between attentive processing that leads to awareness, and processing that does not. Studies currently underway are investigating the relationships between the mechanisms that allow stimuli to enter visual awareness and the mechanisms that underlie only attention and perceptual organization, following the *gestalt* rules for forming configurations.

Q: What are the implications of these findings, studied in normal individuals and those with definite brain lesions causing disturbances of visual perception, for investigations into the mental capabilities of a person in coma or in a vegetative state caused by a diffuse brain lesion? There is an intriguing and specific issue here of whether it may become possible to reveal as yet unknown, masked or covert cognitive propensities in patients who appear to be profoundly unresponsive to their environment. Can the use of visual-perceptual probes that produce errors or illusions, or unconscious responses, in normal subjects provide us with better ways of describing the state of a patient, beyond saying that he or she is in a state of arousal or wakefulness? Can the characterization of a patient's state as "vegetative state" or "locked-in syndrome" be extended to include the level of his or her cognitive abilities? Should we not broaden our assessment of these patients by presenting them repeatedly and insistently with traditional and familiar tests, some of which form part of the batteries used to measure "intelligence" that normal subjects are expected to cope with consciously and explicitly? Needless to say, one would have to carefully limit the tests to whatever restricted responses are within the patient's capacities.

A: Presenting a patient in an altered state of consciousness, even repeatedly, with a stimulus including all the usual attributes that normally elicit the visual system's full-blown capacities would have little chance of producing even a faint, crude response. One could not expect a learning course to start. However, using restricted or fragmented visual displays with prominent features for focal targeting, taking advantage of the growing knowledge about the different strengths of various sensory features and the sequence in which they become dominant, might make it possible to elicit a learned response produced by a patient in the course of emerging from the phase of deep coma.

Q: What about the relationship between emotions and consciousness? The last statements lead directly to this question.

A: The topic of "brain and emotions" is apparently becoming a very high-priority issue at present. Some authors believe that the time is ripe to develop a new field of research alongside cognitive neuropsychology: "affective neuroscience." The affective mind of a person in coma would be the first candidate for this type of study.

Throughout the ages, scholars have disagreed regarding the number and nature of basic emotions. Investigators are not even in agreement regarding the criteria that should be used to classify emotions. A great deal has been written about the topic, but most of it is still controversial. Until recently, this type of question could not be approached from a neurological perspective. Now it can, however, and the increasing interest in the way in which emotions are involved in human cognition and awareness may become particularly relevant in the present context. The need is being felt to advance toward a "computational affective neuroscience" [22]. At present, it appears that a considerable proportion of this type of research is being directed toward the nature of fear. It is believed that consciousness is an important part of the study of emotion and other mental processes. Although we are far from understanding what consciousness is, a number of theorists have proposed that it may be related to working memory, a serially organized work space in which things can be compared and contrasted and mentally manipulated. In the case of an affectively charged stimulus, such as a trigger of fear, the same types of process will be called upon as for stimuli without fear implications; in addition, however, the working memory will become aware that the brain's fear system has been activated. The additional information, when added to perceptual and mnemonic information about the object or event, could provide the conditions for the subjective experience of an emotional state of fear.

Following this line of thinking, the functions of the amygdala and its role in memory consolidation have become a major target of the study of brain mechanisms of memory formation for emotionally arising events. "Various aspects of emotional and motivational behavior require the amygdala, a complex and multifunctional structure" [21]. However, the authors cautioned against a rush to embrace the amygdala as the new center for the emotional brain. It is unlikely that the amygdala is the answer to how all emotions work, and it may not even explain how all the aspects of fear work. There is some evidence that the amygdala participates in positive emotional behavior, but this role is still poorly understood.

Clinical research projects with significant conceptual and practical implications are conceivable. Cognitive and behavioral clinical investigations may contribute to a fuller comprehension of the nature of human consciousness.

Q: All cognitive paths lead to the mechanisms of response. What is the most promising approach to overcoming the problem of output?

A: Currently, the main response to this question deals largely with the topic of motor reactions and motor learning. Rich and quite subtle interactions between brain structures are known to be involved in learning – the production of levels and stratifications of awareness in acquisition and retrieval.

These may serve as a promising, and still not fully explored, basis for a higher level of responsiveness toward wakefulness. The basal ganglia, the cerebellum and the anterior cingulate cortex are now known to have significant roles beyond the motor functioning traditionally ascribed to them. "It is clear that the basal ganglia are involved in a variety of activities that are not unambiguously motor" [23]. Students of the basal ganglia consider that they have a role in processing somatosensory, visual, and auditory information. They have also pointed out basal ganglia functions in attention and nonmotor learning, which are deficient in Parkinson patients before major motor difficulties develop. Finally, it is argued that people with basal ganglia dysfunctions have impaired executive functions – a set of extremely high-level activities that include planning of sequences of movements, and initiating goal-directed behavior. These authors speculate that the basal ganglia are in fact involved in the generation of volitional behavior. Studies have emphasized the role of the basal ganglia in certain types of learning and memory; they support learning in which the organism detects constancies between environmental stimuli and specific behavioral responses. It is therefore a question of stimulus – response or habitual learning. Graybiel and Kimura [24], as well as Kandel and Pittenger [21], have pointed out the role of the striatum for memory of habits. Recent data indicate that behavioral events can be encoded by the activity of single basal ganglia neurons. Finally, there is evidence for the persistence of certain cells in responding to a conditioned stimulus after a behavioral response has been extinguished. This would suggest a mechanism for the spontaneous recovery of a conditioned response.

According to Kandel and Pittenger [21], the cerebellum is necessary for a form of implicit memory: the learning of coordinated motor skills, and in particular for the acquisition of classical conditioning of motor reflexes. Thus, the cerebellum has a role in motor memory. In addition, the cerebellum is thought to be an important neural component in coordination among the joints of one limb, between two limbs, between the eye and hand in reaching, pointing or addressing tasks, and between the eye and leg during walking [25]. Particular attention is being given to coordination between the eye and hand in visually guided tracking tasks. Coordination is defined operationally as "the process facilitating motor performance during synchronous, spatially coherent movement of two effectors"; "the improvement in tracking performance that we observed when eye-hand tracking was almost synchronous must result from involvement of an active coordinating process, because coordinated eye-hand tracking was better than movement of the hand alone" [25].

Q: Are there any practical ways of benefiting from the newly accumulating information about structures such as the cerebellum, in a prospective intervention program?

A: Several points could be made:

- Patients with an altered consciousness or in the vegetative state, presumably due to extensive brain damage, have the lowest responsiveness to environmental sensory stimulation, or any kind of stimulation.
- The structures that are most compromised by this type of damage are the neocortical structures known to be mainly involved in higher cognitive performance, such as predominantly conscious perceptual experiences, explicit and voluntary recall of information, and controlled executive functions.
- Previously less well known cognitive abilities of the supplementary cortical and subcortical structures, notably the basal ganglia and the cerebellum, have been documented in recent years.
- It is increasingly appearing that emotions play a modulating role in memory and learning. The amygdala has quite extensive connections with cortical structures.
- The cognitive limitation resulting from extensive damage is an extreme instance of cognitive reduction, along a continuum of performance ranging from specific induced moments during a generally normal performance, through modular deficits resulting from localized lesions. A tentative evaluation and intervention program can be suggested that focuses on visual experience. This capability is considered to be an elementary manifestation of cognitive awareness, and one that is clearly very accessible to study. A set of tests could be administered by trained speech therapists, occupational therapists, or physiotherapists at the patient's bedside. Conjunctive object stimulation may enhance the neuronal response to a stimulus in a single behaviorally relevant location in the visual field, in a person with low responsiveness. Repeated sensory stimulation at the same spot may be expected to produce a learning effect expressed in physiological responses. There may be a better chance of obtaining some signs of implicit memory or of "priming" memory, for things presented repeatedly in distributed sessions, rather than in massed learning. A consolidation effect of some sort, involving primarily the hippocampal system, might be obtained.
- The components of a visual display have a graded sensory strength – color, orientation, size, etc. – and they stimulate the sensory system in a specific sequence. They may have a different impact in a patient with low reactivity.
- Sensory stimulation should avoid "competition" or "rivalry" from the level of the retina and beyond, to allow better physiological responses.
- As a matter of basic principle, any cognitive stimulation should be enhanced by associating it with emotions believed to originate in earliest part of the person's life.

References

1. Giacino JT. Disorders of consciousness: differential diagnosis and neuropathological features. Semin Neurol 1997; 17: 105–12.
2. Searle JR. Consciousness. Ann Rev Neurosci 2000; 23: 557–78.
3. Gulyas B. "Overlearning": vista into the nature of conscious processes. Neuroreport 2000; 11: i–ii.
4. Paus T. Primate anterior cingulate cortex: where motor control, drive and cognition interface. Nature Rev Neurosci 2001; 2: 417–23.
5. Wilson RA, Kail FK, editors. MIT encyclopedia of cognitive sciences. Cambridge, MA: MIT Press, 1999.
6. Edelman SY, Bulthoff HH. Modeling human visual cortex recognition. Proceedings of the IEEE International Joint Conference on Neural Networks 1992, vol 4: 37–42.
7. Westmacott R, Leach L, Freedman M, Moscovitch M. Different patterns of autobiographical memory loss in semantic dementia and medial temporal lobe amnesia: a challenge to consolidation theory. Neurocase 2001; 7: 37–55.
8. Rees G. Neuroimaging of visual awareness in patients and normal subjects. Curr Opin Neurobiol 2001; 11: 150–6.
9. Olzak LA, Thomas JP. Neural recoding of human pattern vision: model and mechanisms. Vision Res 1999; 39: 231–56.
10. Zeki S, Bartels A. The autonomy of the visual systems and the modularity of conscious vision. Philos Trans R Soc London B 1998; 353: 1911–4.

11. Treisman A. Feature binding, attention and object perception. Philos Trans R Soc London B 1998; 353: 1295–1306.
12. Karni A, Bertini G. Learning perceptual skills: behavioral probes into adult cortical plasticity. Curr Opin Neurobiol 1997; 7: 530–5.
13. Rensink RA. Seeing, sensing, and scrutinizing. Vision Res 2000; 40: 1469–87.
14. Milner AD, Goodale MA. The visual brain in action. Oxford: Oxford University Press, 1995.
15. Posner MI, Rockbart MK. Attention, self-regulation and consciousness. Philos Trans R Soc London B 1998; 351: 1915–27.
16. Crick FHC, Koch C. Toward a neurobiological theory of consciousness. Semin Neurosci 1990; 2: 263–75.
17. Beck DM, Rees G, Frith CD, Lavie N. Neural correlates of change detection and change blindness. Nature Neurosci 2001; 6: 645–7.
18. Lumer ED, Friston KJ, Rees G. Neural correlates of perceptual rivalry in the human brain. Science 1998; 280: 1930–4.
19. Raichle ME. The neural correlates of consciousness: an analysis of cognitive skills. Philos Trans R Soc London B 1998; 353: 1889–1901.
20. Spekreijse H. Pre-attentive and attentive mechanisms in vision: perceptual organization and dysfunction [editorial]. Vision Res 2000; 40: 1179–82.
21. Kandel ER, Pittenger C. The past, the future and the biology of memory storage. Philos Trans R Soc London B 1999; 354: 2027–52.
22. Schmidt LA, Schulkin J. Toward a computational affective neuroscience. Brain Cogn 2000; 42: 95–100.
23. Iversen SD, Muller RU. Cognitive neuroscience: editorial overview. Curr Opin Neurobiol 1997; 7: 151–6.
24. Graybiel AM, Kimura M. Adaptive neural networks in the basal ganglia. In: Houk JC, Davis JL, Beiser DG, editors. Information processing in the basal ganglia. Cambridge: MIT Press, 1995: 103–16.
25. Miall RC, Reckess GZ, Imamizu H. The cerebellum coordinates eye and hand tracking movements. Nature Neurosci 2001; 4: 638–41.

12 Intensive-Care Unit for Vegetative State: Management Guidelines

M. Rachele Zylberman

This chapter aims to present various modalities, parameters, references, and suggestions which in clinical experience have proved helpful and often indispensable for the correct management of a department dedicated to treating patients in the vegetative state. Apart from the directives and detailed obligations that are typical of each country's medical legislation, the setting up of a department of this type should be guided by specific indicative criteria that affect both the structural project and the functional organization – two intertwined and correlated aspects.

General Organizing Criteria

In medical practice and culture, a clear need has emerged that the complex welfare problems of patients in the vegetative state be approached by assigning the patients to qualified teams and including them in specialized programs, characterized by: identification of the prevalent organic pathology; definition of progressive stages; and overall coordination of interventions, starting from the acute state and continuing up until social reintegration.

In this type of department, the process of rehabilitation is given its real status as a holistic approach, ensuring all the diagnostic and therapeutic procedures that are indispensable to guarantee full recovery. Rehabilitation therapy is not carried out in a simplistic way; instead, global care is taken of the person in relation to his or her whole pathological condition, not only by defining and treating the basic illness, but also by avoiding and/or treating complications or associated disorders.

Neurorehabilitation could be described as the end point of a series of complex operations, among which physiochinesy therapy (FKT) is one therapeutic step in the context of the broader and more modern concept of "restorative" medicine, the highest level of health care designed to guarantee the best possible outcome.

Residual disability is often due to primary damage as well as to chains of events that take place after the acute state, ranging from lack of prevention and/or care for resulting impairments, to complications caused by lack of adequate management of patients in a frail condition, for whom immobility itself often produces irreparable clinical disasters.

Prevention, diagnosis, and treatment, integrated into multidisciplinary activities, must be thought of as different steps in a single operation, namely neurorehabilitation; the latter should therefore address everything that precedes, accompanies, and follows the frequent and prevalent phenomenon of severe head trauma.

Clinical departments for patients in the vegetative state were originally regarded as a combination of intensive care and neurosurgical acute-phase treatment in the rehabilitation period (as traditionally considered). The department is highly specialized and provides high-level assistance; it should either be located near a large multidisciplinary hospital or form part of the hospital itself, although distinct from the other operating units. This type of department, the intensive-care unit for patients in the vegetative state, is designed to provide selective care for patients with complex internal medicine problems and severe consciousness alterations. Patients are admitted immediately after they have opened their eyes and have achieved stable respiratory function.

Arousal without (clinical) signs of consciousness, the presence of a tracheostomy cannula, long-term artificial feeding through a gastrostomy, dysautonomia, septic conditions, absence of spontaneous motility problems due to immobility, often complicated in important cranial traumas by various kinds of fractures, a potential for neurologic complications, total inability with regard to all personal needs-all of these situations, as well as others, approximately describe the critical clinical situation that makes these patients almost totally dependent on others and easily prone to complications (especially septic ones).

The clinical management of a patient in the vegetative state is very hard work, and specific departments must guarantee integrated and coherent management. Any activity must follow flow-charts, consistently fulfilling the following fundamental goals:

- Support for vital functions and maintenance of stable systemic conditions
- Support/maintenance of residual organic resources
- Reactivation of autonomous functions
- Help in regaining damaged functions

Standardization of all medical care provided, through the use of periodically revised flow-charts, is necessary to achieve these goals.

The whole management at this stage is guaranteed by a team in which each professional, while maintaining his or her own specific competence, collaborates in identifying personalized models that may suit each specific patient, avoiding the adoption of fixed roles, being well aware that the way in which each action is performed can actually elicit or inhibit a patient's reaction. A complex form of interaction is therefore needed: it is necessary for the whole team to treat patients in order to facilitate the recovery of consciousness, but at the same time, it is also necessary to stimulate environmental contact through multimodal stimulations during everyday care activity.

During the arousal phase after coma, the patient does not seem to perceive external stimuli; it is only at a certain point the during clinical course that this perception appears in a global protopathic modality, without intermediate or discriminating "nuances."

Since the patient is in a state of complete perceptual isolation, the facilitation/promotion of physical experience should be the common feature in all aspects of intervention. Physical experience is the only possibility of "being" – "esse est percipi" (G. Berkeley, *Treatise on the Principles of Human Knowledge*). It is through our own body perception that all new experiences take place and that we build up a consciousness of "self."

It must be borne in mind that mistakes in the early phase may produce irreversible impairments and may be the main reason for therapeutic failure in patients affected by significant difficulties and a slow tendency toward improvement. A combined form of management, with a concentric view of the patient as representing the cornerstone around which different professional figures work to provide global, polymorphic support, appears to be the best type of assistance, targeted at the best possible outcome.

In this team, beyond the boundaries of different medical specialisms, professional nurses and rehabilitation therapists acquire fundamental roles, contributing both to the diagnostic definition and to monitoring of the clinical course. New professional profiles therefore take shape: while dropping traditional roles, staff acquire increasing autonomy, with the new operating model being characterized by team activity and a multidisciplinary approach. From time to time, this multidisciplinary operating model should set achievable objectives for each patient, at each specific moment.

Admission Criteria

The criteria for admission and discharge of patients in an ICU for the vegetative state can be summarized here. The ICU's mission starts when the patient opens his or her eyes and achieves stable respiratory function; it ends as soon as the patient begins interrelating with the outside world. The patient must therefore not be in coma and must have had autonomous and stable respiratory functions and well-functioning vital organs for at least one week. Imminent surgery, or conditions demanding highly specialized clinical treatment such as dialysis or severe hepatorenal failure, or hematological illnesses such as diffuse intravascular coagulation, etc., must not be present.

Discharge Criteria

Discharge generally involves transferring the patient to an intensive neurorehabilitation department to ensure the best possible recovery of motor and neuropsychological sequences, or to a long-term medical department in which basic assistance and maintenance of regained functions is guaranteed.

The patient is ready to be transferred to a new department when, after a mainly reactive phase characterized by reflex motoricity and altered perception, he or she reaches a more selective perception phase and finally a level of motor performance that allows intentional behavior and interacting with the surrounding environment. A patient presenting simple but constant answers, even if restricted to single expression modalities, and with good and stable vital functions must be immediately transferred to a neurorehabilitation department to continue rehabilitation programs with a view to recovering the contents of consciousness and all other damaged functions.

We believe that a patient in post-traumatic vegetative state must receive intensive rehabilitation treatment in an ICU at least for 1 year after the traumatic event. When an evaluation by the whole rehabilitation team shows that the patient has not presented any changes in conscious functions over the last 3 months, the conclusion can be drawn that that patient's potential for recovery is limited. He or she should therefore continue rehabilitation therapy and maintenance support of general conditions in a long-term specialized unit. This decision must be supported by additional preparation and care. A detailed clinical evaluation is written up in the patient's hospital file by the department team and is communicated to the family in advance.

Recovery of conscious activity may become evident even after 1 year or even later, but the longer it takes, the worse the prognosis for recovery is, and the patient often remains in a minimally responsive state (see p. 110).

Direct discharge from hospital to the home for a patient who has not shown a good recovery is a rare occurrence; it would be an extremely difficult situation. The patient's family (especially parents) should have adequate social and economic resources and an adequate and preventive practical and psychological training.

The Department

The functional organization of the facilities described above is the basis for defining the process the patient should follow from the vegetative state to recovery of contact and relationship with environment and people.

The structural equipment and instruments used depend on the kind of patient being treated and his or her clinical condition and potential outcome. Building structures, equipment, and removal of architectural barriers have to follow the legal standards that apply in each country.

The number of beds must be calculated in proportion to those in the intensive-care unit and intensive standard neurorehabilitation unit and long-stay unit, maintaining a ratio of 1 : 4.

The organizational arrangements should make it possible to follow a complete rehabilitation program, thereby achieving the best recovery results and ensuring patient turnover and rapid fulfillment of admission demands. In relation to the cost–benefit ratio and experience in existing units, the ideal number would appear to be not less than eight or more than 16.

As an indication of potential equipment needs, a 10-bed unit can be expected to require:
- A surface area of approximately 500 m^2, subdivided as follows:
  - One or two rooms for in-patients, 150 m^2
  - One or two single rooms, 40 m^2
  - Water therapy area, 50 m^2
  - Gymnasium, 90 m^2
  - Two rooms for special treatment, 30 m^2
  - One prosthesis workshop, 10 m^2
  - Medical and nursing working areas, 30 m^2
  - Dirty and clean depots, 40 m^2
  - Common areas, 40 m^2
  - Service area (kitchen, etc.), 20 m^2
- Specific equipment for each area listed
- Biotechnology facilities
- Human resources
- Specialist competence and reference diagnostic services

Structural Organization

It is necessary to provide an access area where the whole staff can dress up and change clothes at the beginning and at the end of each shift. An electronic checking system at the entrance may be useful. Admittance to the unit is through a filter area in which all staff members, relatives, and any other occasional visitors (consultants or maintenance staff) must ensure a "clean" approach to patients (by wearing uniforms, covering shoes, washing hands, etc.).

The structure must have numerous, user-friendly washbasins.

The residential area must be organized into one or two large areas, and the beds should be located around the perimeter, with a central observation nursing area, in order to maintain direct visual monitoring of each patient, not only using electronic supports (these patients are not able to use any alarm systems properly).

The area for each bed must be calculated so as to ensure easy access from both sides with wheelchairs, lifters, or any other equipment. Each bed must be easily transferable, and each single bed place must be thought of as an independent functional unit, with points for electricity, oxygen, and compressed air, etc. Shelves for monitors, leaning surfaces, nourishment or infusion pumps and various rods must be fixed to the wall or ceiling, using supports that leave the beds free from any anchorage. The patient must be easily transferable on the bed or wheelchair. Beds should preferably work electrically, with blocking devices, and must be capable of verticalizing up to 90°. Latex antidecubitus mattresses must be supported by more complex ones, with computerized air flow.

Electronic monitoring equipment for each single patient's vital functions must be capable of transferring video and numerical data via monitors to an observation and control station. All vital parameters must be retroactively transferable to files. Alarm systems should be constructed in such a way that in each room in the department, a very distinct light signal will show that one of the monitors in the unit is signaling an alarm.

The walls between in-patient areas and common areas must be made of glass.

Single bedrooms are necessary when the patient's clinical condition requires the presence of a relative (in critical situations) or for special infections (for isolation). They are also useful when the patient has regained the contents of consciousness and there is a delay in the transfer process for various reasons. Some centers use single bedrooms to teach relatives about nursing maneuvers and patient management, if a domestic transfer has been planned. Single bedrooms need to have an area large enough to allow the entrance of any kind of equipment that needs to be placed around the bed, which should be easily transferable. Single bedrooms must have a bathroom with shower and a large pool for hydrotherapy, water mobilization, and post-relaxation stimulation.

The hygiene facilities must be regarded as therapeutic areas, and must be subdivided into compartments along one pathway:

- Washbasin area with a mirror wall
- Shower area with a walled WC
- Butterfly pool area

Bathrooms require ultraviolet light for sterilizing the room; they also need a door with a safety device allowing the ultraviolet light to be turned on only when nobody is in.

There should be a doctors' room, with an adjacent visiting room. The infirmary is designed only as a ward sister's organizing room and as a depot for drug and therapeutic preparations. There should also be a staff meeting room.

The gymnasium is one large room dedicated to multifunctional activity, with one mirror wall. It should be large enough to contain 10 patients at the same time, making it possible to carry out different activities simultaneously, such as standing and lying exercises, wheelchair positioning, rolling, and individual deambulator exercises, etc. The following should be provided for inside the gymnasium:

- Occupational therapy area and thermoplastics
- Instrumental therapy area with suitable equipment (for physical therapy, analgesic currents)
- Prosthesis workshop adjacent to the gymnasium

There should be two rooms for individual therapy, sensory stimulating treatment, swallowing and breathing exercises, and cognitive therapy.

Finally, there should be a very spacious and comfortable room for relatives (at least 20 for 10 patients), with refreshments available (including a food dispenser).

There should be an air-conditioned room for hydrotherapy in the butterfly pool.

In addition to the specific rooms described above, it is necessary to organize:

- A clean linen depot
- A dirty linen depot
- A wheelchair depot
- A kitchen for food preparation
- A rubbish drop-off room
- Principal access
- Elevator
- Emergency exit (suitable for this type of patient)

The distribution of rooms should follow an ideal pathway from clean to dirty.

Building Materials

The floor, walls and ceilings must be made of fire-resistant material that easily allows cleaning and disinfection, avoiding inaccessible corners and surfaces. Colors, for example in frames and furnishings, should preferably be pastels or shades that create a pleasant and peaceful atmosphere, avoiding the cold or very medical appearance typical of intensive-care units. The room should be bright in natural daylight but not directly exposed to sunshine.

Equipment and Biotechnology

There should be an air-conditioning system to guarantee thermal stability (21 °C in winter, 24 °C in summer) with a humidification gradient of more or less 65 %, with eight exchanges of sterile air, filtered with eight changes per hour. It is important maintain a slight overpressure in the department to prevent the entry of untreated air or dust.

There should be a ceiling-track lifting system, arranged in different rooms and in the in-patient bedrooms, common areas, gymnasium, and swimming-pool (this reduces work and ensures easy and safe movement of patients). Other items of equipment include:
- Computer system
- Monitor controlling system
- Sound diffusion system
- Eight pulsed oximeters
- Two electrocardiography (ECG) machines
- One defibrillator
- One sterilizer
- One blood gas analyzer for measuring electrolytes and glycemia
- One flexible fibrobronchoscope
- Ten pumps for enteral feeding
- One portable oxygen respirator
- One movable radiography device
- One emergency intubation and tracheostomy trolley
- Centralized vacuum and oxygen installation

Some of the instruments mentioned above are needed to ensure that the unit can function autonomously in emergency situations.

Lying-in Period

- Multi-articulated tilting beds that can be verticalized up to 90°
- Antidecubitus mattresses
- Bed head with centralized O_2 and vacuum equipment, calling system, and lights
- Container modulus for each patient, with various shelves for clean linen, hygienic material, outdoor clothes
- Small and easily sterilizable basket or container next to the bed, in which small prosthetic materials or positioning supporters can be placed; must be individual
- Working shelves
- A U module equipped for nursing observation
- Special wheelchairs
- Ten slings to lift patients
- Two elevators
- Two patient weighing systems
- Two shower stretchers
- One spoon stretcher, one weighing system
- One emergency trolley aspirator
- Three bed-pan washing machines

Gymnasium

- Mirror wall 8 m long
- Three double wall bars
- Carpets of different sizes to cover a total area of 20 m^2
- Two tatami mats
- Two standing devices
- One parallel bar
- Two shaped tables of different sizes for occupational therapy
- Two adjustable stools
- One pool for thermoplastic material
- Teaching materials for occupational therapy
- One electrostimulation device
- Shaped modules of different sizes
- Two kinetic lower limbs
- Two kinetic upper limbs

Sanitary Rooms

- Washbasins fitted for handicapped people, at variable heights, fixed to a single mirror wall
- Butterfly pool
- Material container
- Adequate containers for hydrotherapy
- Two shower stretchers
- Various models of sling

Human Resources

For ten beds, it is necessary to provide:
- Four doctors on internal attendance duty service
- Five therapists
- A sufficient number of nurses and auxiliary staff, excluding cleaning staff, to ensure 10 hours' assistance out of the 24 h for each patient

In view of the complexity of the treatments, the medical staff must have a stable nucleus of doctors on the permanent staff, who may have differing basic areas of expertise, such as internal medicine, resuscitation, neurology, neurosurgery, or physiatrics, but who should also have acquired special experience in this field.

Medical assistance necessarily has to be integrated, with constant collaboration among doctors belonging to different specialized fields, both in surgery and internal medicine. We believe it is important to emphasize again that when a coma ICU department is set up, it should either form part of, or be situated nearby, a specialized multidisciplinary general medical center.

Nurses, physiotherapists, and auxiliary staff must have acquired or should be acquiring specific experience through training courses, refresher courses, and continuous training work, and support for participation in training schemes should be provided by the specialists managing the department.

The specific psychological aspects of the work and the nature of the medical and social relationships involved make it valuable to have a psychologist and social assistants as part of the unit's basic staff.

Twice-weekly meetings are a crucial part of any personnel training program. All staff members should take part in these, and the aim of the meetings is to develop a common professional awareness through continuous assessment of both clinical problems and the inevitable ongoing revisions of working strategies. The group meetings also make it possible to develop a supportive and collaborative working approach through which, with the predominant group dynamics involved, staff can learn to manage and control any individual disruptive dynamics.

Epilogue and Future Prospects

Giuliano Dolce and Leon Sazbon

Some 35 years have passed since we first started research on the vegetative state (although different terms were used for the condition in those days). At the end of life-long and dedicated research careers, we hope our studies may have contributed to the progress observed in recent decades. In this concluding section we would like to provide an overview of the achievements, problems still to be solved, and future developments foreseen on the basis of the constant advances being made neurology, neurobiology, and neuroscience.

A few facts outline the achievements made and indicate limitations that still exist. Advances in emergency care have significantly increased the chances of survival after severe brain injury; more patients now survive severe trauma, and with better outcomes, than in the past. In addition to survival, the quality of recovery after brain damage has also improved, mostly due to the reduction of secondary neuronal damage through proper treatment of edema and intracranial hypertension during the first weeks following trauma. The increasing availability of immediate and fast transportation (e. g., by helicopter) and of highly specialized centers for emergency care has also proved crucial. Nowadays it is unusual to observe damage due to inadequate nursing or, more specifically, nutrition, and emaciation has therefore largely disappeared among patients who have been in vegetative state for several months. Inadequate nutrition can impair metabolism in the peripheral nerves and cause polyneuropathies, or may lead to often significant worsening of brain pathology. In the latter case, the resulting worsened effects of primary and secondary brain damage further inhibit recuperation of conscious functions. Interference with the immune system is also possible, and this can contribute to the occurrence of bedsores, infections, sepsis, and shock or death. Prolonged sensory loading (often causing damage rather than benefiting the patients) has now fallen out of favor, and early rehabilitation (in the initial months after brain injury) now involves regulated procedures, rather than depending on improvisation. This has significantly contributed to better recovery of conscious activities, even after a prolonged vegetative state. We have emphasized the evidence that there is no unique pharmacological action or rehabilitation procedure that has particularly good effects. Instead, positive rehabilitation results from an ensemble of treatment modes and rules (the "therapeutic milieu") that are applied in specialized units for patients in the vegetative state as elements of each therapeutic strategy or procedure.

This approach (and the rules and procedures it helped develop) allowed us to produce rewarding results, with about one-third of patients recovering conscious functions to a stage allowing work or study at levels comparable to those prior to brain injury. Based on these results, it should be clear that the post-traumatic vegetative state should be regarded as resulting from a pathological condition in the brain, which, although severe, can improve and develop to a significant extent with the help of an appropriate "therapeutic milieu."

The first lesson to be drawn is therefore for those responsible for planning the organization of health care. Health authorities should be urged to build and operate highly specialized intensive-care units for patients in the vegetative state. A requirement of about 10 beds per 4–5 million population should be considered, as indicated by epidemiology and the available guidelines (see Chapter 12). At the same time, it is also necessary to give the patients' families appropriate education regarding their relatives' clinical condition, and about the predicted outcome and selected rehabilitation procedures. The family should also be involved in therapeutic and rehabilitative programs and trained to perform all complementary actions that may help rehabilitation. A program should also be designed to provide the patients' relatives with professional psychological support. However, such psychological support should never involve members of the team caring for the patients themselves, although operating in collaboration with it.

Despite hopes for unexpected breakthroughs in neurology and neuroscience, a substantial improvement in the prospects for rehabilitation (due to new and more effective procedures) can hardly be expected in the near future. Accordingly, the rehabilitation of patients in the vegetative state is unlikely to improve significantly. It is therefore our personal hope that this handbook may be helpful for many years to come to the young professionals who will be taking responsibility for patients in the post-traumatic vegetative state in dedicated care units that will be established in developed countries to face the expected incidence of this condition.

Today, the treatment of patients in the vegetative state is mostly based on promoting and facilitating the development of a new functional arrangement to replace the damaged one. It should be noted that this process occurs spontaneously. It depends on residual learning mechanisms and is strongly limited in pathological conditions in which large neuronal populations have been severely damaged.

Anatomical replacement and reorganization of damaged central nervous system structures now seems possible, and this could expand the range of potential recovery of lost brain functions. However weak the experimental evidence regarding the gray matter of the brain may appear today, the potential of neural stem cells implants may suggest new perspectives. Based on this, some of the principles concerning the regulation of growth in neuronal aggregates may need to be substantially revised.

The regrowth of damaged white matter appears to be more promising in the short run. Diffuse axonal damage is certainly a major factor determining the development of post-traumatic brain pathology into the vegetative state. In the future, the recovery of conscious functions might be able to reach levels unimaginable today if axonal damage could be restored, and this unprecedented goal may now be closer than we expect.

In the central and peripheral nervous systems, axonal growth is a rapid, efficient, and aggressive mechanism of repair. In contrast to the peripheral system, however, the growth of damaged axons at the central level ends quite quickly, and never expands beyond the lesion. The "empty" synapse of a severed axon is a potent mechanism of axonal growth, because of the attraction exerted on the axon by the disconnected synaptic sites. The growth of the axon specific to a synaptic site (homotopic), however, is inhibited, and the site is occupied by an unaffected axon through sprouting phenomena and heterotopic innervation. This process results in two negative effects – namely reinnervation that does not respect the highly selective neuronal organization and permanent inhibition of the growth of the axon specific to the synapse.

Neuroscientists have been familiar with these mechanisms for several years now, but it was only recently that the amyloid beta precursor protein was identified as a major factor inhibiting the growth of severed axons. The evidence for such a mechanism is a major breakthrough in research on pharmacological methods potentially favoring the repair of damaged white matter in the brain or spinal cord. Partial reorganization of the white matter would make it possible to reestablish the functional connections between neuronal aggregates or structures, with unprecedented perspectives for the recuperation of damaged brain functions.

These novel, unexpected prospects for recovery also require better skills in the care of patients and protection of their residual neuronal functions after brain damage. To a significant extent, this achievement is already possible today, if the indications and guidelines outlined in this book are adhered to and the knowledge and expertise acquired over a lifetime of research can be cherished and passed on, in the expectation of yet more brilliant and rewarding therapies in the future.

Index

Note: Page numbers in *italics* refer to figures and tables. 'VS' refers to vegetative state

A

acidosis, secondary brain damage   7
active abandonment   121, 123
activity, minimal   110
Addison's disease   23
adductor hypertonus   104
cyclic adenosine monophosphate (cAMP)   60
adult respiratory distress syndrome (ARDS)   19
aerosol therapy   97, 108
affective neuroscience   137–8
age   4–5
 outcome   43
akinesia   16
 absolute   15
akinetic mutism   3, 14
 anterior cingulate cortex lesions   132
 corpus striatum lesions   38
 VS differential diagnosis   35–6, 38–9
alarm reactions, neurovegetative   98
albuminoglobulins, inversion   60
alcohol use   43
alertness
 minimal response syndrome   114–15
 staff members   127
alkaline phosphatase   60, 107
aluminium hydroxide antacid   23
amantadine   77
American Medical Association (AMA)   122
American Task Force   2
γ-aminobutyric acid (GABA) *see* GABA
amphetamines   77, 89
amygdala functions   138
amyloid beta precursor protein   148
anemia   23
anesthetic block   105–6
anger   126, 127
anoxia   42, 43
anterior cingulate cortex   132, 138
anterior communicating artery aneurysm   39
anterior tibialis muscle, lateral transposition of part of tendon   106
antidiuretic hormone (ADH)   23
anxiety   126
apallic syndrome   1, 3
apolipoprotein Eε4 allele   60
apperception processes   13–14
arm rotation   104
arousal
 anterior cingulate cortex role   132
 disturbance in minimal response syndrome   114
 phase   142
arrhythmia   18
arthrodesis   106
ascending reticular activating system (ARAS)   16
 functional blocking   16–17
assessment tools   46–52
astrocytic reaction, secondary   7
atelectasis   19
athetoid movements   34
atropine   77
attention   133
 recognition in minimal response syndrome   114
 stimulation   96
 visual   135, 137
attentiveness loss   2
auditory comprehension recovery   45
auditory evoked potentials   69
auditory-tactile sensory stimulation   89
auto-eroticism   35
automatism   29, 31, 103
 oral   32
autonomic disturbances   25–6
autonomy, partial   91
avoidance by staff   127
awakening without awareness   31
awareness   16
 clinical evaluation   112
 generalized   111
 metacognitive   111
 sensory   111
 thalamus role   7
 visual   135, 136
axon(s)
 growth   148

repair   6
 separation   6
 sprouting   148
 see also diffuse axonal injury
axonal injury
 brain injury   16
 centrum semiovale   *64*
 severity   7
axonal regeneration   148
 inhibition   7
axonal retraction bulbs   6
axotomy   6

B

Babinski sign, bilateral extensor   36
baclofen   105
 intrathecal administration   106–7
bacterial overgrowth   20
balled-up movements   34
basal ganglia   16
 cognitive abilities   139
 lesions   20
 roles   138
basilar artery
 ischemia   36
 thrombosis   37
basilar tip occlusion   40
bathing   91, 92
bathrooms   144
bed hygiene   92
bedrooms   144
beds   143, 144, 145
 electric   97, 98
 mattresses   92, 145
bedsores *see* decubitus ulcer
behavioral performance recovery   32
behavioral responses   28
behavioral signs, value assignment   28
Bland, Tony   122
blepharoptosis, hypersomnia   40
blink reflex   34
blood, occult   60
blood proteins   92
blunt injury   5, 6
body position   33

body weight monitoring 94
botulinum toxin 106
brain
  activity 120
    event-related potentials 70
  anoxic damage 117
  coherence model 16
  emotions 137–8
  functional interaction between systems 11
  functional organization in vegetative state 16–17
  functional residual plasticity 11–12
  higher functions 16
  neuropsychological assessment of function 65–7, 68, 69–72
  primary pathology 2, 3
  swelling with secondary brain damage 7
brain death 120
brain injury
  acute 6
  altered consciousness 132
  autonomic disturbances 25–6
  axonal damage 16
  cognitive limitation 139
  deep vein thrombosis 24–5
  dysautonomia 25
  family comprehension of consequences 128
  hydrocephalus 22
  imaging 61
  ischemic 7
  minimal response syndrome 112
  outcome prediction with EEG reactivity 66
  perception 134
  postlesional organization 12
  recovery of comatose patients 117
  recovery of function 44–6
  residual neuronal function protection 148
  sensory stimulation programs 81–3
  severity 76
  somatosensory evoked potentials 69
  surgical outcome 81
  surgical therapy 79–81
  survival 147
  ventricular enlargement 22
  wakefulness without awareness 71
brainstem
  diffuse axonal injury 61
  evoked response to auditory stimulation 69
  functional disconnection from cortical control 29

lesions and sensory stimulation 82
  preservation 6
breathing, ataxic 19
bromocriptine 77
bronchial secretion drainage 101
bronchoscopy, fibrotracheal 108
building materials 145
bulbopontine loop 28–9
bulldog reflex 29, 31, 35, 103
bupivacaine 105
butterfly pool see hydrotherapy

C

cachectic patients 94
calcium 23
caloric requirements 94
calorie supplementation 22
cannulas, permanent 91
car accident 5, 64
carbidopa 77
cardiac rate 18
cardiovascular system
  complications 18–19
care, passive 84
carers
  anxiety 126
  bond with patient 120
  depression 126
  minimal response syndrome 115
  see also family members; staff members
catabolic processes 93
catatonia 38
catecholamines 60
catheterization, urinary bladder 19, 93
cellular immune function depression 24
central nervous system (CNS) 148
central venous catheters 91
  feeding 94
centrum semiovale, axonal injury 64
cerebellum 138–9
  cognitive abilities 139
cerebral blood flow
  neurostimulation 79
  perfusion studies 65
cerebral cortex see cortex
cerebrospinal fluid (CSF)
  absorption resistance 80
  dynamic change with hydrocephalus 80
  enzyme levels 60
  homovanillic acid 77
  hydrocephalus 22
  pressure and hydrocephalus 79–80
cervical myotactic reflex 29, 35

cervical spinal cord stimulation 79
change blindness 136
chest trauma, myocardial damage 19
chewing
  automatism 29, 31
  uncoordinated movements 103
children
  mental delay 116
  mental recovery 45
  outcome 43
    functional 5
    recovery of function 44
chloride 23
choreiform movement 34
ciliospinal reflex 28, 34
cingulate gyrus 15
cingulum 12
circadian rhythms, recuperation 89
citicoline 78
clonidine 105
Clostridium difficile bacterial overgrowth 20
clothes 91
coagulation cascade activation 23
cognition, thalamus role 7
cognitive abilities, covert 131–9
cognitive elements of VS 134
cognitive malfunction, minimal response syndrome 114
cognitive processes 133
cognitive reduction 139
cognitive significance of brain potential 120
cognitive status fluctuation 32, 42, 46
cognitive stimulation 139
coherence, theory of 11, 89
coherence model 16
collagen production in trauma 7
collar 101
color perception 134–5
coma 36
  arousal phase 142
  chronic 1
  differentiation 3
  EEG 66
  masking VS 3
  minimal response distinction 112
  minimal response syndrome 110
  non-traumatic origin 3
  outcome prediction 67, 69
  progression 2, 30
  prolonged 3
  sensory stimulation 82
  sleep patterns 67
  somatosensory evoked potentials 67, 69
  traumatic origin 3
  unconsciousness 111

Index

visual evoked potentials 69
VS development 2
Coma Exit Chart 50–1, 83
Coma/Near Coma Scale 48, 83
Coma Outcome Scale 111
Coma Recovery Scale 48–9
communication
  electronic 37
  establishment 32
  family members with staff 129
  hydrotherapy 98
  hygiene procedures 91
  hypersomnia 40
  inner life determination 46
  minimal response syndrome 116
  promotion 96
  quantitative scale 28
  recovery 45
  speech 16
communicative behaviors 116
complementary therapy 115
computed tomography (CT) 61, 65
congenital bilateral aplasia of frontal area 8, 14
conscious activity 133
  recovery 30–2, 143
  recuperation 89
consciousness 12
  altered state 110, 131, 132, 133
    recovery 116
    stimulus presentation 137
  concept 111, 131
  contents 2, 11
  emotions relationship 137–8
  gradation 132
  loss 15, 131
  metaphorical model 14
  minimal response syndrome 110
  phenomenal content 133
  reactive 31
  recovery 42
  state transitions 132
  surgical outcome 81
consent of patient 120
constipation 20, 93
contingent negative variation (CNV) 70, 71, 120
contractures 20
control issues 128
coordination 138–9
corneal reflex 28–9, 34
corneo-chin reflex 29, 31, 35
corneomandibular reflex 29, 33
corona radiata 61
corpus callosum
  diffuse axonal injury 61
  injury causing VS 61, 62–3, 64
corpus striatum lesions in akinetic mutism 38

cortex
  anterior cingulate 132, 138
  atrophy 22
  damage 6
  extended contusions 61
  frontoparietal 136
  functional disconnection of control from brain stem 29
  functional relationship with hippocampus/limbic system 11
  information recall 11
  medium-frequency neuronal discharge 12
  perceptual transitions 136
  postcomatose unresponsiveness 110, 111
  processing 134
  visual 133
corticospinal tract, spasticity 20
cortisol 60
cost of care 121, 122
cough reflex 96, 103, 104
court rulings 121
cranial nerve impairment 28
creams, hydrating 91, 92
creatine phosphokinase 60
Crotone Document (1998) 122
Cruson, Nancy 122
cultural evolution 121
cytidine diphosphate choline 78

dantrolene sodium 105
death, concept of 120
decerebrate crisis 27
decerebrate position 33
decorticate crisis 27
decorticate position 33
decubitus ulcer 26
  hypercaloric diet 93
  local treatment 93
  medications 91
  prevention 92
  risk reduction 101
  treatment 92
deep brain electrical stimulation 78–9
deep vein thrombosis 24–5
defecation 93
defense mechanisms 28
  family members 126
  staff members 128
degenerative disorders 3
dementia
  severe post-traumatic 6
  thalamic 41
dendrite growth 115
denial 126
dentate gyrus 15
depression 126

depressive stupor 38
dermatological changes 19, 26
developmental malformations 3
dextroamphetamine 77
diabetes insipidus 23, 24
diapers 19, 93
diarrhea 20, 93
  water loss 23
diazepam 105
diencephalon lesions in akinetic mutism 38
diffuse axonal injury 6, 61
diffuse intravascular coagulation (DIC) 23
disability
  persistence 44
  residual 141
Disability Rating Scale 47–8, 49, 83, 117
diuresis 23
documentation of observations/procedures 92
doll's eye sign 29, 34
dorsal column stimulation 79
dressing 91, 92
drooling 33
drug therapy 76–8, 90–1
  access route monitoring 91
  complications 26
  dosage 105
  minimal response syndrome 114
  modes 90–1
  spasticity 105
dysautonomia 25–6

electrical stimulation
  deep brain 78–9
  functional 102
  oral 104
  spasticity 105
  spinal cord 106
  thalamic structures 89
electroencephalography (EEG) 66–7, 68
  brain activity 120
  coma 66
  interhemispheric coherence 66
  K-complex 83
  quantitative analysis 66
  reactivity 66
  sleep 67, 68
  sleep-wake cycles 30, 68
electrolyte balance 22–3
  disturbances 76, 94
electrolyte imbalance 60
electromyography (EMG) biofeedback 105
electronic monitoring equipment 144

Index

emergency care provision   147
emotional functioning   123
  family   125, 126
  minimal response syndrome   115, 116, 117
  stubbornness   120
emotional reactions   16
emotional states, behavioral expression   15
emotional stress in staff members   127–8
emotions
  brain   137–8
  consciousness relationship   137–8
  inner world   16
  learning   132, 139
  memory   132, 139
encephalopathy, hypoxic–ischemic   3, 4
enemas   93
energy consumption   22
enteral feeding   94
enterocyte glutamine metabolism   94
enteropeduncular nucleus of Montanalli-Hassler   12, 13
environment, stimulation-rich   114–15
environmental stimulus   132
  responsiveness   139
epilepsy   21
  fits   34
  post-traumatic   76
  premorbid   43
  ventricular shunting   81
  see also seizures
epileptic event EEGs   66
equipotentiality, theory of   16
erection episodes in REM sleep   67
esophageal peristalsis   103
esophageal sphincter insufficiency   101
ethical issues   120–3
  late recovery   44
  minimal response syndrome   116–17
ethyl alcohol   106
euthanasia   121, 123
event-related potentials   70, 71
evoked potentials
  auditory   69
  somatosensory   67, 69
  stimulus-related   67, 69–72
  visual   69
exercise
  facilities   144
  rolling   96
exploration of blanket   35
extension of limbs   27
extrapyramidal syndrome   20
eye-hand tracking   139
eye movements   28–9, 34
conscious visual experience
  suppression   137
  normal   34
  response to an order   34
  spontaneous   34
  see also gaze
eye tracking   32, 34, 139
eyes, perceptual dominance   136

facial nerve   28–9
facial spasms   103
family assessment   125
family members   84, 120
  boundaries with staff   127–8
  communication with staff   129
  complaints   127
  contribution to recovery   124
  defense mechanisms   126
  discharge of patient   143
  education   147
  emotional needs   125, 126
  expectations   101, 128
  facilities   144
  helplessness   126
  minimal response syndrome   114, 115
  needs   124, 128
  physical needs   125
  psychological reactions   125–7
  psychological support for   147
  psychosocial intervention   129
  rehabilitation process   127, 128–9
  spiritual needs   125
  staff interactions   124–9
  stress   128
fat embolism   19
fear   138
feeding
  administration routes   94
  interruption   122
  program   104
  see also nutrition
feelings   2
femoral abduction   102
fetal position   33–4
fever   25
fibroblasts   7
fibrosis in trauma   7
fibrotracheal bronchoscopy   108
finger following   34
fingers
  clubbing   19, 26, 34
  deformation   34
flaccidity   27, 102
flexion of limbs   27
flexor hypertonus   20
flushing   33
food intake   93
forced vital capacity   19
France   122
free fatty acid mobilization   25
frontoparietal cortex   136
function recovery   44–6
functional electrical stimulation   102

GABA analogs   105
GABAergic neurotransmission   13
galanthamine   77
gastric reflux   20
gastric tubes   94
gastrointestinal tract
  complications   19–20
  hemorrhage   19–20, 23
gaze   28
  akinetic mutism   38
  conjugated   101
  lateral conjugate deviation   34
  movements   31
  orientation   15, 95
  recovery of conscious activity   31
  skew deviation   34
  see also eye movements
general state observation   90
Germany   123
Glasgow Coma Scale   47, 49, 111, 132
  cognitive scores   83
glial proliferation   7
glial scar   7
globus pallidus lesions in akinetic mutism   38
glutamic oxaloacetic transaminase   60
glutamine   94
glycosphingolipids   78
grasping reflex   35
gravity
  postural realignment opposing   105
  response to   101
gray matter   148
growth hormone   21
Gudden fasciculus   16
Guillain-Barré syndrome   37
gymnasium   144, 146
  treatment   94–6

half-moon pucker mouth   29, 32
haloperidol   77
head
  alignment   101
  flexion   27
  hyperextension   27
  support   101

Index

head-retraction reflex 29
head trauma 3–4, 5
  blunt 5, 6
  cure 120, 123
  direction of motion 7
  epilepsy 21
  hyperdynamic cardiovascular reactivity 18–19
  motor control disturbances 20–1
  movement disorders 20–1
  visual system damage 69
  see also brain injury
health authorities 147
health care organization 147
helplessness feelings of staff 127
hematological alterations 23
hematoma, intracranial 7
hemiplegia 20, 21
hemosiderin 6
hepatitis, viral 20
hip flexion 104
hippocampal formation 15
hippocampus 15
  functional relationship with cortex/limbic system 11
homicide 121
homovanillic acid 77
hormonal disorders 23–4
hostility 126
human resources 146
humidification 97
  tracheostomy 108
humoral deficit 24
hydration 93
  discontinuing 121
  tracheostomy 108
hydrocephalus
  akinetic mutism 39
  communicating 22, 80
  diagnosis 80
  ex vacuo 80
  normal-pressure 22, 39, 76
  obstructive 22
  onset 79
  post-traumatic 22
  shunting 22, 39
  surgical therapy 79–81
  treatment 80–1
hydrotherapy 98–100
  facilities 144, 146
  spasticity 105
hygiene 91–3
  facilities 144
  minimal response syndrome 113–14
  oral 91, 92
hyperbaric oxygenation 78
hypercaloric diet 93
hyperglycemia, stress-induced acute 60
hyperkalemia 23
hyperlipidemia 60

hypermylasemia 60
hypernatremia 23
hypersomnia see paramedian diencephalic syndrome
hypertension, neurogenic 18
hypertonia 27, 104
hyperventilation, central 19
hypoalbuminemia 23
hypoglycemia 60
hypokalemia 23
hyponatremia 23
hypopituitarism 24
hypoproteinuria 60
hypotension 19
hypothalamus
  hormonal disorders 23–4
  hyperdynamic cardiovascular response 19
  preservation 6
  thermoregulatory system failure 25
  VS 67
hypothyroidism 23
hypoxia 19, 60
hypoxic–ischemic encephalopathy 3, 4

ideas 2
illusory conjunctions 136
imagination 2
immunodeficiency 92
immunoglobulins 24
immunological disorders 24
inappropriate antidiuretic hormone syndrome (IADHS) 23, 24
infections
  nosocomial 24
  ventricular shunting 81
information processing 11
inner world
  determination difficulty 46
  emotions 16
  relationship 15
innominate artery erosion 19
intensive care unit 124
  admission criteria 142
  admittance 144
  biotechnology 145
  building materials 145
  discharge criteria 143
  equipment 144, 145
    needs 143
  human resources 146
  management
    demands 128
    guidelines 141–6
  organization 141–2
  provision 147
  sanitary rooms 146
  structural organization 143–5

International Classification of Diseases (ICD) 4
interstitial nuclei of Cajal 96
intracortical connection damage 6
intracranial pressure, high 7, 19
intraoral sensitivity 103
ischemia
  secondary brain damage 7
  see also hypoxic–ischemic encephalopathy
Italy 122

joint deformities 20
judgment making 127

Klebsiella 24
Klippel signs 33, 34

L-dopa 77
labiomental reflex 29
lactic dehydrogenase 60
laminin 7
lamotrigine 78
laryngeal reflex 103
larynx, lifting 104
lateral thalamic geniculate body 29
lazaroids 78
learned response eliciting 137
learning 133
  basal ganglia 138
  emotions 132, 139
  motor 138
  residual mechanisms 148
legal issues in late recovery 44
lergotrile mesylate 77
leukocytosis 60
lidocaine 105
life cycle 125
lifting systems 145
light reflex 34
limbic lobe 15
limbic system 16
  functional relationship with cortex/hippocampus 11
limbs 29–30
  coordination 138
  extension/hyperextension 27
  flexion 27
    progressive 20
  motility 29–30
  movement in response to painful stimuli 34
  posture 27
  upper 102

lip-chin reflex 35
liver function, impaired 20
living will 121, 122, 123
localized function, theory of 16
locked-in feelings 127
locked-in syndrome
  akinetic mutism differential
    diagnosis 38
  VS differential diagnosis 35–7
locked-out syndrome 11, 15
lockjaw 103
locomotion
  backward 12
  forward 13
Loewenstein Communication Scale
  for the Minimally Responsive
  Patient 51–2
low-awareness state 110
lung capacity improvement 101

macrobronchial aspiration 19
macroelectrodes, electrophysiological signals 65
macrophages 6
magnesium 23
magnetic phenomenon 35
magnetic pulse stimulation 105
magnetic resonance angiography
  61, 65
magnetic resonance imaging
  (MRI) 61, 62–4, 65
  diffusion-weighted imaging
    (DWI) 62–4, 65
  fluid-attenuated inversion re-
    covery (FLAIR) 62–3, 65
  perfusion studies 61
magnetic resonance
  spectroscopy 61
  mesencephalon 65
maintenance therapy in long-term
  specialized unit 143
mamillary tegment 16
management of patients 89–109
  clinical 142
  goals 18
  maintenance therapy 143
  minimal response syndrome
    113–15
  treatment 91–107, 122
  see also intensive care unit
Marinescu-Radovici reflex 35
mastication 103
  see also chewing
mattresses, anti-decubitus 92,
  145
meclofenoxate hydrochloride 78
media 121, 122
medical care standardization 142
medication see drug therapy

memory 2, 133
  basal ganglia 138
  black-out 11
  consolidation 133, 138, 139
  disorders in minimal response
    syndrome 114
  emotions 132, 139
  hypersomnia 40, 41
  implicit 139
  priming 139
  REM sleep 67
  working 138
meninges, adhesions 22
mental life continuation 2
mepivacaine 105
mesencephalic reticular formation
  lesions in akinetic mutism 38
  stimulation 79
mesencephalon
  injury causing VS 64
  interstitial nuclei of Cajal 96
  lesions in akinetic mutism 38
  magnetic resonance spectros-
    copy 65
mesna 108
metabolic imbalance 93–4
metacognitive awareness 111
methylphenidate 77
microaspiration, recurrent 19
mimicry 35
minimal response syndrome
  110–17, 143
  alertness 114–15
  assessment tools 111–12
  care-givers 115
  care of patients 113–14
  clinical management 113
  clinical treatment providers
    115–16
  communication 116
  communicative behaviors 116
  complementary therapy 115
  complication prevention 114
  diagnosis 111–12
  drug therapy 114
  emotional functioning 116,
    117, 123
  ethics 116–17, 123
  family members 115
  family support 114
  functional progress 115–16
  health policy implications
    110–11
  hygiene 113–14
  incidence 112–13
  management 113–15
  medical monitoring 114
  minimal movement 116
  motor control 115
  nutritional intervention 113
  pain control 114
  physiotherapy 115
  policy 116–17

prediction tree 113
prevalence 112–13
recovery process 116
rehabilitation 116, 117
respiratory tract 114
satisfaction feelings 115
seizure prevention 114
sensory stimulation
  programs 116
sexuality 114
skin care 114
sleep control 114
spiritual maintenance/spiritu-
  ality 114
stimulation-rich environment
  114–15
therapy 114–15
tonus control 115
touch 114
treatment objectives 113
minimally responsive state 46–7
mismatch negativity 120
mobility, spontaneous 31, 32
mobilization of patient 92, 93
  passive 95
moral consciousness 120
moral issues 128
motility
  limbs 29–30
  voluntary 16
motor activity, routine daily 114
motor control
  disturbances 20–1
  minimal response
    syndrome 115
motor planning 16
motor reactivity 21, 138
motor reflexes, classical conditioning 138
motor response
  learning 138
  recovery 31
  refusal 28
motor skills 16
  learning 138
motor systems 15
  contralateral 12–14, 15
    functioning 101
    passive induction 89
    synchronization 97
  ipsilateral 12, 13, 15
    functioning 101
    passive induction 89
    synchronization 97
  primitive 12–14, 15, 16
  problems 20–1
mourning process 125–7
mouth
  half-moon pucker 29, 32
  opening 35
movement
  abnormal 34
  involuntary 21

contralateral turning 12–14
disorders in head trauma 20–1
minimal 116
normal uncontrolled 21
passive 27
pathological 27
primitive motor systems 12–14, 15
slow-motion 34
spontaneous 27
stereotypic 33
tongue 103
see also mobility; mobilization of patient; motility
mucolytic compounds 108
Multi-Society Task Force 5
multidisciplinary operating model 142
multimodal stimulation 142
muscles
  hypotony 20
  tone 27
muscular contractions, myoclonus 22
music stimulation therapy 82, 83
myasthenic crises 37
mydriasis 28
myelotomy 106
myocardial damage, chest trauma 19
myoclonus 22
myotactic cervical reflex 29, 35

nasogastric tube 20, 103
  feeding 94
neocortex 16
  damage 139
nervous system
  damaged structure replacement/reorganization 148
  information processing 11
Netherlands 121
neural stem cell implants 148
neural synchrony 111
neural system dishabituation 82
neuroendocrine disorders 76
neurological examination 26
neurological signs 26
  definitions 33–5
  late 32
  prognostic value 27, 29, 32–5
neurolysis 105–6
neuronal population damage 148
neurons
  primary damage 16
  sprouting induction 7
neuroradiology 61, 62–4, 65
neurorehabilitation 141
neurostimulation therapy 78–9
neurosurgery, spasticity 106–7

neutrophil dysfunction 24
nitrates 94
nociceptive stimuli, limb response 34
non-traumatic conditions 3, 4
  prognosis 42–3
norepinephrine 60
nuclear aspartic acid (NAA) 65
nutrition 93
  discontinuing 121, 122
  evaluation 93–4
  minimal response syndrome 113
  see also feeding
nutritional recovery syndrome 23
nystagmus 28
  optokinetic 38
  retractory 35
  spontaneous 67

occlusive bandages 106
ocular motility 28–9
oculo-oral reflex 29, 31, 103
oculocephalic reflex 29
oleic acid 94
onanism 35
opisthotonos 20, 27
opsoclonus-myoclonus 22
optic-oral stimulation 35
oral electrical stimulation 104
oral expression recovery 45
oral feeding 94
oral hygiene 91, 92
oral reflexes 29
organ donation 120–1
orientation gaze 15, 95
orienting reaction 34
oropharynx, videofluoroscopy 103
orthopedic surgery 106
orthosis 95–6
orthotherapy 106
ossification, heterotopic see periarticular new bone formation (PNBF)
osteotomy 106
outer world relationship 11–15
  absence of contact 28
  recovery 31
oxygen, peripheral saturation 97

P250, pain-related 79
P300 70, 120
pain control 114
palatal myoclonus 22
pallidum
  external 13

internal 12, 13
Q-bundle 12
panagnosis 1
panapraxis 1
pants, absorbent 19
Papez circuit 15
parahippocampal gyrus 15
paramedian diencephalic syndrome 35–6, 39–41
paraplegia in flexion 33
paravertebral muscle hypertonus 20
paresis 20–1
passive care 84
patient
  bond with staff members 120
  care skills 148
  dependence 141–2
  living will 121, 122, 123
  see also management of patients
pelvis
  positioning 101–2
  rotation 101
perception 16, 133, 134
  blindness 136
  brain injury 134
  capability assessment with auditory evoked potentials 69
  color 134–5
  control 135
  opposite motor system association 14
  phenomena 15
  taste 103
  visual 133, 134–5
    development 135–6
    suspension 137
perceptual isolation 142
percutaneous endoscopic gastrostomy 20, 94, 103
periarticular new bone formation (PNBF) 21, 60
  spasticity 104, 107
peripheral vasodilatation 98
persistent vegetative state 3
person, potential form 120
pharmaceuticals see drug therapy
pharynx, posterior 103
phenol 105–6
phonation 45
phosphorus 23
phrenic nerve, traumatic paralysis 19
physical experience 142
physicians
  duties 123
  obligations 121
physiotherapy
  botulinum toxin 106
  minimal response syndrome 115
physostigmine 77
piracetam 78

Index

pituitary dysfunction 23–4
plegia 20–1
pneumoencephalography 80
pneumonia 19, 20, 24
  locked-in syndrome 37
pneumothorax 19
poliomyelitis 37
polyneuropathy 37
pons lesions in locked-in syndrome 36
positioning of patient 93, 95–6
  dynamic 96
  verticalization 97–8
  wheelchair 100–2
positron emission tomography (PET) 61
postcomatose unawareness 111
postural drainage 97
postural reactions 96
postural realignment 105
posture 27
postvegetative state 110
potassium 22–3
pre-attentive mechanisms 137
Preliminary Neuropsychological Battery 51
pressure volume index (PVI) measurement 80
prognosis 41–6
  neurological signs 27, 29, 32–5
Prognostic Model of Emergence from Vegetative States 49–50
protein supplementation 22
pseudomembranous colitis 24
Pseudomonas 24
pseudosyndrome of Balint 14
pulmonary embolism 19, 25
pulse dosimeter 97
pupils 28
putamen 12, 13

Q-bundle 12
quality of life 44–5
Quinlan, Karen Ann 122

rabbit-snout phenomenon 29, 32
radionuclide cisternography 80
Rancho Los Amigos Levels of Cognitive Functioning Scale 47, 83
rapid eye movement (REM) sleep 30, 67
  memory 67
re-innervation 148
recovery
  altered state of consciousness 116
  brain damage severity 76

communication function 45
conscious activity 89
family contribution 124
function 44–6
late 32, 43–4
mental 45
normal pattern 112
slow 110, 112
recovery unit 18
reflexes 30
  blink 34
  bulldog 29, 31, 35, 103
  cervical myotactic 29, 35
  ciliospinal 28, 34
  corneal 28–9, 34
  corneo-chin 29, 31, 35
  corneomandibular 29, 33
  cough 96, 103, 104
  grasping 35
  head-retraction 29
  labiomental 29
  laryngeal 103
  light 34
  lip-chin 35
  Marinescu-Radovici 35
  motor 138
  oculo-oral 29, 31, 103
  oculocephalic 29
  oral 29
  primitive 105
  rolling exercises 96
  snout 29, 33
  sucking 35
  swallowing 103
  tactile-oral 29, 35
  tendons 30
regression signs 103
rehabilitation 29, *30*
  cardiovascular complications 18–19
  early initiation 83
  family members
    education 147
    involvement 127, 128–9
  intensive care unit 141
  long-term specialized unit 143
  minimal response syndrome 116, 117
  outlook 147–8
  resources 117
  swallowing 103–4
rehabilitation-ready status 117
relaxation 89
resources, distribution 121
respiratory tract
  complications 19
  minimal response syndrome 114
  water loss 23
respiratory treatment 96–7
restlessness 33
reticulobulbospinal fibers, descending 12

reticuloendothelial system, defective 24
reticulospinal tract, spasticity 20
rhizotomy 106
rib cage expansion 97
rib fractures 19
  respiratory problems 96
rigidity 20
road accidents 5, *64*
rolling 96

saccadic suppression 137
saline intrathecal bolus injection 80
sanitary rooms 146
satisfaction feelings 115
scratching 35
sedatives 78
sedimentation rate 60
seeing 136
seizures 21–2, 34
  prevention 114
  see also epilepsy
self, awareness of 2
sensory awareness 111
sensory function loss 2
sensory information channels 135
Sensory Modality Assessment and Rehabilitation Technique 51, 83
sensory regulation 82
sensory stimulation 89
  assessment 83
  auditory-tactile 89
  competition avoidance 139
  duration 83
  evaluation scales 83
  frequency 83
  interpersonal relatedness of therapist 84
  learned effect 139
  multimodal 82–3
  outcome 83–4
  programs 81–3, 116
  techniques 82–3
  unimodal 82–3
Sensory Stimulation Assessment Measure 49, 83
sensory systems 15
  cortical regulatory motor apparatus 14
  information processing organization 135
  visual display 139
sexuality 114
shearing injuries 61
  imaging 65
shoulder hyperadduction 104
showering 92

signs, observation 89
sinusitis 24
sketchy movements 34
skin
  care 114
  changes 19, 26
  damage 92
  hygiene 91
sleep
  control in minimal response syndrome 114
  hypersomnia 39
  patterns 30, 67
  phase classification 66
sleep EEG 67, *68*
sleep-wake cycles 3, 30
  EEG 30, *68*
  outcome 67
slow-motion movements 34
snout reflex 29, 33
sodium 22-3
soft palate 103
solitary tract nucleus 19
somatosensory evoked potentials 67, 69
soul 111
spastic tetraplegia 36
spasticity 20, 27, 102
  anesthetic block 105-6
  botulinum toxin 106
  evaluation 104
  neurosurgery 106-7
  orthopedic surgery 106
  periarticular new bone formation 104, 107
  physiotherapeutic measures 104-5
  treatment 104-5
spatiotemporal orientation loss 2
speech 16
sphincter activity
  management 93
sphincter function 101
sphincteral incontinence 93
spinal alpha motor neurons 20
spinal cord stimulation 79
  electrical 106
spirituality
  family needs 125
  minimal response syndrome 115
split anterior tibial tendon (SPLATT) 106
staff members 84
  bond with patient 120
  boundaries with families 127-8
  communication with family 129
  emotional stress 127-8
  family hostility 126
  family interactions 124-9
  human resources 146

meetings 146
supportive interventions 129
teams 142
tension sources 127-8
treatment program involvement 91
see also physicians
status epilepticus 22
step mechanisms, automatic 29, *30*
stimulation techniques 81-4
  monomodal 98
  simple 89
stimulus-related evoked potentials 67, 69-72
stress
  family members 128
  staff 127-8
subcallosal gyrus 15
subcortical connection damage 6
sucking 103
  automatism 29, 31, 103
  reflex 35
support groups for staff 129
supraliminal stimulation, persistent 89
surgical therapy 79-81
swallowing
  automatism 29, 31
  disturbance treatment 102-4
  oral feeding 94
  reflex mechanism 103
  rehabilitation 103-4
  tracheostomy 108
sweating 25
  baclofen effect 107
  excessive 33
  water loss 23
synaptic conductivity 115

tactile-oral reflex 29, 35
tactile stimulation 91
taste perception 103
teeth evaluation 103
tendinoplasty 106
tendons
  reflexes 30
  retraction 20
tenotomy 106
tensions in staff members 127-8
terminally ill patients 122, 123
tetraplegia 20-1
  spastic 36
thalamic dementia 41
thalamic structures, electrical stimulation 89
thalamocortical system 11, 15
  coherence changes with activation 66
thalamus 16

anterior ventral nucleus 12
damage 6
injury mechanisms 6-7
lesions
  akinetic mutism 38
  hypersomnia 40
neuronal loss 6
posterior lateral nucleus 12
retrograde degeneration 6
ventral intermediate nucleus 12
ventral medial nucleus 12
therapeutic goals 89
therapeutic milieu 147
therapeutic plan 89
therapy rooms 144
thighs
  padding 102
  supports 101
thought process 133
tizanidine 105
tongue evaluation 103
tonus control 115
touch 114
tracheal stenosis 108
tracheobronchial infection 19
tracheobronchial secretion
  aspiration 107-8
tracheoesophageal fistula 19, 108
tracheomalacia 19, 108
tracheostomy
  cannula 103, 107
    removal 108-9
  complications 108
  countercannula disinfection 107
  humidification 97
  inhalation 107-8
  locked-in syndrome 37
  patient management 107-9
  swallowing 108
tracheotomy 37
transplant procedures 120
transportation of patients 147
trauma 3-4, 5
  collagen production 7
  fibrosis 7
  prognosis 42-3
  secondary brain damage 7
  secondary effects 127
treatment
  discontinuing 122
  program 91-107
tremor 34
trigeminal pathway 28-9
trunk 29-30
  alignment 101

unawareness 2
  postcomatose 110, 111

unconsciousness
  coma 111
  duration 43
undernutrition 22
uninhabited body 120
United Kingdom 122
United States 122
urinary bladder
  catheters 19, 93
  globoid 93
  neurogenic 19
urinary retention 93
urinary tract
  complications 19
  hospital-acquired infection 19, 24
urine collector, external 93
urolithiasis 19

value of life 122
vegetative state
  assessment 46–52
  causes 3–4
  characterization 2
  circumstances 5
  clinical outline 1
  clinical picture 18–52
  clinical progression 11
  complications 18–26
  concept 1–2, 3–7
  definition 1, 2, 3
  differential diagnosis 35–41
  duration 4
  epidemiology 4–5
  etiology 3–4, 42–3
  functional organization of brain 16–17
  gender 4
  incidence 4
  irreversible 3
  laboratory findings 60
  medical aspects 18–26
  minimal response distinction 112
  mortality 41, 42
  natural history 41

  neurological aspects 26–30
  neuropathology 6–7
  outcome 6, 41–6
  pathological anatomic lesions 11
  prevalence 4
  progression 18
  recovery 30–2
    rate 4, 5
  residual function 15
  seasonal variability 5
  survival 41
    time 41–2
  time of day 5
  see also prognosis
vegetative storm 25
ventral intermediate nucleus (VIM) 12
ventricular enlargement 7, 22, 79
  progressive 80
ventricular shunting 22, 80–1
  akinetic mutism 39
  complications 81
ventriculoatrial shunting 81
ventriculoperitoneal shunting 81
verbal command response 28
verticalization 97–8
vestibular nuclei 12
vestibulospinal fibers, descending 12
vestibulospinal tract, spasticity 20
vibration, spasticity 105
videofluoroscopy of oropharynx 103
vigilance 2
  absence 16
vision, conscious experience 136
visual attention 135, 137
visual awareness 135, 136
visual change detection 136
visual comprehension
  recovery 45
visual cortex 133
visual display 139
visual evoked potentials 69
visual orientation 135–6
visual patterning information processing 134

visual perception 133, 134–5
  development 135–6
  subjective experience 135
  suspension 137
visual system damage 69
visuomotor response 136
vital capacity 19
vital parameter survey 90
vital signs
  instability 94
  monitoring
    during verticalization 98
    in wheelchair 100
vocalization, spontaneous 35
voice recognition 16
volitional behavior 138

wakefulness 2, 3
  ipsilateral motor system 12
  without awareness 71
Walton of Detchant, Lord 122
washing 92
water balance 22–3
water intoxication 23
water loss 23
wedges 101
weight loss 22
Western Neuro-Sensory Stimulation Profile 48, 51, 83
wheelchair
  mobilization of patient 93
  positioning of patient 100–2
  verticalization of patient 97
white matter
  damage 6, 148
  injury causing VS 61
  regrowth 148
  wasting 22
working memory 138

zinc
  serum levels 60
  supplementation 78

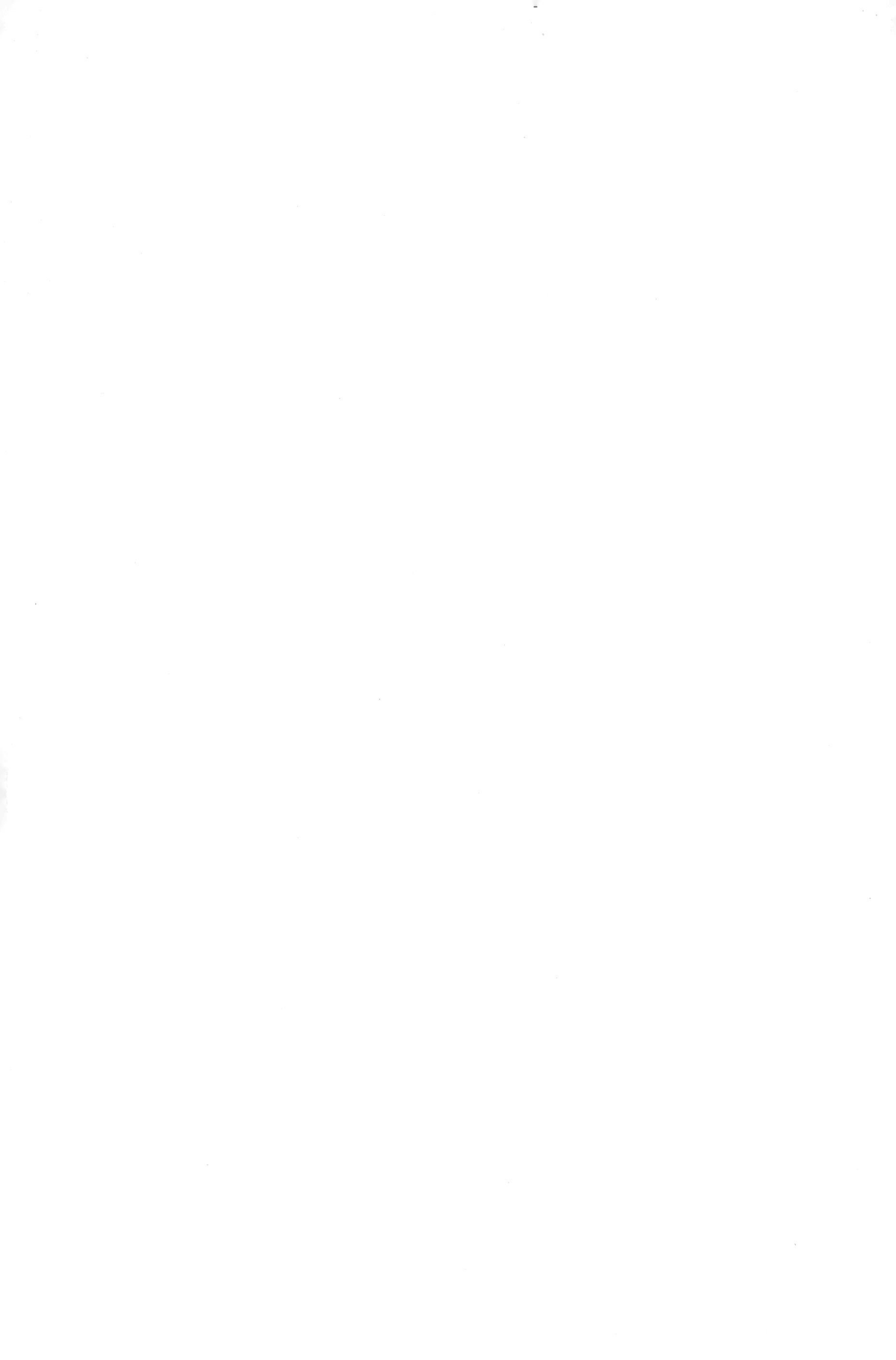